Fit & Active

The West Point Physical Development Program

Maureen K. LeBoeuf
Lawrence F. Butler

Editors

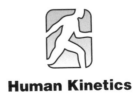

Human Kinetics

Library of Congress Cataloging-in-Publication Data

Fit & active : the West Point physical development program / Maureen K. LeBoeuf, Lawrence
F. Butler, editors.
     p. cm.
  Includes bibliographical references.
  ISBN-13: 978-0-7360-6074-5 (soft cover)
  ISBN-10: 0-7360-6074-X (soft cover)
  1. Physical education and training--Study and teaching. 2. Physical fitness--Study and
teaching. 3. United States Military Academy. I. LeBoeuf, Maureen K., 1953-   II. Butler,
Lawrence F.   III. Title: Fit and active
  GV361.F49   2008
  613.7'1--dc22

                                        2007025491

ISBN-10: 0-7360-6074-X
ISBN-13: 978-0-7360-6074-5

The Web addresses cited in this text were current as of August 24, 2007, unless otherwise noted.

Acquisitions Editor: Scott Wikgren; **Developmental Editor:** Bethany J. Bentley; **Assistant Editor:** Anne Rumery; **Copyeditor:** Joyce Sexton; **Proofreader:** Anne Meyer Byler; **Permission Manager:** Dalene Reeder; **Graphic Designer (interior and cover):** Robert Reuther; **Graphic Artist:** Kathleen Boudreau-Fuoss; **Photographs (cover):** © Human Kinetics and © Stockbyte (bottom right); **Photographs (interior):** Courtesy of the United States Military Academy, unless otherwise noted. Photos on pages 93, 98, 99, 175, 176, 178, and 179 by Neil Bernstein; **Photo Office Assistant:** Jason Allen; **Art Manager:** Kelly Hendren; **Associate Art Manager:** Alan L. Wilborn; **Illustrator:** Accurate Art, Inc.; **Printer:** Sheridan Books

Printed in the United States of America   10   9   8   7   6   5   4   3   2   1

Human Kinetics
Web site: www.HumanKinetics.com

United States: Human Kinetics
P.O. Box 5076, Champaign, IL 61825-5076
800-747-4457
e-mail: humank@hkusa.com

Canada: Human Kinetics
475 Devonshire Road Unit 100, Windsor, ON N8Y 2L5
800-465-7301 (in Canada only)
e-mail: orders@hkcanada.com

Europe: Human Kinetics
107 Bradford Road, Stanningley, Leeds LS28 6AT, United Kingdom
+44 (0) 113 255 5665
e-mail: hk@hkeurope.com

Australia: Human Kinetics
57A Price Avenue, Lower Mitcham, South Australia 5062
08 8372 0999
e-mail: info@hkaustralia.com

New Zealand: Human Kinetics
Division of Sports Distributors NZ Ltd.
P.O. Box 300 226 Albany, North Shore City, Auckland
0064 9 448 1207
e-mail: info@humankinetics.co.nz

**Dedicated to the
United States Corps of Cadets
at
West Point**

Contents

Preface

As our nation moves toward a work foundation based primarily on intellectual ability and knowledge, the emphasis on fitness has dramatically decreased in our public school system. Over half of the adult population in the United States are overweight, and almost a third are clinically obese. This trend is of particular concern because it is occurring in our youth as well as in adults. Our young adults need to become more physically active, even in a world that focuses more and more on intellectual ability. There is no doubt that a solid fitness foundation helps prepare our students both for success in the academic realm and for active, healthy lifestyles long after they graduate.

With this mission in mind, we wrote this book to serve as a practical, ready-to-use resource for physical educators at the high school and higher education levels, as well as for youth sport directors who are committed to inspiring our youth to be more physically active. In each chapter we describe what has worked for us in the West Point program and have provided detailed strategies for modifying our approach for a variety of ages and environments.

At West Point, we believe that physical fitness serves as a foundation for emotional and intellectual well-being. We have developed a program that is carefully coordinated to achieve our objectives, and it has proven to be very successful. It's important to note that while we are a military academy, we do promote the importance of participating in enjoyable physical activities along with knowledge, skills, and fitness activities. As physical educators we believe that it is vital to inspire our students to make physical activity and fitness an integral part of their lives long after they leave our program.

To meet this objective we need to reach students and young adults in their own worlds. Recently we received an e-mail from a public school physical education teacher who noted that "many schools still teach physical education using a curriculum from the 1960s." The value of this book is that it provides a great deal of specific, current information that will give teachers new ideas for improving their programs.

Overview

The first chapter provides an overview of the Physical Development Program at the U.S. Military Academy (USMA) and describes the philosophical and conceptual underpinnings for the structure, process, and content of our physical education program. This provides some context for readers as they proceed through other chapters. Chapter 2 focuses on the unique contribution that sport education can make in enhancing the leadership skills of our students. *"Every cadet an athlete, every athlete challenged"* is a phrase coined by General Douglas MacArthur when he was the superintendent at USMA following World War I, and captures the essence of this discussion. The chapter describes how the sport education approach can be modified to suit the needs of the public school teacher. It also provides strategies for physical educators who are interested in developing leadership skills and promoting positive character traits and values through sport experiences. The critical process of program assessment in West Point's Physical Development Program is discussed in chapter 3. West Point has a rather extensive and continuous assessment program both within the Department of Physical Education and across the Academy. The author provides a general overview of assessment and then suggests strategies and ideas for readers to consider in their programs.

Chapters 4 through 7, in part II of the book, describe "core activity courses," including Basic Movement, Swimming, Self-Defense, and Fitness Boxing. We consider these essential in developing the types of motor skills that our future leaders will require. Chapter 8 discusses how West Point uses obstacle courses to develop certain traits normally associated with the affective domain. The purpose of these activities is to promote students' self-confidence, self-esteem, and ability to work together effectively as a group—and sometimes they are just plain fun to do! The chapter describes the purpose and design of the obstacle and adventure-type courses used to promote psychomotor and affective development.

Diagrams for our core fitness challenges, the Indoor, Balance Sequence, Confidence, and Adventure Obstacle Courses, are provided, along with suggested strategies to modify these activities for both indoor and outdoor settings.

In part III, chapter 9 focuses on fitness and the various fitness assessments used at West Point. It provides strategies for teachers to use to physically challenge their students through activities that are enjoyable. Sample workout designs will help teachers modify these programs to meet the needs of their students. Chapters 10 and 11 focus on our academically oriented courses in Wellness and Personal Fitness. All of the topics in these two courses are essential for future leaders who will be entrusted with the care of young as well as older soldiers. The Wellness chapter includes topics such as emotional and spiritual health, coping with stress, communication and conflict resolution, basic nutrition and supplements, fitness assessment, eating disorders, reducing the risk for cancer, preventing sexually transmitted diseases, drinking responsibly, and understanding addictive behaviors. The Personal Fitness chapter includes energy systems, sport nutrition, body composition, cardiorespiratory and muscular endurance, and exercising in extreme environments.

In part IV, chapters 12 through 19 provide detailed descriptions of our Lifetime Activity courses, including Tennis, Golf, Ice Skating, Rock Climbing, Soccer, Volleyball, Group Fitness, and Cross-Country Skiing. For all activities, the authors describe the course, its purpose, the instructional area, risk management strategies, and primary skills and techniques, as well as present sample lesson plans. In addition, course modifications are suggested so that teachers can tailor the material to their own students.

The Department of Physical Education at USMA has a unique program, developed to meet the needs of Army leaders for the 21st century. We hope that you will be able to tailor some of these concepts to meet the physical development needs of your students—who are also future leaders of our country.

On a more personal note, we hope that this book will be a valuable resource for you as you work to inspire and motivate your students toward a lifetime of physical activity and wellness.

Acknowledgments

The editors wish to thank their teaching colleagues in the Department of Physical Education at West Point who volunteered to share their expertise with the teaching community. These individuals are truly subject matter experts in their sport or activity. In addition, we would like to thank Mrs. Jeanne Hunkapiller, Ms. Lindsay Kennedy, and Mrs. Stacy Schaefer for their assistance in gathering information and editing. We would also like to thank Jon Liba and Lynn Fielitz for taking the photos for many of the chapters.

Finally, we are indebted to those New York State secondary school teachers who volunteered to review the final document for content accuracy and as a reality check. Their contribution was significant in making this a better text that will indeed be helpful to in-service teachers. We want to express our sincerest gratitude to Cathy Haight, former "secondary school teacher of the year" and former president of the New York State Association for Health, Physical Education, Recreation and Dance, for coordinating the efforts of our superb secondary school teachers and editors, Jason Lehmbeck, Linda Joyce, and Cathy Dodd, and of course Cathy Haight. Thank you all!

PART I

Program Development and Assessment

Introduction to the Physical Development Program

Maureen K. LeBoeuf and Lawrence F. Butler

West Point is the only university in the nation whose sole responsibility is to prepare each student for professional service as a regular Army officer. The Physical Development Program, like the other aspects of the 47-month West Point experience, is designed to foster development in leadership, moral courage, and integrity essential to such service. An integrated, concurrent, and progressive process is integral to leader development in the Academic, Military, and Physical Programs. These programs are distinct, yet highly complementary. Each program serves to reinforce the fundamental values, ideals, and principles that are the core for leaders of character. Moral-ethical development is integrated throughout all programs that comprise the West Point experience—the process that strives to develop cadets into leaders of character for a lifetime.

From the first day of a cadet's West Point experience, the Physical Development Program complements the Military Program by introducing physical training and preparing cadets for the physical rigors that they will face as future Army officers. The Physical Development Program supports the Academic Program by challenging cadets to learn and think critically and creatively about physical fitness and physical education, as well as maintain a high standard of health essential for effective military service.

The Physical Development Program is a 47-month educational experience that begins on Reception Day, when a new cadet enters Cadet Basic Training, and ends on Graduation Day when the cadet is commissioned as a second lieutenant in the United States Army. The Physical Program comprises three complementary performance components:

instructional coursework, sport education participation, and physical and motor fitness assessment and evaluation.

The Physical Development Program is based on the philosophy that physical development occurs through progressive and sequential experiences that incorporate all domains of learning. The initial phase of the Physical Development Program focuses on the development of skills and concepts of basic movement patterns and physical fitness. Underlying this phase is a focus on developing moral-ethical behaviors, managing fear, and promoting a "will to win the right way" attitude necessary for Army officers. As cadets progress through the program, greater emphasis is placed on applying basic skills and knowledge in a military environment. This process is particularly evident in the two-course Fitness Leader sequence (Wellness and Personal Fitness) that initially focuses on individual wellness and fitness and culminates with a capstone experience in unit fitness.

The Department of Physical Education has established specific goals and objectives that are aligned with the mission of West Point and meet the needs of the United States Army.

Physical Development Program Pathway

West Point graduates must be able to respond quickly in a wide variety of environments and situations such as waking up at near sea level at Fort Bragg, North Carolina, and in less than 35 hours being at 10,000 feet (3,050 meters) in Afghanistan. West Point graduates must be agile in order to be able to move efficiently and effectively in close spaces. They also need to be versatile, to be able to balance, vault, jump, land, move with heavy loads, climb ropes, crawl, and negotiate natural and man-made obstacles (Headquarters Department of the Army, 1993).

"Officership is the practice of being a commissioned Army leader, inspired by a unique professional identity that is shaped by what an officer must KNOW, & DO, but most importantly, by a deeply held personal understanding and acceptance of what an officer must BE. This unique self-concept incorporates four interrelated roles: Servant of the Nation, Member of a Profession, Warrior, and Leader of Character" (USMA Circular 1-101, 2002).

The West Point experience is developmental. Each year approximately 1,300 civilian men and women arrive, and during the 47-month experience we strive to develop them into commissioned Army officers who are leaders of character. In order to accomplish this development, West Point has adopted a developmental learning model commonly referred to as the "BE, KNOW, DO" model.

The "KNOW" is the educational or knowledge piece, and the "DO" is the skills and training component. The "BE" is the facilitation of the development of cadets into mature adults. The challenge at West Point is to tailor the experience to the needs of the individual cadet. "Facilitating cadets' development is challenging work that requires striking a fine balance among several competing objectives; tailoring experiences to cadets' needs and abilities, encouraging cadet ownership, and learning from successes and failures" (USMA Circular 1-101, 2002).

West Point graduates represent some of the very best that America has to offer. They are bright, articulate, and physically fit and are leaders of character. They stand ready to lead their soldiers into combat to maintain the freedom and security that all Americans enjoy.

The physical education program at West Point is accomplished through participation in the core courses and a variety of Lifetime Activity courses. The core courses consist of Survival Swimming, Boxing (men and some women), Self-Defense (women), Basic Movement (known as military movement at West Point), and Combatives. Additional core courses include Wellness and Personal Fitness/Unit Fitness. The Lifetime Activity course program is designed to stimulate individual development through participation in a wide variety of physical activity classes. Cadets can learn a sport or activity that they have never had the opportunity to experience. The following detailed discussion of the 47-month physical education program is ordered chronologically to provide the reader with a perspective on the overall program.

All 4,000+ cadets participate in physical education, physical fitness assessment and evaluation, and a sport education or intercollegiate athletic experience for all four years. The summer physical fitness program is developed and supervised by the Department of Physical Education; however, the execution of the fitness program is the responsibility of the junior or senior cadets. These cadets serve in the leadership roles during Cadet Basic Training (CBT) and Cadet Field Training (CFT). Being a member of the CBT/CFT cadre is a tremendous leadership opportunity for these cadets, one in which they can

- develop leadership skills through exposure to a variety of physical fitness training methods and experiences;
- improve and maintain their fitness levels as well as the fitness levels of the cadets in their units; and
- enhance morale, cohesion, and teamwork through rigorous physical activity and friendly competition.

Daily physical fitness is conducted six days a week from 5:30 a.m. to 7:00 a.m. This program prepares a cadet for the physical demands of cadet and military service life and the combat environment; introduces the new cadets to the Army physical conditioning program; and strives to foster a positive attitude and positive behavior toward physical fitness. Physical fitness activities allow the upperclass cadets to apply their knowledge and model the psychomotor skills, attitudes, and behaviors that will result in a sustained high level of physical fitness and ultimately enhance future combat readiness.

Freshman Year

During the academic year, the freshmen take three physical education core courses: Self-Defense for the women and Boxing for the men; Survival Swimming, conducted on four levels from elementary through advanced; and Military (Basic) Movement. Self-Defense is designed to introduce the women to an integrated set of basic self-defense skills and strategies and tactics necessary to avoid, escape, or break a physical assault. The course includes methods of falling, stances, movement, striking, kicking, and blocking skills. This course exposes a woman to potential physical threats and enables her to protect herself as a soldier in time of conflict and as an individual in today's society.

The Boxing course taken by the men (and some women who volunteer) is designed to develop offensive and defensive skills of boxing. The course includes stances, movement, basic punches (e.g., cross, jab, hook, and uppercut), defenses, strategies, and tactics. Instruction in refereeing, judging, and serving as a corner second is part of the course content. The course exposes men to the coping strategies necessary to deal with physical threat. Because of the risk management associated with boxing, it is not presented as an option within this book. At West Point, boxing is conducted in the safest way possible. Before taking Boxing, cadets are screened for prior closed head injuries. Headgear, a mouth guard, and an athletic cup are worn to mitigate the risk of injury to the cadet. For additional safety, the cadets wear 16-ounce (.45-kilogram) gloves. National Athletic Trainers' Association–certified athletic trainers are located in close proximity to the boxing venue when the classes take place.

The placing of a cadet into a particular section in the Survival Swimming course is based on his or her performance on a 150-yard swim test that is conducted during the summer. A cadet who cannot swim is placed into Aquatic Foundations. The Aquatic Foundations course is an introductory swimming exploration program designed to prepare nonswimmers for success in the elementary-level course. The foundations program is arranged sequentially to help cadets acquire in-water experiences and gradually refine the basic motor skills needed to be comfortable, safe, and effective while engaged in and around a water environment.

All cadets must successfully complete a Survival Swimming course. The course is designed to develop aquatic proficiency. The cadets who swam 150 yards in 4 minutes are placed in Elementary Survival Swimming. The low intermediate course is for the cadets who swam 150 yards between 3:16 and 3:59. The high intermediate section is for those cadets who swam 150 yards between 2:20 and 3:15; and the advanced course is for swimmers who swam 150 yards in less than 2:30 during their initial entry swim classification test.

Aquatic instruction is divided into two areas: basic swimming and combat-survival swimming. Emphasis in all levels is on the military application of swimming and survival skills including the elements of breath control, buoyancy positions, stroke assessment, and swimming endurance.

Military or Basic Movement is designed to provide cadets with a comprehensive movement experience in all directions, rotations, and ranges of motion. The course is developmental and is intended to cultivate optimal physical capability and potential for movement so that each cadet can meet the physical requirements of the military profession and the broader demands of a healthy, active lifestyle. This course provides a foundation for other athletic and military activities encountered at West Point and in one's Army career. Focus is placed on applied movement tasks. The following skills are emphasized:

- Agility, including fast movement in enclosed spaces
- Balance and managing fear of heights
- Jumping, vaulting, and landing safely
- Strength development for rope climbing, pull-ups, and resistance exercises
- Low crawling
- Negotiating natural and man-made obstacles in the form of confidence and obstacle courses

Sophomore Year

The Physical Program for the sophomores actually begins during the summer prior to their sophomore year, when cadets participate in CFT. Cadet Field Training is eight weeks of military field training. It is designed to be physically and mentally challenging and in many instances simulates actual military field training. Cadets participate in daily physical training and take Combatives. In the first module of Combatives III the basic movements, blocking, striking, and kicking combative skills, are reviewed. Cadets are then taught falling, throws, takedowns, and situational self-defense techniques needed for survival in unarmed combat. Instruction also promotes the development of an aggressive combative mind-set and increases cadets' confidence in their ability to defend themselves in a combative situation.

During the academic year, sophomores take two courses, Combatives and Wellness. Combatives IV is an 18-lesson gender-integrated course in which students are exposed to a comprehensive set of unarmed combat skills, as well as the strategies and tactics needed to neutralize a physical attack. Responses to a striking, kicking, joint-locking, choking, throwing, and ground grappling attack are taught with an emphasis on submission holds applied on the ground as finishing techniques. The course is designed to increase cadets' confidence in their ability to defend themselves from all forms of striking and grappling attacks and to foster the development of a combat-survival mind-set. Students are evaluated on their demonstration of required skills and their performance in simulated combat and self-defense scenarios.

Wellness is the first course in a two-course lecture and lab sequence. The purpose of this course is to introduce the various dimensions of wellness that create and foster a healthy lifestyle. As a result of this course, cadets gain the knowledge and skills to shape their personal well-being. They begin to develop a sense of self-responsibility for a lifetime of fitness and wellness. The course promotes an increased understanding of basic nutrition, nutritional supplements, basic fitness training principles, weight management, eating disorders, injury prevention and management, the cardiovascular system, cardiovascular disease, spiritual and emotional wellness, stress management, cancer, substance abuse, and sexually transmitted diseases. Cadets complete two major projects, a nutrition analysis and a behavior change plan, during Fitness Leader I.

Junior Year

During the junior year, cadets take Personal Fitness and may elect to take a Lifetime Activity course. The focus of the Personal Fitness course is to prepare cadets to develop effective personal and unit physical fitness programs. As leaders it is imperative that cadets know how to take care of their soldiers. Future Army leaders must be knowledgeable about all aspects of personal and unit fitness and about how to address those issues with their soldiers. The fitness topics include energy systems, sports nutrition, cardiorespiratory system and training, muscular system and training, developing a unit physical fitness program, and battle-focused physical training.

Senior Year

A Lifetime Activity course is required for all seniors. Each course consists of 18 lessons, each 55 minutes long, conducted over half of a semester. The program is designed to further develop a foundation of skills, knowledge, and personal attributes that will enable cadets to successfully develop an active lifestyle. Cadets can choose from a wide variety of courses, such as Advanced Close Quarters Combat, Combatives Instructor Certification, Aerobic Fitness, Basketball, Cycling, Emergency Water Safety, Golf, Ice Skating, Judo, Rock Climbing, SCUBA, Alpine Skiing, Snowboarding, Cross-Country Skiing, Soccer, Strength Development, Tennis, and Volleyball. Several of the lifetime sport courses are described in greater detail in part IV.

Assessing and Evaluating Physical Fitness

Physical fitness is a vital part of Army readiness. Throughout our Army's history there have been times when soldiers were not physically prepared to perform their jobs. To promote general physical fitness among soldiers and to establish performance benchmarks, fitness tests were developed to assess the various components of fitness.

All cadets take two fitness tests throughout their four years at the U.S. Military Academy (USMA). Twice each year the cadets take the Army Physical Fitness Test (APFT). The APFT is a three-event physical performance test used to assess muscular and cardiorespiratory endurance. The APFT is a simple way to measure a soldier's ability to effectively move the body by using major muscle groups and the cardiorespiratory system (Headquarters Department of the Army, 1992). The APFT is the fitness test that all soldiers take in the Army. The test consists of 2 minutes of push-ups, 2 minutes of sit-ups, and a timed 2-mile run.

The Indoor Obstacle Course Test (IOCT) is a fitness test that is learned in the freshman Military (Basic) Movement course. The three upper classes take the IOCT as a stand-alone test. The IOCT is probably one of the best overall fitness tests given at USMA. The IOCT has been administered for well over six decades and is both physically and mentally challenging. It is designed to evaluate a cadet's muscular strength, muscular endurance, flexibility, agility, coordination, anaerobic capacity, balance, and decision-making skills while under pressure. The IOCT consists of 11 obstacles.

The USMA is an institution that places great emphasis on physical fitness activities, and at times cadets do get injured. However, we expect cadets to stay physically fit within the limits of their injury. Several alternative fitness tests are available if a cadet is on an extended medical excusal and is unable to take a regular fitness test.

Participating in Sport Education

Every cadet participates in sport and thus must participate at one of three levels each academic term: Intercollegiate, Sport Club, or Intramural. This requirement is designed to provide each student with the opportunity to develop his or her physical and leadership skills. Participation in the sport education program provides cadets with the opportunity to

- exhibit those personal qualities deemed indispensable for leaders of character,
- learn and demonstrate fair play and sportsmanship,
- gain an appreciation for the level of fitness required to participate in sports and in the military lifestyle,
- participate in a level of sport consistent with their ability,
- gain an appreciation for the importance of winning the right way in sport and military life, and
- develop effective teamwork needed to attain team success.

The Department of Physical Education provides oversight for the intramural program and has operational control over the competitive club teams.

Adapting the West Point Physical Development Program for Other Settings

You are probably asking yourself, How does all this apply to my setting? You may think that because our physical education program is located at the USMA, we have exceptional facilities and unconstrained resources. Nothing could be farther from the truth. We struggle with the same types of facility, logistics, and resource issues and concerns that you do. For four years, our 500,000-square-foot (46,450-square-meter) facility underwent a major renovation. The front of the building is historic and could not be demolished; the back section was completely razed. Our offices were moved, and most of the fitness facility was not available for use; we were literally spread out and teaching all over West Point. We had to make significant adjustments to the way we delivered and administered our program. The majority of our program was fully administered during this time.

Within most of the following chapters is a section with the title "Adapting This Course for Your School" or a similarly worded title. Hopefully you will find a number of creative ways to tailor what we do at West Point to your unique setting.

How to Use This Book

Certainly you can start from the front and read this book to the end, which of course we hope you do. However, you can also go directly to chapters or sections of the book you are interested in, such as those on core activity courses, sport education, or wellness.

Key Terms

At the end of most of the chapters is a section on terminology. Terms that may require further explanation are associated with many of the activities. Additionally, West Point uses some unique terminology that many people may not be familiar with.

References

The reference section at the end of most chapters provides additional resources that you may find useful as you develop and revise your unit, curriculum, or lesson plans, including books, journal articles, and Web sites. Many chapters also list the national governing bodies of the various activities.

We hope that you find this book useful as you work to provide your students with the best physical education program possible.

References

Headquarters Department of the Army. (1992). *Physical fitness training.* FM 21-20. Washington, DC: Government Printing Office.

Headquarters Department of the Army. (1993). *Training in units.* AR 350-41. Washington, DC: Government Printing Office.

USMA Circular 1-101. (2002). *Cadet leader development system.* West Point, NY: U.S. Military Academy.

2

Sport Education

Joseph Doty, Bart Woodworth,
Jon Alt, and Joseph LeBoeuf

Sport education programs emphasize much more than just the psychomotor domain of sport and fitness. They also focus on the cognitive and the affective domains. In the sport education model, the mental and emotional aspects of fitness are emphasized along with such attributes as teamwork, perseverance, and the will to win the right way. Sport also has the potential to contribute to a student's moral and ethical growth by providing opportunities to focus on values, fair play, selflessness, and sportsmanship.

A fundamental part of the sport education model is the idea that every student is an athlete. Inclusion of all students is a must. A sport education program can be designed to meet the needs of each student. Such a program can help students acquire skills in individual and team sports; develop physical ability; engage in healthful, vigorous recreation; and enjoy maximum opportunities for development of positive citizenship and lifetime fitness. Students should be encouraged to participate in a sport and receive some sort of feedback or assessment (or both) for their participation. Sport education programs should require that students meet a specified minimum participation requirement because participation gives them the opportunity to come face to face with situations that develop some of the attributes (i.e., responsibility, teamwork, respect, conflict management) of a citizen-leader. In a sport education program, students have many opportunities to administer and coach, as well as to be members of a team.

This chapter is divided into four parts. In the first two parts we discuss the purposes of sport education and the rationale for values education. The third part is an examination of leader development through sport. The fourth and final part provides suggestions on how to adjust the West Point sport education model to fit your school setting.

Purpose of Sport Education

The ideals of good sportsmanship, ethical behavior, and integrity permeate our culture. However, most of the research in this area shows that participation in sport, especially at higher competitive levels, results in a *decrease* in sportsmanship and ethical behavior (Silva,

1983; Beller & Stoll, 1995; Bredemeier & Shields, 1984; Hahm, 1989; Priest, Krause, & Beach, 1999). The values of good citizenship and high behavioral standards should apply and should be taught in all activity disciplines. In perception and practice, good sportsmanship is defined as behaviors that are characterized by respect for others, generosity, fair play, and genuine concern for others. In addition, individuals should understand the influence of their behavior on others. West Point views good sportsmanship as a critical, essential behavior that focuses on a commitment to fair play, ethical behavior, respect, and integrity.

The purpose of the sport education program at West Point is to promote the education and development of students through intercollegiate sports, club sports, intramural sport participation, or some combination of these. This development involves a commitment to high ethical standards and to the principle that participation in athletics serves as an integral part of the total educational process.

The mission of the Competitive Sports office (Sport Education) at West Point is to coordinate intercollegiate club and intramural activities that enhance the students' educational experiences. These are provided through equitable opportunities, positive recognition, and learning experiences for students while the achievement of educational goals is maximized.

As mentioned in chapter 1, the purpose of West Point is to provide the nation with "leaders of character." For the Army, the ultimate test of military leadership is in combat. On the athletic fields and in varsity, club, and intramural sports, participants may encounter conditions similar to those they may face in combat. Among the similarities between athletic competition and combat situations are the mental, emotional, and physical stress; the fluidity and uncertainty of the situation; and the absolute necessity to work as a team (Anderson, 1988; USMA Circular 1-101, 2002).

In athletic competition at West Point, the qualities of mental and physical toughness, aggressiveness, personal courage, confidence, and determination, and the ability to think and act quickly and effectively under pressure, can be developed in order to prepare future Army officers for combat. This is why the Academy's leadership and faculty embrace the motto, "Every cadet an athlete, every athlete challenged." Students who do not participate on a varsity intercollegiate team must participate in the intercollegiate club sports or intramural athletic programs. An outcome goal of these athletic experiences is to contribute to the overall West Point purpose and mission—developing leaders of character.

Participation in athletics has the potential to increase each student's leadership skills (Siedentop, 1994). When properly conducted, and through adherence to the principles of fair play, these activities fully support and contribute to the basic purpose and mission of the Academy. Such quali-

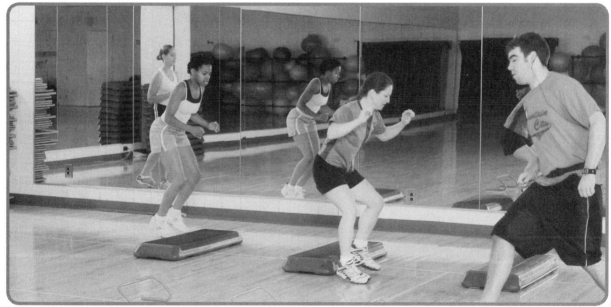

A student-led sport conditioning class.

© Human Kinetics

ties, expressed in action, are the traits that compose the traditional Army Values—loyalty, duty, respect, selfless service, honor, integrity, and personal courage. Because athletic activities involve many of the deepest and most powerful of human emotions, athletics offers the potential development of desirable leader qualities. Herein lies the true value of the sport education program at West Point, in which every student is a participating athlete.

Since every student participates in a sport at West Point, all are educated through the sport education model. There are three levels of competitive sport at West Point—Intramural, Intercollegiate Club, and Intercollegiate Varsity—and every student must participate in a sport during each academic term. This requirement is designed to provide each student with the opportunity to participate in sport, to develop leadership qualities, and to develop morally and ethically.

West Point's content and performance standards are similar to the National Standards for Physical Education (National Association for Sport and Physical Education, 1995). As a result of participation in competitive sport education, a sport leader of character (1) has learned the skills necessary to perform a variety of sports; (2) is physically fit; (3) participates regularly in sport; (4) knows the implications of and the benefits from involvement in sport; and (5) values sport and its contributions to leader development. In order to help clarify these values-based standards, the Academy has developed outcome and process goals. The outcome goals are what West Point wants its students to be able to do as a result of participating in the sport education program.

Outcome Goals

As a result of participation in sport education, students will

- exhibit those personal qualities deemed indispensable for "leaders of character,"
- demonstrate fair play and sportsmanship,
- gain an appreciation for the fitness required to participate in sport and the military lifestyle,
- participate in a level of sport consistent with their ability,
- gain an appreciation for the importance of "winning the right way" in sport and military life, and
- demonstrate effective teamwork and social interaction needed to attain team success.

The process goals provide the context within which the students will participate. In addition, to help translate broad program goals, program performance objectives are included that are more specific to achieving desired goals and end states.

Program Process Goals

- Provide challenging competitive sport experiences designed to promote the Army Values, personal growth, and a "warrior ethos" (*warrior ethos* is a military term meaning to never quit and to have an intense desire to win the right way)
- Provide students with opportunities to serve in leadership roles
- Provide a safe environment and appropriate resources to execute the program
- Program Performance Objectives
- Promote Army Values: loyalty, duty, respect, selfless service, honor, integrity, and personal courage
- Promote the roles of an officer—war fighter, leader of character, servant of the nation, and member of a time-honored profession
- Promote fair play and sportsmanship
- Ensure that every student is an athlete
- Provide opportunities for students to compete
- Develop a will to win the right way and the warrior ethos
- Provide leadership opportunities
- Develop leader attributes, skills, and actions:
  - Attributes: mental, physical, and emotional
  - Skills: conceptual, interpersonal, and sport skills
  - Actions: influencing (communicating, decision making, and motivating); operating (fitness, fair play, and winning attitude)

Values Education in Sport

While "Duty–Honor–Country" and "respect for others" provide the underpinnings of the West Point moral ethos, the sport education program is one of the vehicles for character development. Students get firsthand experiences testing these bedrock values in a relatively safe environment. West Point attends to the moral development of students, a process "inexorably integrated throughout all activities that comprise the West Point Experience" and "integral to the physical program" (USMA Circular 1-101, 2002). In order to develop an atmosphere of integrity and respect in sport, the Competitive Sport Education program at West Point has adopted the "Champions of Character" model from the National Association of Intercollegiate Athletics. This program includes pursuing victory in competitive sport while learning five core values—respect, responsibility, integrity, servant leadership, and sportsmanship (National Association of Intercollegiate Athletics, 2005).

To that end, the purpose of sport education is to illustrate and teach the principles of honor and respect for others on athletic fields—that sportsmanship, fair play, and honoring the rules are inherent in true victory. Success in this or any program does not guarantee that students always exercise their moral insights and apply their ability to reason ethically. But a sport education program exposes students to situations that often require them to act publicly when moral and ethical dilemmas arise. Students cannot escape encountering ethical dilemmas on the athletic fields. The Physical Program at West Point works with the other developmental programs (Academic and Military) to help students engage meaningfully with their emerging understanding of appropriate moral and ethical behavior. Through sport education, students can develop their ability to examine ethical issues and to act appropriately. Society needs educational institutions to furnish citizens of character who recognize the moral complexity of life, reflect on ethical matters, act on their moral convictions, and understand the moral implications of their decisions.

The sport education program at West Point seeks to educate students to be players in the fullest sense and to help them develop in the psychomotor, cognitive, and affective domains. The sport education program uses the U.S. Army's leadership doctrine of "Be (who you are), Know (what you know and understand), and Do (how you act)" as the framework to define the characteristics necessary for student leaders. This construct frames leaders in terms of their character, skills, and actions. Sport attributes and values help reveal one's character, "Be"; knowledge reveals itself in one's sport skills, "Know"; and the manifestation of the "Be" and the "Know" is ultimately in one's actions, "Do." The whole "Be, Know, Do" construct, however, is greater than the sum of its parts. Essentially,

students must possess a sound set of principles, know what to do in any given situation, and then apply the principles they have learned, both on and off the athletic field.

In the following section we describe how sport can be used to promote the development of leaders and leadership skills.

Leader Development Through Sport

Sporting activities not only have the potential to develop physical skills and promote well-being in participants; they also offer powerful opportunities for leader development. A way to understand development through sport participation is to examine leadership through two important developmental lenses:

1. Emerging leader development theory
2. The importance of the individual and the collective nature of leader developmental contexts

This section provides a brief explanation of the key aspects of these development perspectives, and then connects them to the leader development opportunities available in sport programs.

Emerging Leader Development Theory

For a long time, effective leader development was thought to be generated through simple experiences—the more experiences an individual had, the better he or she was thought to be developing as a leader. Our understanding of leader development has increased significantly over the last decade, and we now recognize that leader development is not just about experiences. Although experiences are still the foundation of all leader development, there is much more. Experiences must be intentionally designed as developmental and must be coupled with other important considerations (see figure 2.1).

Experiences will always be the hallmark of any developmental process. These experiences, to be developmental, must be intentionally constructed to be challenging; to create the possibility of loss or failure; and to move individuals outside of their intellectual, behavioral, and emotional comfort zones. Competitive sport does this by placing people in stressful, challenging situations that stretch individual and collective skills and provide

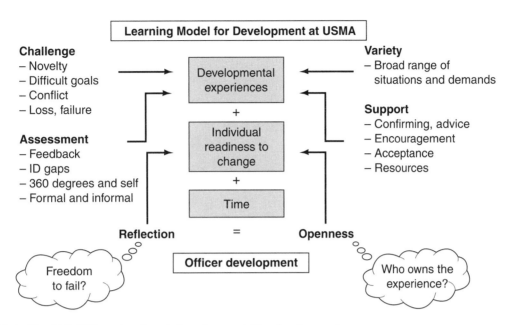

FIGURE 2.1   The U.S. Military Academy's learning model for development.

for the possibility of success, failure, or loss. Sport educators can purposefully create these challenging situations and learning experiences for students in many ways, such as

- skills assessments against an established standard,
- competitions,
- leadership positions (coaches, referees, timekeepers, etc.), and
- specific tasks and responsibilities.

A key aspect of any effective leader development system rests on the importance of reflection. Reflection is of critical importance for making sense out of experiences in order to turn them into something meaningful. Reflection is a learned process that can range from simple questions to complex journaling based on a set of targeted questions around the experiential context. Students should have the opportunity to think about and make sense of their experiences in a manner that facilitates learning and leadership growth. Professionals should provide opportunities for their students to reflect on their learning experiences on a regular basis.

In addition to reflection, support and feedback and subsequent developmental efforts should also be provided. As described earlier, developmental experiences provide challenges and move individuals outside of their comfort zones. Developmental experiences should cause individuals to confront

their personal limitations and must "stretch" them beyond what they think they can handle. At the same time, students need to feel empowered to take risks, to actually get outside of their comfort zones and think and behave in different ways. Physical education professionals must be willing to underwrite failure while holding individuals accountable for development through constructive criticism and meaningful feedback. Finally, students must be given sufficient time to develop. Each student is on his or her own developmental journey. Some take more time than others to reach developmental milestones. But given time, appropriate readiness, challenging experiences, and regular reflection with support and feedback, each student can reach established developmental goals.

Leader Development: An Individual and Collective Process

Student development is predominantly seen as an individual process focusing on building intrapersonal competencies. Competencies such as self-awareness, self-regulation, self-confidence, and self-motivation are normally associated with leader development as an individual process. West Point is integral in its involvement in the building of leaders of character for the Army; and this development, for the most part, occurs one student at a time. The Academy's development system requires that instructors "meet students where they are" in their

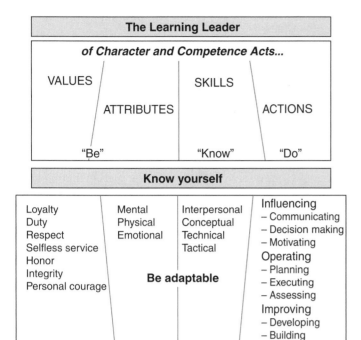

FIGURE 2.2 The Cadet Leader Development System.

developmental levels and then guide them along through the six domains of development (academic, physical, military, social, moral-ethical, spiritual) as outlined by the Cadet Leader Development System (see figure 2.2) (USMA Circular 1-101, 2002).

Leadership development primarily occurs in the context of associations with others, focusing on what the leader is doing. It is about expanding the collective capacities of organizational members to perform effectively in assigned roles and in their interaction with others. Competitive sports, many of which are team sports, provide a wonderful opportunity for leader and leadership development. Sports not only provide the context for developing valuable *individual* knowledge, skills, and abilities in participants, but also provide a *collective* context for leadership development. Team-based sports create opportunities to learn about a number of important life skills including teamwork, cohesion, conflict resolution, and putting team needs ahead of individual preferences.

What is important in this discussion is that competitive sports are *not* just about the development of specific knowledge, skills, and abilities within a given athletic venue. As suggested by emerging leader and leadership development theory, sporting activities provide a rich opportunity for development if they are viewed as developmental venues. Competitive sporting activities, if properly organized and constructed, can have significant long-term impacts beyond the athletic playing fields, not only in building leadership skills but also in preparing students for their roles as productive citizens and community leaders.

Making the Connection to Your School Setting

Although every school has its own unique situation and setting, what follows are suggested guidelines to implement an intramural or recreational sport program using the sport education model. Supervisors and program directors can use this section as a guide to plan and execute their own programs.

Choosing a Sport

It is important for educators to choose a sport that they know well and that is appropriate for the age levels of their students. This will help teachers in evaluating the students as well as in modifying the game to meet the objectives of the unit. The teacher can create a student sport "council" to assist in modifying the game to meet various ability levels. The council does not have to be a formal organization, just a forum for getting input from the students. One of the keys to the success of the sport education model is empowering students in many aspects of the program. The teacher can also give students a set of constraints and limitations imposed by facilities, time, and level of experience and can allow them to come up with their own solutions to the sport's challenges. The teacher does not have to use the students' ideas, but by listening to students and selecting the best of their work, the teacher gives them ownership of the activity.

For example, the teacher can provide students with a selection of six sports and then allow them to vote on the sport they wish to play. Again, this process can increase the students' sense of ownership of the sport and may further motivate them and engage them in the activity.

Other considerations in choosing a sport include ensuring that the sport is age appropriate and that it enables students to experience a variety of activities. The complexity of the sport and its rules should gradually increase as students get older. When the rules of a sport are simplified, students who might not have understood the sport or may have been reluctant participants may feel less intimidated or more willing to participate. There is also a benefit to exposing students to a variety of sports. New or novel sports will often "level the playing field" with more skilled or coordinated students, and can help students develop coordination and confidence in a new activity. By using a sport that most students are unfamiliar with, the teacher can create a challenge for those students familiar with traditional sports and can ease the fear of failure of those who do not have a competitive sport participation background.

The use of elimination sports is not recommended. Elimination sports are sports in which participants are removed from the game as part of the rules of the game. Dodge ball is a common example. Elimination sports are counter to the philosophy of sport education.

Modifying the Sport

Changes to the game can be implemented to suit both the students' and the teacher's needs. Modifications made to the game can be a key component to a successful season and can often maximize student participation. While the modifications possible are limited only by the instructor's imagination, the following are several possibilities:

- Small-sided games
- Smaller fields
- Short-duration games
- Equipment variations (e.g., larger scoring areas, nets, goals)
- Scoring variations
- Rules simplification
- Mandatory player touch (every player on a team must touch the ball before the team can score)

Smaller-sided games allow more players to become actively engaged. Smaller fields serve the same function, can often speed up the play of the game, and create more opportunities for the active engagement of all students. Short duration allows for games that can more realistically fit in a physical education class time frame. Instructors can modify the game to fit their particular classroom or field space situation. Equipment variations, such as the use of a smaller-sized soccer ball and goal, can help level the playing field by creating a more challenging setting. Simplification of game rules allows the game to flow more smoothly. If rules are more readily understood by less experienced students, less time will be spent awarding penalties or interpreting calls, and more time will be spent on involvement in the sport.

Selecting Teams

In the sport education model, the method of team selection depends largely on the instructor's particular setting and goals. Every technique will not work for every teacher or every setting. Allowing students to select the teams, coaches, and game officials, as well as any other roles an instructor might find necessary to execute the program, can maximize student ownership. Again, this allows students to realize that this is their sport season, not the instructor's.

Several techniques exist for determining teams. A lottery system may be used. A student sport council may be established to select teams and possibly also to select coaches. Some teachers utilize a tryout system. A common check that must be performed following the selection of teams is to ensure that players are distributed as evenly as possible according to their skills. Either the students, the sport council, or the teacher can do this. If the teacher empowers the students to select teams, then the teacher must carefully and diplomatically ensure that skilled players are equally distributed.

When establishing the guidelines for team selection, the teacher must identify any special concerns with his or her particular group of students. Are there students who will be physically unable to participate because of temporary or long-term injuries? Students with temporary injuries could be utilized in nonplaying roles such as scorekeeper or statistician. Those with long-term injuries precluding participation could fill the same roles if it is determined that there is no way to adapt the game to allow them to participate safely. Have the students been introduced to the sport in a lead-up unit? In most settings it is appropriate to conduct a lead-up unit or series of lessons prior to the actual start of the sport season. This establishes a base of knowledge that the student coaches can build upon.

Implementing Student Roles

A variety of roles can be used in a sport education season. The selection of the roles themselves and students to fill these roles is a pivotal piece of the establishment of the sport season. The teacher and students can work together to accomplish both of these tasks. The teacher can lay out a basic framework of roles to be filled and can allow the students to add or delete positions. Again, this empowers the students and gives them a sense of ownership. The amount of ownership in filling roles will largely depend on the age of the students. The teacher should establish clear criteria for those students who are to be placed in leadership positions. The following are possible roles, along with a brief description of the duties associated with each.

- Coaches: responsible for planning and conducting team practices
- Assistant coaches or captains: aid coaches and captains in fulfilling their duties
- Captains: assist coach, lead team onto the field
- Referees and officials: maintain order and discipline during record contests, enforce rules fairly and impartially
- Scorekeepers: keep track of the score during record contests or scrimmages
- Statisticians: keep team and individual statistics throughout the season
- Publicists: publicize team or league results in school newspaper or fliers; advertise contests; increase student body awareness of sport season
- Managers: assist with equipment issue, aid in the creation of a team identity
- Trainers: plan and conduct physical training and conditioning for the team
- Sport council: liaise between the students and the teacher, aids in selection of students to fill various roles and in team selection, settles any disputes or protests related to record contests, plans season, sets record contest schedule
- Sportscasters: announce at record contests, announce at award ceremonies, disseminate results of record contests with daily announcements on the school public address system

Teachers may use as many or as few of these roles as they deem appropriate. The key is making certain that all students are included and feel that they are a valuable part of the sport season. To that end, teachers should tailor the roles provided and the duty description for each of those roles to fit their unique instructional situation.

Appropriate Competition for Your Students

One of the goals of most sport education units is to maximize students' participation or time on task. In order to facilitate this, teachers should keep elimination tournaments and double elimination tournaments to a minimum or should simply not use them. Competition schedules should be set to allow all teams to continue to participate, regardless of a winless record. If a league champion is desired, the teacher can select the champion based on overall records for the season. The following are types of competition schedules:

- Round robin: Every team plays every other team in the league.
- Two or four leagues: The teacher sets up as many leagues as needed; a league could be established for each class hour.
- Multiple competitions: Each team plays multiple competitions on each record contest day.
- Performance standards versus competitions: Teams compete against a known standard, for example running a cross-country course in an established time.

Promoting and Teaching Sportsmanship and Fair Play

Teachers should be especially concerned with the issue of sportsmanship and fair play when planning a sport season. The research shows that youth sports often tend to neglect this area to a great extent and that students may end up bringing a "win at all costs" attitude to the physical education setting (Bredemeier, 1995; Rudd & Stoll, 2004; Wandzilak, Carroll, & Ansorge, 1988). However, there are examples across the country of youth sport programs that focus more on sportsmanship and fair play than on winning and losing (Coakley, 2004; Hellison, 2003).

Several techniques may be utilized to create this type of atmosphere. One such technique might entail establishing a code of conduct. The teacher can utilize the students' sport council to develop a code of conduct and allow officials and coaches to enforce the code during practices and games. Rules and consequences can be developed and enforced by the sport council. The code of conduct should address not only player behavior, but also the behavior of the coaches and spectators.

A fair-play system could be used to help determine a team's standing for the year or to assist in the determination of the winner of a game. Regardless of the type of system used, some common themes for success in implementation do exist. First, the instructor or the sport council (or both) should make sure that specific behaviors related to fair play are made clear and are understood by the students. The officials and the sport council can assist in helping to implement and enforce this. Second, the instructor should reward positive behaviors and penalize negative behaviors through some type of accountability system. This sort of system utilizes student officials to assess each team's behavior as well as address specific instances of poor conduct. This action could consist of a point (or points) reward for good sportsmanship or a deduction for poor sportsmanship, depending on how the class and the instructor choose to set up their particular system. Other enhancements that may aid in the promotion of fair play are awards for individuals and teams demonstrating the best sportsmanship and the establishment of rituals that promote sportsmanship, such as shaking hands at the conclusion of a game.

Another technique to teach sportsmanship and fair play is for each team to establish two or three themes or goals they will emphasize during their season. For example, a team may have a goal that they will never taunt or trash talk their opponent. Instructors can have teams write these goals down and refer to them during the season.

Teachers can use their sport education setting to teach values and attributes that can result in fair play and good sportsmanship. Opportunities to take advantage of "teachable moments" will present themselves often in a sport setting and will allow educators to discuss and show students what certain attributes look like in a sport setting. The following are some examples.

Responsibility—keeping commitments, performing one's duty and fulfilling obligations, and exercising self-discipline

- Being where you are supposed to be
- Being on time and prepared
- Following directions and listening carefully

Respect—having regard for the fundamental worth and dignity of every human being

- Taking turns
- Cooperating and listening to what others have to say

- Being fair
- Not taunting or trash talking
- Not making fun of others
- Sharing
- Saying "I'm sorry"; "nice play"; "good job"; "good game"
- Controlling your temper and your language

Honesty—being truthful, forthright, and sincere

- Telling the truth
- Keeping your word
- Being trustworthy

Courage—facing adversity, challenges, and fears

- Greeting a new student or player
- Asking for help when you are afraid to do so
- Telling a peer or friend to stop doing something that is hurtful or bothering to someone else
- Trying something you don't think you are very good at

Gratitude—understanding and being appreciative of what you have, who you are, and what others do for you

- Saying "thank you"
- Helping those in need or less fortunate than you
- Avoiding envy and jealousy
- Being grateful for your uniqueness

When situations arise in a teacher's educational sport environment that allow these and other attributes to be modeled, taught, or reinforced, teachers should take advantage of them. They should also allow time for reflection and discussion. What happened? Why did it happen? How can we prevent this from happening in the future?

Facilitating Sport Education

The role of the teacher at all levels should be as a facilitator for the students' sport season. The teacher enables the students to be successful during the season by conducting a lead-up unit on the sport, by establishing clear criteria for the selection of students to fill various roles, and by assisting and aiding in the development of a manual for the sport. How much additional guidance and support the teacher provides depends largely on the students' experience with the sport, their age, and their maturity level. Middle school students often require more input from the teacher while secondary school students might require only minimal input. Good advance planning by the teacher sets the students up for success.

Coaching clinics before the start of the season are key to well-run games, and it is important that they be maintained throughout the season as well. Crucial to the empowerment of the team's student coaches and officials is teacher feedback, filtered through the student coach or official rather than given directly to the student players. Every age level requires varying levels of guidance from the teacher. As a rule, the teacher should try to allow students to take on as much responsibility as pos-

sible. Doing this serves to increase their ownership of the sport season and allows them to learn valuable leadership and organizational skills that will increase their overall level of confidence. This "hands-off" approach is often difficult for active teachers, especially novice teachers. However, teachers must make a conscious effort to work through the student leadership and allow their students to make decisions. It is also imperative that teachers monitor all games for any unsafe or unwise decisions.

What follows is an example of taking an existing game, soccer, and modifying it to meet the goals and resources available to an intramural program. The result, known as "sockey" (soccer with a little bit of hockey), has been enjoyed in West Point's intramural sport program for several years.

Sockey

Seven-versus-seven soccer is a small-sided variation of the real 11-sided game. The rules have been modified to increase the pace and score of the game. The game should be adjusted to fit your school's unique situation. A recommended time for a contest is two 10-minute halves with a 5-minute half-time break. At approximately the 5-minute mark of each half, during a natural stoppage of play, the referee will turn to each coach and ask for substitutes. This should be a 15-second process with no time-out for coaching.

INSTRUCTIONS

A coin flip determines which team kicks off to start the game and which team attacks and defends at which end of the field. Both teams will attack and defend their respective ends of the field until half-time, when the directions will change. The team that kicks off to begin the game will change at half-time. The kickoff begins each half. The game is restarted after every goal is scored; it is restarted from a team's own 25-yard line. All members of the attacking team must stay behind their 25-yard line until the ball has been kicked and has traveled one revolution. At that point, all attacking players may step up and play. All players on the defending team must stay behind their 25-yard line until the attacking team has put the ball in play. Once the ball has traveled one revolution, the defensive team may step up and defend.

SETUP

- Dimensions: 75 by 40 yards (69 by 37 meters)
- Field divided into playing thirds (offensive, middle, and defensive), 25 yards (23 meters) in length
- Team handball goals centered on end lines
- Restraining arcs, 5-yard (4.5-meter) radius, centered in the middle of each goal
- Penalty kick spot: 12 yards (11 meters) from goal line, centered with middle of goal (see figure 2.3)

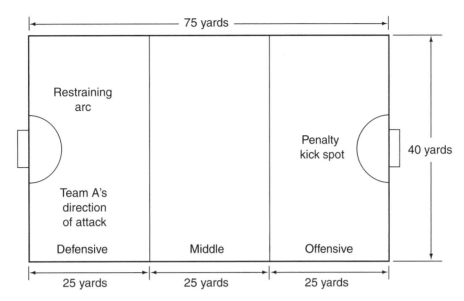

FIGURE 2.3 Sockey setup.

SCORING

- Goals scored from a team's offensive third count as 1 point.
- Goals scored from a team's middle third count as 2 points.
- Goals scored from a team's defensive third count as 3 points.

The winner of a game is the team with the most total points at the end of the game, which include fair-play points subtracted for yellow and red card infractions.

FOULS

All fouls are treated as direct-kick violations (on the restart, the ball may be kicked directly into the goal). Fouls committed by the defensive team in the offensive team's middle and defensive third result in a direct free kick from the point of the infraction. There are no offsides on the initial restart kick. After the initial kick, the offsides rule comes back into play. The defensive team is required to be 10 yards away from the ball until after the kick is taken. Fouls committed by the defensive team in the offensive team's final third result in a penalty kick taken by the offensive team from the 12-yard line.

POSSIBLE FOULS

- Spitting
- Kicking or attempting to kick opponent
- Tripping or attempting to trip another player (includes stooping in front or behind)
- Charging an opponent in a violent or dangerous manner
- Charging an opponent from behind unless the latter is obstructing
- Striking or attempting to strike another player
- Holding
- Pushing
- Handling the ball intentionally (except by the goalkeeper in his or her penalty area)

- Playing in a dangerous manner
- Intentionally obstructing when not playing the ball
- Charging the keeper (exceptions are discussed)
- Slide tackling

Misconduct is punished by either a caution (yellow card) or a send-off (red card). Teams receiving cards lose fair-play points—5 points for a yellow card and 10 points for a red card. Players are cautioned (given a yellow card) for the following incidents of misconduct:

- Entering or leaving the field without permission
- Persistent infringements of the rules
- Dissent
- For the coach if his or her team reports 5 or more minutes late for any contest

Five "cumulative" yellow cards, given over the course of the season, equal one red card. Players are given a red card for the following:

- Violent conduct, such as striking someone
- Serious foul play, usually against the rules of play
- Foul or abusive language or gesture
- Second yellow card offense after having received a previous yellow card during the same game
- Receiving two yellow cards in one game
- Receiving five cumulative yellow cards

RESTRAINING ARC

At both ends of the field, a restraining arc, 5 yards (4.5 meters) in radius, is drawn and centered from the center of each goal. Only the goalkeeper is allowed to defend the ball inside of this arc. Should the ball touch or strike any other defensive field player within this restraining arc, a penalty kick is awarded to the offensive team. It is permissible for attacking players to run through or into the restraining arc and to play the ball. The purpose of the restraining arc is to discourage defensive packing in front of the goal and to encourage offense and scoring.

OUT-OF-BOUNDS

A ball must be completely over the sideline or the end line in order to be considered out-of-bounds.

The team that touches the ball last before it goes out-of-bounds loses possession of the ball. The new attacking team puts the ball back into play with a direct free kick from the point where the ball went out-of-bounds. There are no offsides during the initial kick on kick-ins. After the initial kick, the offsides rule applies.

If the defensive team last touches the ball before it goes over the end line, the offensive team takes a corner kick (direct free kick) from the side of the field where the ball went out-of-bounds. If the offensive team last touches the ball before it goes over the end line (i.e., a missed shot), the ball is put back into play by the new offensive team (a goal kick) with a direct free kick from the end line, on the side of the goal closest to where the ball went out-of-bounds. The defensive team must retreat back outside the 25-yard (23-meter) box (their final third) until the ball has been put back into play.

OFFSIDES

The offsides rule is similar to that in hockey. All attacking players must stay behind the 25-yard (23-meter) line that separates their attacking and middle third of the field until after the ball has entered the final attacking third. Once the ball has entered the final third, attacking players may be anywhere inside that zone and must not be offside. Should the defensive team clear the ball into the middle third, all attacking players must leave the final third and wait until the ball reenters the zone before reentering it themselves. Violations of the offsides rule result in a direct free kick for the defensive team from their own defensive 25-yard line. Players on the offending team must be 10 yards (9 meters) away from the ball when it is put back into play. There are no offsides on kick-ins.

PENALTY KICK

Any rules infraction committed by the defensive team inside their defensive third of the field results in a penalty kick taken by the opposing team. A penalty kick is a direct free kick taken from the 12-yard (11-meter) spot. Only the goalkeeper is allowed to defend inside the restraining arc. All players are required to stand behind the end line or 25-yard line until after the penalty kick has been taken. Players lining up behind the end line must do so outside the restraining arc. The order in which players can line up is defensive player next to the arc, then alternating offensive, defensive, and so on (the way basketball players line up for foul shots). Once the kick has been taken, the game resumes, and all rules apply.

SHOOTOUTS AND PENALTY KICKS (PLAYOFF GAMES ONLY)

If the game is tied at the end of regulation time, fair-play points are used to determine the winner. Should the two teams have equal fair-play points, penalty kicks are taken for declaring a winner. Teams alternately take penalty kicks until each team has taken three kicks. Only players on the field at the end of regulation time are permitted to participate in the initial shootout. If the score is still tied after the six total kicks, the remaining eight players from the field shoot in sudden death format. If the game is still tied, teams take alternating kicks using the remaining players on the sideline, in sudden death fashion. After all players on a team have taken a kick, then the same rotation of kickers is used until a winner has been declared.

GOALKEEPER

The goalkeeper is identified by a colored armband. Only goalkeepers are allowed to defend within the restraining arc. Goalkeepers are expected to play the field and are considered a goalkeeper only when they are inside the restraining arc. Goalkeepers are not allowed to pick up with their hands any ball that is passed back off the foot of a teammate. They may handle any ball that is passed back from any other body part.

POINT SYSTEM FOR STANDINGS

- Winner: 3 points
- Tie: 1 point
- Loser: 0 points

At the end of all regulation contests, the following system determines who will advance to the playoffs:

- Point total
- Head-to-head competition

- Goal differential
- Fair-play point total
- Most goals scored
- Least goals allowed
- Flip of coin

Using the sport education model as a guide to plan and execute a sport program in a school setting is a superb and effective way to get all students involved and to teach them more than just how to play a sport. The sport education model allows teachers to challenge both themselves and their students to develop in the psychomotor, cognitive, and affective domains, and offers wonderful opportunities to teach and develop positive character traits and to learn about sportsmanship and fair play.

References

Anderson, J. (1988). Competitive sports and character development. Unpublished manuscript. West Point, NY: U.S. Military Academy, Department of Physical Education.

Beller, J.M., & Stoll, S.K. (1995). Moral reasoning of high school student athletes and general students: An empirical study versus personal testimony. *Pediatric Exercise Science, 7(4),* 352-363.

Bredemeier, B.L. (1995). Divergence in children's moral reasoning about issues in daily life and sport specific contexts. *International Journal of Sport Psychology, 26,* 453-463.

Bredemeier, B.J., & Shields, D.L. (1984). Divergence in moral reasoning about sport and life. *Sociology of Sport Journal, 1(4),* 348-357.

Coakley, J.J. (2004). *Sport in society: Issues and controversies.* (8th ed.). Boston: McGraw-Hill.

Hahm, C. (1989). Moral reasoning and development among general students, physical education majors, and student athletes. Unpublished doctoral dissertation, University of Idaho.

Hellison, D.R. (2003). *Teaching responsibility through physical activity.* (2nd ed.). Champaign, IL: Human Kinetics.

National Association of Intercollegiate Athletics. (2005). Champions of character. Retrieved 20 April, 2005, from http://naia.org.

National Association for Sport and Physical Education. (1995). *Moving into the future: National standards for physical education.* Reston, VA: American Alliance for Health, Physical Education, Recreation and Dance.

Priest, R.F., Krause, J.V., & Beach, J. (1999). Four-year changes in college athletes' ethical value choices in sports situations. *Research Quarterly for Exercise and Sport, 70(2),* 170-178.

Rudd, A., & Stoll, S. (2004). What type of character do athletes possess? An empirical examination of college athletes versus college non athletes with The RSBH Value Judgment Inventory. *The Sport Journal, 7(2),* 1-10.

Siedentop, D. (1994). *Quality PE through positive sport experience: Sport education.* Champaign, IL: Human Kinetics.

Silva, J.M. (1983). The perceived legitimacy of rule violating behavior in sport. *Journal of Sport Psychology, 5(4),* 438-448.

USMA Circular 1-101. (2002). *Cadet leader development system.* West Point, NY: U.S. Military Academy.

Wandzilak, T., Carroll, T., & Ansorge, C.J. (1988). Values development through physical activity: Promoting sportsmanlike behaviors, perceptions, and moral reasoning. *Journal of Teaching Physical Education, 8(1),* 13-22.

Suggested Readings

Clifford, C., & Feezell, R.M. (1997). *Coaching for character.* Champaign, IL: Human Kinetics.

U.S. Department of the Army. (1999). *Army leadership.* Field Manual 22-100. Washington, DC: Government Printing Office.

National Governing Organization

American Sport Education Program
P.O. Box 5076
Champaign, IL 61825-5076
800-747-5698
E-mail: asep@hkusa.com

3

Program Assessment

Susan Tendy

Assessment is an evaluation of worth. An assessment initiative can have meaning only if there is a measure of worth or effectiveness guiding the process. Any approach to program evaluation should focus on a measure of effectiveness based on predetermined benchmarks or goals. Program assessment evaluates goal accomplishment and is often referred to as "outcomes assessment." This goals-based approach tells us where we want to go before we make a judgment concerning our progress toward that goal. These outcome goals or *tasks* are the guiding tenets that give us direction. It is important to note that we must be attentive to the process as well as to the outcome. The sequence of learning activities through which a student travels forms the pathway to goal attainment. Assessment of the teaching–learning model and assessment of the curriculum design are also important aspects of an integrated assessment system.

The primary *tools* that we have at our disposal are various measurement techniques, many of which are already in place and which may be unique to an organization. Taking advantage of these already existing indicators (performance scores, surveys, written reports, etc.) from multiple perspectives helps to maximize efficiency and minimize disturbance to the normal routine. Every effort should be made to collect and identify data that accurately present the program being examined. These relevant data allow those responsible for the program to make an informed decision based on credible and relevant information.

A calendar or *timeline* of measurement tools set out beforehand will enable program evaluators to prepare for these events and to troubleshoot any issues involving data identification or collection. Additionally, using measures from multiple points in time increases the reliability of the information gathered, as well as the validity of the conclu-

The author would like to acknowledge former visiting professors Dr. Larry Hensley, University of Northern Iowa, and Dr. Jerry Krause, Gonzaga University, for their mentoring and expert guidance, as well as their contributions to the foundational activities of the Assessment Division of the Department of Physical Education at the United States Military Academy.

sions. An ongoing assessment program should be responsive to decision makers. In contrast to the negative connotation often associated with accountability procedures, periodic assessment affords an opportunity to receive assistance for improvement. It also promotes informed decision making when change is necessary, in addition to ensuring that resources are appropriately allocated.

Purpose of Program Assessment

The purpose or mission of the assessment section is to evaluate our program in terms of stated goals in order to improve programs and to respond to both internal and external agencies. This goals-based evaluation plan enables our program leaders to create an assessment process that generates information that may be used to guide program development and improvement, as well as to demonstrate accountability and program impact. Our assessment system must generate information that measures the Physical Program's outcomes for internal use, as well as for reporting back to external agencies such as the Department of the Army, the Department of Defense, the United States Congress, or the Middle States Association of Colleges and Schools as requested.

The structure consists of a director of assessment and committee members representing each of the areas within the Physical Program. In our department, those areas are the instruction, facilities, research, competitive sports, and assessment divisions. The director provides oversight of the assessment process. This person has responsibility for the overall management of the Physical Program assessment system, compiles all external assessment data, and makes this information available to all directorates as needed. With committee input, the director assembles an annual assessment report. The division representative helps the director establish a focus for the overall assessment process for the department and the divisions within. Additionally, the representative provides advice relevant to their area of interest in order to help determine the degree to which division and department goals are attained. Committee members synthesize all annual division findings and recommendations and provide input to the assessment director relative to the annual report.

Initiating an Assessment Program for Your School

The first step in the process of initiating an assessment program is to establish a representative group of stakeholders who will be able to demonstrate to decision makers the linkage between program goals, program design, modes of implementation, and desired outcomes. Once this group has been established, develop a general strategy and methodological procedures for gathering assessment information. The following steps are a general blueprint that you might find helpful.

Goal Development

1. The design (or revision) and acceptance of program or department goals. These should be linked to larger institutional goals.
2. The design (or revision) and acceptance of the subgoals of the respective divisions or groups within the program (for example, instruction, competitive sport, facilities, operations, assessment). These division goals must be linked to the program goals.
3. Operationalization of the goals-based program assessment effort. This means that an established goal must be defined in such a way that it is an observable or measurable event.
4. Conducting a periodic review, affirmation, and adjustment of the program and division goals as needed.

Develop a strategic assessment plan that considers the following:

1. Program goals. A periodic review of goal statements should be conducted in light of changes in program and institutional needs, national educational trends, state mandates, and locally obtained assessment results.
2. Design of the program. As program goals and desired outcomes are formulated, assessing your program design might involve examining the appropriateness of current physical education courses, competitive athletic experiences, physical fitness testing procedures and results, and other supporting activities. Such an assessment should include an examination of the alignment of course goals with program components. It is important to develop course goals based on faculty input

and perspectives, as well as considering the students who are served by the program.

3. **Implementation of the program.** Assessing how your program is executed requires an examination of course syllabi, instructional materials, pedagogical practices, students' course products, students' course feedback, faculty perspectives, and relevant summative reports.

4. **Desired outcomes.** Assessing the achievement of outcome goals is largely based on student performance data; attitudinal surveys of various constituencies; and department chair, principal, or superintendent feedback.

Procedures for Gathering Assessment Information

Your starting point should be to determine the *institutionalized data collection systems* that are already in place (see table 3.1). Examples include opinion surveys of stakeholders (students, parents, faculty, and administrators), self-report questionnaires looking for trends within a population, and focus group interviews to establish recommendations for change. Maximizing the use of this existing information is an important part of an efficient assessment process.

Embedded indicators within a program, such as fitness performance tests, student portfolios, performance reports, summative reports, and course or instructor evaluations by students, are other valuable tools currently in existence in most programs that provide another view of goal attainment. Summative reports, which are conducted immediately after an event or course has been completed, serve as documented feedback to both participants and program administrators. A recommended summative report format consists of suggestions for improvement and should be written under the following headings: *Issue, Discussion,* and *Recommendations.* This enables quick identification of the problem, affords an opportunity for the person giving feedback to discuss confounding issues, and provides decision makers with a recommendation from the stakeholders' point of view.

External visitors, consultants, and inspectors, such as visiting professors, exchange students, or accreditation review committees, will offer observation opportunities that provide an outside perspective. Scheduling regular exit interviews as part of a program involving these participants will enable comparison of external opinions over time.

Graduate performance data such as the percentage of students who successfully achieve established program goals are an excellent indicator of a program's success. Colleges and universities naturally follow their graduates. However, there may be smaller, accessible units within your elementary or secondary school that can be easily identified. One example is members of an athletic team who have maintained contact with their former coach.

Tasks, Tools, and Timelines

It is important to identify program elements (tasks) that will be evaluated during an assessment period and that will help determine the assessment methodology (tools). The determination of an assessment schedule (timeline) permits a realistic collection of information and reporting of results. Knowing where to go for data already collected as part of your school's normal procedures will avoid repeating work already completed. As illustrated in the examples in figure 3.1, program assessment is an ongoing activity that does not stop at the end of the assessment period. The process is continuous, with various pieces of the puzzle being examined as time goes on. Recommended benchmarks for assessment activities might include the following:

- Conduct an initial assessment-planning meeting with your division working group or committee members.
- Establish your assessment focus for the current academic year.
- Identify potential assessment tools and verify that these tools are developed and in place.
- Establish a data collection or retrieval and analysis timeline.
- Committee chair prepares an initial report format, with committee input.
- Final report is submitted to assessment committee for review.
- Establish assessment prospectus for the next assessment or academic year.

Applying Assessment Information

Your final assessment report is a feedback tool for decision makers that can be diagnostic, formative, or summative. Periodic in-progress reviews are

Table 3.1 Methodologies for Gathering Assessment Information

Tools	Timeline	Data source
Student surveys	Annual	Institutional
Course surveys	Annual	Institutional
Graduate surveys	Annual	Institutional
Supervisor surveys	Annual	Institutional
Interviews with students	As needed	Department
Interviews with faculty and staff	As needed	Department
Interviews with graduates	As needed	Department
Interviews with current students	Annual	Institutional
Command climate survey	Every other year	Institutional
Student demographics inventory	Annual	Admissions
Athletic surveys	Periodic	Athletic department
Special needs surveys—various groups	As needed	Target group
Admissions data	Annual	Admissions
Examination of fitness scores	Annual	Physical education
Course grades	Each round	Instructional division
Course products	Annual	Instructional division
Course/Instruction student evaluations	Each round	Instructional division
Certification reports	Annual	Instructional division
Examination of course content and alignment	Periodic	Instructional division
Summative reports	Continuous	All divisions
Injury reports	Periodic	Athletic training
External evaluation team reports	As needed	Ad hoc
Visiting professor reports	Annual	Visiting professor
Division assessment reports	Annual	All divisions
Facilities inspection reports	Annual	Operations
Review of faculty portfolios	Annual	Department chair

Reprinted from United States Military Academy, Department of Physical Education, 2001, *Physical Program Assessment Committee Report* (West Point, NY: United States Military Academy), 40.

important to ensure that the assessment process is on track. It is important that the information be returned in a timely manner and that any recommended changes and improvements involve several courses of action. For example, suggestions for change should consider the lead time required for changes within the operational abilities of an organization to effect those changes. Offering more than one solution may increase the possibility that your recommendations can be implemented. With

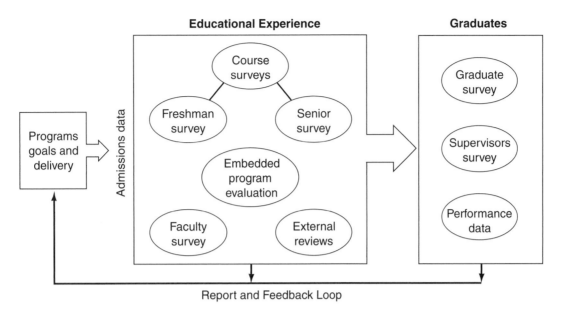

Educational Experience

Course surveys

Freshman survey

Senior survey

Embedded program evaluation

Faculty survey

External reviews

Admissions data

Programs goals and delivery

Graduates

Graduate survey

Supervisors survey

Performance data

Report and Feedback Loop

FIGURE 3.1 The program assessment loop.

Reprinted from United States Military Academy, Department of Physical Education, 2001, *Physical Program Assessment Committee Report* (West Point, NY: United States Military Academy), 35.

this in mind, your report should allow time for the information to be processed, analyzed, discussed, and reflected upon by all concerned, both internal and external to your assessment division. Scheduling face-to-face assessment briefings with involved decision makers will highlight and clarify essential findings.

Report development should be based on the results of assessment efforts limited to the preceding assessment calendar year. However, comparative data from prior years will alert leaders to important trends and changes. The following format may be helpful in preparing your assessment report:

- Review of established goals
- Summary of assessment activities
- Findings in relation to goal attainment
- Recommendations
- Appendix (including supporting data, information, charts, etc.)
- Assessment prospectus for next year (tasks, tools, timelines)

One final thought: The benefits of forming an assessment division or committee in your school for the purpose of evaluating your program are well worth the time and effort. Your ability to make a statement about the level of accomplishment of goals in your program, and backing it up with hard data, place you in a powerful position when

you are asking for additional resources, protecting your program, or responding to external agencies. You will not be queried on your program based on your years of experience, but on the facts that are in front of you. If you don't have an assessment program in place, start small by examining and perhaps refining your program goals, and build from there. It is imperative that as you assess your program, you link it to your program goals. The result of a quality outcomes assessment process may possibly be the key to protecting your program and may result in an improved physical education program for the students you teach.

Reference

United States Military Academy, Department of Physical Education. (2001). *Physical Program Assessment Committee report.* West Point, NY: United States Military Academy.

Suggested Readings

American Association for Higher Education. (1992). *Principles of good practice for assessing student learning.* Washington, DC: AAHE.

Joint Committee on Standards for Educational Evaluation. (1994). *The program evaluation standards: How to assess evaluations of educational programs.* (2nd ed.). Thousand Oaks, CA: Sage.

Metzler, M., & Tjeerdsma, B. (2000). *Assessment of physical education teacher education programs.* Reston, VA: NASPE.

Middle States Association of Colleges and Schools. (1996). *Framework for outcomes assessment.* (2nd ed.). Philadelphia: Commission on Higher Education.

Middle States Commission on Higher Education. (1999). *Report by the Commission on Higher Education of the Middle States Association of Colleges and Schools.* Philadelphia: Middle States Commission on Higher Education.

Middle States Commission on Higher Education. (2002). *Characteristics of excellence in higher education: Eligibility requirements and standards for accreditation.* Philadelphia: Middle States Commission on Higher Education.

National Association for Sport and Physical Education. (1995). *Moving into the future: National standards for physical education.* Reston, VA: NASPE.

PART II

Core Activity Courses

Basic Movement

Jeffrey Coelho

Military academies have a long history of gymnastics and movement instruction. Gymnastics, in one form or another, has been offered at West Point since 1838. The present Basic Movement course at West Point is a gymnastics-oriented, movement fundamentals experience with a focus on selected military physical challenges and applications.

Participating in movement fundamentals and gymnastics-related activities is an important part of every student's overall experience in physical education and can make significant contributions to the goals of physical education (Pangrazi & Dauer, 1992). Students use basic movement skills (supporting, swinging, hanging, jumping, vaulting, rolling, climbing, crawling, landing, etc.) in their everyday lives and in many sports. The benefits of participating in a basic movement course include improved body control; development of locomotion and manipulative skills; and the promotion of strength, power, flexibility, balance, agility, coordination, social interaction, and teamwork. Other benefits include opportunities for problem solving, skill analysis, error recognition and correction, understanding of body mechanics, and developing an appreciation for the aesthetic significance of sport.

The design of a gymnastics program can include the traditional model, educational gymnastics, stations and circuits, and rhythmic gymnastics (Werner, 1994). The infinite variety of teaching situations, program goals, time constraints, and equipment are just some of the factors that determine the type of gymnastics approach that can be offered. Often, a combination of approaches may effectively meet the needs of students and the goals of most programs.

Educational gymnastics is a movement education method that allows for individual differences, focuses on problem solving, and develops body control. The development of skills involves multiple correct solutions to open-ended movement patterns (Nilges, 1997). Students perform and progress within their ability levels while developing body management skills. Skills are broadly defined to encourage individual creativity and versatility. Students progress and explore their own unique ways of completing the movement tasks. Educational gymnastics is especially appropriate for elementary-age students.

Stations and circuits offer the advantage of keeping students active while allowing for the general supervision of many students at one time. Circuits or stations are set up to allow students to move from one station to another in a timely and efficient manner. Ideally, the activities included in a station model should not require spotting and should consist of basic movements that allow for little risk for injury. Stations may be designed to develop muscular strength and endurance, skill, or flexibility. Many gymnastics skills help develop muscular strength and endurance because they require pulling, pushing, supporting, and swinging. Utilizing stations increases student activity and minimizes waiting time.

Purpose of the Course

The Basic Movement course at West Point is developmental and serves as a foundation for other athletic and lifetime physical activities. It focuses on applied movement designed to prepare students for a broad application of physical tasks. Emphasis is on the following attributes: agility, including fast movement in enclosed spaces; balance and controlling fear of heights; vaulting, jumping, and landing correctly; strength development activities and skills such as rope climbing, pull-ups, and resistance exercises; crawling; and negotiation of natural and man-made obstacles. The course objectives are as follows:

1. Demonstrate basic competency in selected movement skills
2. Exhibit a minimal level of kinesthetic sense in selected motor skills (i.e., jumping, climbing, vaulting, mounting, supporting, dismounting, falling, swinging) that prepare students for military activities
3. Demonstrate a sufficient level of upper body and trunk muscular strength and endurance
4. Exhibit a minimal competency level of motor fitness (coordination, agility, balance)
5. Demonstrate basic spotting techniques and utilize them while assisting others
6. Demonstrate personal safety behaviors while performing gymnastics tasks
7. Demonstrate teamwork and cooperation
8. Enhance self-confidence by successfully overcoming fear and completing challenging tasks

Instructional Area

A basic movement course requires a gymnasium or room with ample height, plenty of floor space for safety, and satisfactory lighting and acoustics. A floor plan should be developed for effective utilization of space, the maintenance of a safe and functional traffic flow pattern, and maintenance of good visibility for supervision. Several factors to consider when developing the instructional area are (1) the nature of the planned activity; (2) the number of participants; (3) the type of equipment used (some typical gymnastics apparatus, such as freestanding horizontal bars or uneven parallel bars, requires floor plates, weights, and cables in order to be secured to the floor); (4) room in the landing and activity areas for plenty of matting; and (5) equipment storage areas for equipment when not in use (USA Gymnastics, 1998).

Equipment

The equipment used for a basic movement course can include typical gymnastics apparatus such as parallel bars, rings, side horses, vaulting boards, horizontal bars, uneven parallel bars, balance beams, trampolines, vertical and horizontal ropes, and competition landing mats. Other equipment options consist of a variety of blocks, wedges, octagons, spheres, and apparatus shaped in other ways that can be used for teaching basic movement skills. Regardless of the equipment used, USA Gymnastics recommends that equipment and matting be appropriate for the age, size, and ability of the students and that the equipment be continuously maintained and inspected (1998).

Risk Management

Basic movement and gymnastics courses include activities that have potential to cause injury. Safety in any sport depends on sound risk management procedures. To develop safe and appropriate teaching and learning environments, it is necessary to answer the following questions (USA Gymnastics, 1998):

1. What are the abilities, sizes, ages, and experience levels of the participants?
2. What is the planned activity?
3. What equipment is available?
4. What is the instructor's knowledge and experience?

The ability to answer these questions facilitates sound decision-making procedures.

Teachers must have sufficient knowledge and abilities in spotting, lead-up activities, skill progressions, and class management techniques to conduct a safe program. Using appropriate progressions and ensuring proper equipment and teaching aids may greatly reduce the risks of injury. Specific strategies to enhance safety include the following:

- Teachers must be knowledgeable and properly trained.
- Instructors must provide plenty of room for students to perform.
- Students should be allowed to perform only those skills that they have been taught.
- Instructors should insist that students behave appropriately and conduct themselves according to classroom rules.
- Adequate mats and padding for equipment must be provided.
- Instructors must ensure that equipment is stable and properly set up, spaced, and maintained.
- Students should know and understand proper spotting and self-spotting techniques, including ways to "bail out" of skills safely by rolling and landing to avoid injury.
- Teachers must instruct students in proper progressions and skills that meet each student's abilities.

See table 4.1 for possible risks and strategies for reducing them.

Course Overview

Movement courses are designed to provide the facilities and resources necessary to expose students to gross motor coordination in all directions, rotations, and ranges of motion. The activities in table 4.2 are developmental and are intended to help begin cultivating students' optimal physical capability. Additionally, the activities aid in developing the potential for movements that serve as a basis for healthy living and daily and athletic activities.

Skills and Techniques

This section highlights skills and activities from selected lessons of the Basic Movement course at West Point. A typical lesson provides instruction in two or more skills, routines, or activities and follows the general sequence of (1) student accountability; (2) instructor demonstration of the skills and activities; (3) dividing students into two or three groups; (4) rotation of students through teaching stations while providing feedback and conducting skill assessment; (5) recording of daily grades; and (6) lesson closure and dismissal. Lesson plans are developed to provide maximum time on task by limiting transition time, maintaining an appropriate student–teacher ratio, and having plenty of equipment available. Skills are taught in a carefully designed, sequential progression from basic to more advanced lessons. Students must become proficient in key skill areas to progress to more advanced skills.

Table 4.1   Possible Risks in the Basic Movement Course

Risk identification	Reduction strategies
Collisions with other students	• Establish a functional and safe flow pattern. • Space equipment properly.
Collisions with equipment	• Establish a functional and safe flow pattern. • Space equipment properly.
Falls from apparatus	• Provide spotting and assistance when necessary. • Teach appropriate spotting techniques. • Provide plenty of well-placed matting. • Keep equipment as low to the ground as possible.

(continued)

Table 4.1 *(continued)*

Risk identification	Reduction strategies
Slipping on floor surface, tripping over equipment	• Instruct students to remove socks. • Cover slippery floor surfaces with matting. • Regularly check the floor for slippery spots. • Establish a functional and safe flow pattern. • Space equipment properly.
Engaging in skills beyond ability	• Instruct students to do only the skills demonstrated in class. • Demonstrate proper technique for all skills. • Place students in ability groups. • Provide proper progressions for all skills. • Provide a variety of skills that are appropriate for all students. • Supervise all activities and intervene when necessary.
Horseplay	• Instruct students about rules prior to activity. • Maintain a safe environment through a specific discipline plan. • Warn students that they will be asked to cease activities if horseplay occurs.
Equipment failure or malfunction	• Conduct periodic inspections of equipment. • Conduct periodic maintenance of equipment. • Repair equipment when necessary.
Student attire	• Ensure that students wear proper attire for gymnastics. • Direct students to remove shoes and socks. • Instruct and enforce that students not wear jewelry. • Request students with long hair to tie it back.

Table 4.2 Overview of Basic Movement Lessons

Lesson	Skills
1	• Two forward dive rolls—backward roll • Vertical rope lock climb—instruction and practice • Chin-up test
2	• Side horse vault flank vault series • Vertical rope lock climb—instruction and grade • Ankles-to-the-bar test
3	• Indoor obstacle course test (IOCT) instruction
4	• Handstand on floor • Vertical ropes clinch and lock • Dips test • IOCT
5	• IOCT instruction

Lesson	Skills
6	• Side horse vault squat sequence • Knee swing on horizontal bar • IOCT
7	• Cartwheel on floor • Vertical rope grapevine climb • IOCT
8	• Horizontal rope safety brief • Horizontal rope feetfirst • Inverted hang routine on rings • IOCT
9	• Practice and testing • Midcourse grade calculations • Deficiency reports • IOCT
10	• Applied movement sequence • Applied balance sequence • IOCT
11	• Round-off on floor • Horizontal rope headfirst side swing • Vertical rope hands only • IOCT
12	• Horizontal rope hands only • Handspring (instruction only) • IOCT
13	• Side horse vault squat sequence and elephant squat • Handspring (review instruction and grade)
14	• Seat drop on trampoline • Straight-body inverted hang/L-hang routine on rings • IOCT
15	• Swivel hips on trampoline • Pullover on horizontal bar • IOCT
16	• Front drop on trampoline • Long horse vault straddle vault • IOCT
17	• Big-three sequence on trampoline • Knee swing—drop back to knee swing on horizontal bar • Knee circle on horizontal bar • IOCT
18	• Team movement challenge
19	• Practice and testing • IOCT • Final grade calculations

Two Dive Rolls and Backward Roll

Forward dive rolls are considered advanced rolls and require the student to demonstrate flight and distance as well as a smooth and safe landing. Students should master basic tucked forward rolls before attempting a dive forward roll. Being able to roll correctly can help students avoid injury when falling or landing improperly.

TEACHING CUES

- Begin forward roll with arms stretched overhead.
- Lean and spring forward.
- Feet and knees remain together.
- Head should not touch floor on dive forward rolls.
- Arms act as shock absorbers—body should not land hard.
- Hands and arms are extended forward on the roll-up phase; hands should not be used to support or push the body to stand on roll-up phase.
- Forward dive roll should be smooth and controlled.
- Squat down with legs and feet together on backward roll.
- Sit back in a tight, round position.
- Use the momentum of sitting back to roll over.
- Hands are near the ears with fingers pointing toward the shoulders.
- Elbows are up.
- Chin is on the chest.
- Hands and arms should support body weight.
- Backward roll should be in a straight line.
- All rolls end in a controlled standing position.
- Shoulder rolls can be performed in place of the backward roll.

SUGGESTED LEARNING ACTIVITIES

- Demonstrate basic tucked forward rolls, and then add distance and some flight for the development of the dive forward roll.
- Emphasize absorbing body weight with the arms, round body position, and smoothness on the rollout.
- Start the backward roll from a squat or tucked position and then roll backward. The backward roll will eventually be done from a standing position.
- Demonstrate the optional shoulder roll for students having difficulty with the backward roll.
- Generally no spotter is required. For students having difficulty, emphasize tight tuck positions on forward and backward rolls and utilize wedge mats.

Lock Climb on Vertical Rope

The lock climb is a fundamental technique for ascending the vertical rope. The lock is also used as a descending and resting technique for all other vertical rope climbs. It allows a slow, controlled descent with minimal use of the arms. An effective lock is necessary to conserve upper body strength (see figure 4.1).

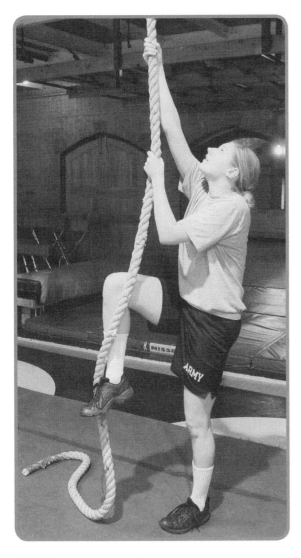

FIGURE 4.1   **Lock position.**

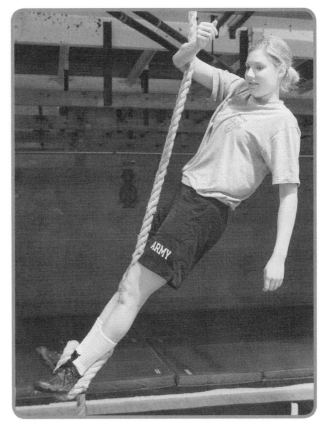

FIGURE 4.2   **Clinch.**

TEACHING CUES

- Address rope with right leg.
- Addressing leg is lifted high—knee flexed and above hip level.
- Rope passes on inside of thigh, over front of shin, and across top of foot.
- Grasp rope high above head.
- Squeeze rope between feet.
- Raise the knees high between locks.
- There are three ways to form the lock on the rope:
  1. Clinch: Cross legs and trap rope between feet. Then drag rope over to lock position (see figure 4.2).
  2. Gap: Externally rotate the right leg, forming a gap so that the left heel goes right into the lock.
  3. Underhook: Underhook the right leg under the setup left foot (rope runs behind the left calf muscle and across the outside of the left heel), forming a "sideways S."

SUGGESTED LEARNING ACTIVITIES

- From a standing position on the floor, students should cross their left leg over the right leg and bring the edges of their shoes together. They should then drag their left heel over their right foot to simulate the application of the lock.
- Check effectiveness of the lock by hooking an elbow.
- Ascend the rope with two or three locks in a row. Hook elbow and pause. Descend; touch lightly and put on the lock.
- An instructor spotter can help when a performer is in distress by using verbal coaching and physically catching the student by the hips.

Flank Vault Series Over Three Horses

The flank vault over a series of horses requires students to demonstrate coordination, power, and agility. The flank vault technique can be used for clearing a variety of obstacles while moving swiftly in a forward direction. The flank vault requires the performer to spring from two feet, support with two arms, and lean to the side while the side of the body passes over the horse or obstacle. It is an elementary method of getting over a stationary obstacle.

TEACHING CUES

- Approach horse from a running start.
- Place two hands on one side of horse—hands should be placed approximately shoulder-width apart.
- Spring off two feet approximately 1 to 2 feet (.3-.6 meters) away from horse.
- As body passes over horse, lean to the side.
- Push down with both arms; lead with head and shoulders over the horse.
- The lower leg lands first; step out into run with other leg.

SUGGESTED LEARNING ACTIVITIES

- Have students assume flank position on floor.
- Allow students to jump up to flank position on top of horse.
- Over low horse, execute flank vault without a run.
- Practice landing and stepping out on one foot.

Handstand

The handstand is a primary support and balance skill that serves as a prerequisite for the cartwheel, round-off, and handspring. The handstand requires the student to demonstrate the ability to support body weight, maintain orientation, and control and balance the body in an inverted position. A free handstand without the support of a wall or spotter is an advanced balance skill.

TEACHING CUES

- Start from a standing position with arms stretched overhead.
- Step forward on one foot to a deep lunge position.

- Place hands on the floor, shoulder-width apart, fingers pointing forward and elbows straight.
- Kick up toward an inverted position with head up and back arched.
- Look at the hands and floor during the handstand.
- Keep legs together.

SUGGESTED LEARNING ACTIVITIES

- Have students start with arms overhead, step forward, and kick several 3/4 handstands, keeping legs apart but supporting and balancing momentarily.
- Students kick handstand against wall with or without spotter. Only the heels touch the wall; the eyes are fixed on the hands, and the back is arched.
- Students should work in pairs and help each other balance in the handstand by holding the thigh near the knee.
- Spotting technique: As performer kicks up to handstand position, have the spotter lift (or grab) the lower thigh near the knee. Spotter should make proper corrections and alignments.

Cartwheel on Floor

A cartwheel is essentially a traveling-sideways handstand. It requires a powerful leg kick and push, coordination, balance, and rhythm. Cartwheels develop students' ability to move through an inverted position while supporting and balancing body weight. The cartwheel is a prerequisite for the round-off and other more advanced skills.

TEACHING CUES

- Step forward to a lunge position.
- Place hands in line directly in front of lead foot.
- Kick vigorously through the handstand position.
- Maintain a wide-open "straddled" leg position.
- Keep head up and arms straight.
- Hand and foot placements form a straight line.

SUGGESTED LEARNING ACTIVITIES

- Practice 3/4-kick handstands with straight arms.
- With arms overhead, kick fast cartwheels across mat, covering as much distance as possible.
- If students are having difficulty, have them do cartwheels on a curved line or circle (body faces inside of circle).
- Have students do fast cartwheels to maintain balance.
- Have students count out loud the 1, 2, 3, 4 rhythm of the cartwheel.

Inverted Hang Sequence on Rings

The inverted hang sequence on rings combines elements of strength, balance, and coordination. Students must use muscular strength to pull their body to an inverted pike and straight-body inverted hang and balance to maintain proper body position. The sequence is as follows: From a straight-arm hang, pull legs up to a pike inverted hang position for 1 second. Extend legs up toward ceiling until body is fully extended into a straight inverted hang (3 seconds) (see figure 4.3*a*). Return to a pike inverted hang for 1 second, and slowly lower to a straight-arm L position for a 3-second hold (see figure 4.3*b*). Lower to straight-arm hang and drop off.

TEACHING CUES

- Legs remain straight throughout the entire exercise.
- The inverted pike hang is balanced with the legs horizontal to the ground.
- Keep the chin in and eyes on the knees.
- The arms are extended along the outer thighs.
- Extend the legs up between the straps to a straight-body inverted hang.
- Extend into a slight arch with head up and eyes focused on the floor below.

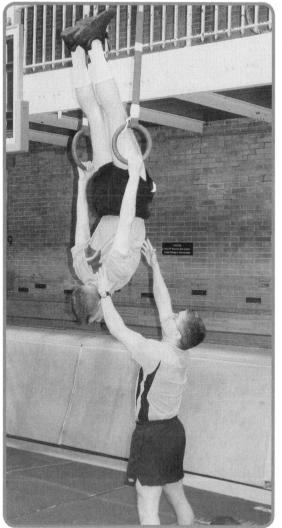

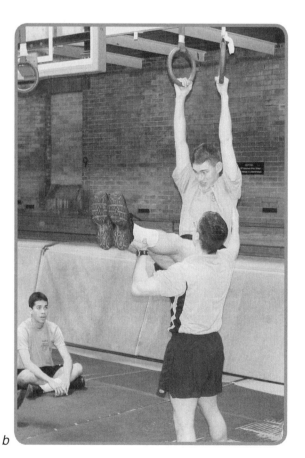

FIGURE 4.3 *(a)* Piked hang position and *(b)* L position.

- The thumbs should be on the thighs in the inverted hang.
- Arms should be fully extended along the side of the body.
- The exercise is smooth, continuous, and done at a moderate pace.
- Slowly lower to a straight-arm L position.
- Lower the legs to a hang and dismount.

SUGGESTED LEARNING ACTIVITIES

- On the floor, before mounting the rings, students should lie on their backs and assume the pike position.
- Have students do the straight-body inverted hang by lying on their stomachs and arching up with the arms alongside.
- They should place feet against inside of the ring straps for support to learn the inverted hang.
- Spotting techniques: Spotter lifts and "stills" the performer. The spotter assists the performer into the basic body positions by verbally coaching and physically manipulating the performer's body.

Round-Off

A round-off is a movement that is used to change direction from a forward run to a backward movement. It is an essential skill that students must master in order to progress to more advanced backward tumbling skills. It requires students to demonstrate power, agility, balance, and the muscular strength to support their body weight. It is similar to a cartwheel, except that the torso and hands turn more and the feet are joined together at the top. It passes quickly through the handstand position and is completed by extension through the shoulders while the feet and legs are directed toward the floor (handstand snap-down).

TEACHING CUES

- Start from a short controlled run.
- Execute a deep lunge with arms extended overhead.
- Place hands on floor (similarly to cartwheel).
- Kick trailing leg.
- Push off forward leg as the body passes through an extended handstand position.
- Head is up and arms are generally straight.
- Feet and legs come together through the handstand phase.
- "Snap down" (move from arched, extended body to slightly piked, round position).
- Land on both feet simultaneously.
- Rebound off two feet to a controlled landing.

SUGGESTED LEARNING ACTIVITIES

- Have students perform handstands and fast cartwheels as a warm-up.
- Have them do cartwheels, with the feet and torso finishing as in the cartwheel on a balance beam.

- Teach the hurdle (hop-step) with arms overhead and landing in the kick handstand lunge position.
- Emphasize a fast kick and powerful leg push into the handstand phase.
- Emphasize fast hands (spending only a brief time on hands).

Pullover on Horizontal Bar

The pullover is a method of mounting a bar that requires students to demonstrate muscular strength and timing. The students jump to a regular handgrip and pull themselves through an inverted position to a support position above the bar. To dismount, students bend forward and roll down through a piked position to an extended hanging position.

TEACHING CUES

- Focus eyes on the bar with chin forward.
- The pull-up and leg lift (pike) actions occur simultaneously.
- The elbows remain bent at a 90-degree angle or greater throughout the entire pullover.
- Pull the hips to the bar and get the body up and over the bar in one smooth, continuous motion.
- Show a straight-arm, shoulder-shrugged support position above the bar.
- Bend forward and slowly roll down (forward roll) to hang before dismounting.

SUGGESTED LEARNING ACTIVITIES

- Have students work in groups to assist each other on the pullover.
- Spotting technique: Spotter or spotters put the performer through the exercise by pushing the performer up and over by lifting the legs, pushing the lower back, and grabbing the shoulder to rotate.

Adapting This Course for Your School

There are ways to design a basic movement course or unit to fit almost any setting or age group. To offer quality movement and gymnastics programs, there are some important factors to consider. Some of these factors are (1) teacher education, (2) risk management (liability concerns), (3) equipment and facilities, and (4) class size and time constraints.

Teacher Education

Teachers can improve their skills and gain knowledge by participating in workshops and conferences, referring to the many new books now available, and copying successful programs. Observing and analyzing gymnastics skills, developing an awareness of proper progressions and safety, and improving spotting skills can increase teacher confidence in teaching basic movement and gymnastics.

Equipment and Facilities

If possible, equipment should remain set up throughout the entire unit and should be inspected on a regular basis to ensure that it is set up properly. If keeping the equipment set up is not feasible, equipment transporters or dollies need to be available for moving heavy or bulky equipment. To set up the equipment, teachers may also recruit the assistance of the custodial staff, other teachers, or, on a limited basis, students.

Many schools cannot afford to purchase multiple sets of gymnastics apparatus. Therefore, teachers should develop a long-term plan to procure equipment by purchasing one or two pieces of equipment each year. Other items such as tables, chairs, crates, boxes, stacked mats, hula hoops, and jump ropes can also be used (Nilges, 1997; Werner, 1994).

Physical education classes are often taught in cramped or multiuse facilities. Gymnastics requires a room with ample floor-to-ceiling height and plenty of floor space for safety. A floor plan should be developed to assist in using space effectively. To maximize activity and efficient use of space, teachers may have to split students into two or more groups and plan additional activities for each group.

Class Size and Time Constraints

Short class periods and lack of equipment to accommodate large numbers of students make it difficult to keep all children active and on task. Students often spend more time waiting in line than actively performing skills. Teachers can maximize available time for practice by using effective class routines, setting up mats and equipment prior to class, and using effective techniques to get students' attention.

Teaching Elementary and Middle School Students

Appropriate basic movement curriculum choices for elementary and middle school age children can include educational gymnastics (movement education), stations and circuits (obstacle courses), and other noncompetitive age- and developmentally appropriate activities. Programs can be developed around broad skill themes such as rolling, balancing, vaulting, traveling, hanging, climbing, landing, crawling, and supporting. Students can explore a variety of basic movement skills from each of the skill themes. In addition, the environment in which a skill is done can be manipulated to challenge the student and broaden the movement experience. For example, students learning a simple forward roll on the floor may learn to roll up and down hills using a wedge mat, or learn to roll over objects, under ropes, through hula hoops, fast or slow, and so on. Changing and manipulating the environment expose students to a broader range of rolling skills.

Since the skills offered in the Basic Movement course at West Point are essentially based on move-ment themes, much of the content in the West Point Basic Movement course can be modified to safely meet the needs of elementary and middle school students. Adjustments to the West Point course model may include (1) changing the environment in which the skills are performed; (2) modifying the assessment procedures; (3) eliminating skills requiring spotting or assistance; and (4) moving toward a more student-centered, educational approach by placing more emphasis on exploration, problem solving, and group work.

The following activities represent only a small number of skills and movement experiences that can be taught to elementary and middle school students. The activities selected are based on many of the skills offered in West Point's Basic Movement course.

Rolling

Rolling skills are appropriate skills for children of all ages. However, for younger children, dive rolls or any type of roll demonstrating height or distance should not be taught, for obvious safety reasons. Basic rolling on the floor (forward, backward, and sideward) should be preceded by allowing children the opportunity to explore basic body positions such as tuck, pike, straddle, and stretched body (layout). The use of wedge mats or mats set up on an incline can provide opportunities to roll up and down, forward, backward, and sideways. Rolling activities can be done on the floor and on mats, beams, wedges, low horizontal bars, parallel bars, rings, and other apparatus.

Rope Climbing

Vertical and horizontal rope climbing can be offered to elementary and middle school students if proper matting is used and safety precautions are taken. On a vertical rope, students should not be allowed to climb more than 6 feet (1.8 meters) high—ropes should be marked or a safety stop should be attached to keep students from climbing higher. Appropriate matting should be used under the ropes. As a minimum, 4-inch mats should be used, but thicker "crash" mats are preferable if they are available.

Horizontal ropes can be secured at low heights (3 to 5 feet [.9-1.5 meters] off the ground) and provide an excellent climbing experience for young children. Children can learn and explore a variety of ways to hang and travel along a horizontal rope.

For all rope climbing activities, the focus should be on development of effective climbing technique, the ability to support body weight on the rope, and confidence while exploring different ways to climb ropes. Children should be taught how to descend and dismount ropes properly to avoid injury.

Vaulting and Landing

Vaulting activities can be an important part of a basic movement course for students of all ages. Basic vaulting movements can be learned on the floor prior to moving to a spotting block, folded mat, or, if available, a vaulting horse. Vaulting apparatus can be set up in series to allow students to do vaults at different heights, from short or long running approaches, from standing positions, and so on. Vaulting can be done with or without the use of a springboard. For younger students, a low vaulting platform without a springboard is recommended.

Landing safely is an important skill in many gymnastics, movement, and sport environments. Jumping and landing from a raised platform such as one used for vaulting can be an important teaching emphasis. Students should learn how to properly absorb shock, balance, and maintain control during landings. Jumping forward to two feet followed by a forward or shoulder roll is an excellent way to develop safety "bail-out" techniques. Modifying this drill to include twisting jumps, tucked jumps, and backward and sideward rolling proficiency will increase students' range of safe landing skills.

Obstacle Courses and Movement Sequences

Obstacle courses may be a great way to use a movement education approach by allowing students the opportunity to solve problems and explore different ways to negotiate obstacles. The choice of obstacles or movement challenges is limitless; however, a keen awareness of safety and some minimal guidance are necessary to ensure that students do not attempt risky solutions to the obstacle. It is not recommended that students compete or race on the obstacle course. Instead, the emphasis should be on cooperation, teamwork, and the development of unique and creative ways to solve movement problems and negotiate obstacles.

Balancing Skills

Balance is an extremely important component of motor fitness. Students can explore their balance capabilities by attempting to balance in a variety of body positions: on one leg, on their hands, on hands and feet, and on top of mats and other appropriate equipment. A familiar gymnastics balance skill, the handstand, may be too difficult for many students. Prerequisite skills such as the tripod and headstand should be introduced first. Students can do modified handstands, in which they place their legs up on a folded mat with hands supporting their weight (wheelbarrow position). A 3/4-kick handstand (kicking up toward a handstand) is also an important progression toward developing the balance and support requirements for a handstand. As students progress, they can kick a handstand against a wall for assistance.

Hanging, Swinging, and Supporting

Hanging, swinging, and supporting are natural activities for children and can be done in a variety of body positions. Children can explore hanging from a tuck, pike, or straddle, with bent arms, straight arms, upside down, and so on. Basic muscular strength exercises can also be incorporated into the lesson. Chin-ups, pull-ups, ankles-to-the-bar, flexed-arm hangs, and dips are some of the exercises that can be done from hanging and supporting positions. Apparatus used for hanging, swinging, and supporting should be low to the ground and equipped with appropriate matting for safety.

There are many different approaches to basic movement and gymnastics instruction that can be combined, modified, and developed to meet the needs of students of any age and ability and to suit any school setting. The creative use of teaching methods, time, equipment, and space is necessary for the development of any high-quality physical education program.

Physical education teachers should be willing to explore and utilize a wide array of resources, instructional strategies, and assessment techniques to offer a complete, developmentally appropriate gymnastics program for students of all ages.

Key Terms

balance—State of equilibrium.

center of gravity—The weight center of the body; the point at which the force of gravity is centered on the body.

hanging—Position in which body weight is below the point of support.

jumping—Springing from and landing on both feet.

landing—The controlled stop of the body's descent.

pike—Position in which the body is bent at the hips.

rolling—Turning the heels over the head in a tuck, pike, straddle position, forward, or backward.

straddle—Position in which legs are straight but apart.

support—Body position with shoulders above the apparatus.

swinging—A movement in which the body creates an arc about the point of support.

tuck—Position in which the body is bent at knees and hips.

vaulting—Springing onto or over an apparatus.

References

Nilges, L.M. (1997). Educational gymnastics: Stages of content development. *Journal of Physical Education, Recreation and Dance, 68(3),* 50-55.

Pangrazi, R.P., & Dauer, V.P. (1992). *Physical education for elementary school children.* New York: Macmillan.

USA Gymnastics. (1998). *USA Gymnastics safety handbook,* 1998 ed. Indianapolis, IN: Author.

Werner, P.H. (1994). *Teaching children gymnastics: Becoming a master teacher.* Champaign, IL: Human Kinetics.

Suggested Readings

Fodero, J.M., & Furblur, E.E. (1989). *Creating gymnastic pyramids and balances.* Champaign, IL: Leisure Press.

Malmberg, E. (1995). *Kidnastics: A school appropriate model for the teaching of gymnastics.* (2nd ed.). Cortland, NY: State University College at Cortland.

Ward, P. (1997). *Teaching tumbling.* Champaign, IL: Human Kinetics.

Sport-Specific Organization

USA Gymnastics
Pan American Plaza
201 S. Capitol Avenue, Suite 300
Indianapolis, IN 46225
317-237-5050
Fax: 317-237-5069
USA Gymnastics Online: www.usa-gymnastics.org

5

Swimming

John McVan and Raymond Bosse

Swimming is an ideal activity for students to learn because it contributes to several of the health-related components of fitness. Once mastered, it can be done either alone or in a group. Swimming eliminates the impact on joints caused by so many other aerobic offerings, thus making it a true lifetime activity. Indoor and outdoor pools all over the country enable people to enjoy the sport year-round.

The ability to swim also gives students the opportunity to participate in numerous other aquatic activities such as water polo, scuba diving, water skiing, and triathlons. People who can swim learn these activities more easily. The proliferation of adult swimming classes and masters swimming groups in the United States has been tremendous. Many of these masters swimmers, surprisingly, are not former competitive swimmers, but rather adults who are new to the sport and who learned the basics of swimming as a youngster.

Having the ability to swim enables people to enjoy the aquatic environment safely as they participate in a lifetime fitness activity that has tremendous physiological advantages.

Purpose of the Course

Swimming has been part of the curriculum at West Point since 1885. It was recognized long ago that the ability to swim would not only be crucial to the effective operation of officers on the battlefield, but also be a means to improve and maintain physical fitness.

After many soldiers drowned in the landings at Normandy during World War II, it was determined that swimming courses for military personnel should include some focus on "tactical"-type swimming. Besides learning the elements of basic locomotion, students learn how to operate in the water while wearing military gear. Students at West Point must not only learn to swim to save themselves, but must come to understand that they may be the "aquatic expert" among the soldiers they are leading. This is a sobering thought for a group of weak swimmers who feel uncomfortable in the water. The focus on both basic swimming instruction and operating effectively in the water while wearing military gear is what drives the design of the program in place today.

Instructional Area

These skills can be taught in a typical high school or YMCA pool. An ideal pool has six lanes and is about 25 yards (23 meters) long. It should have a shallow end (3 to 4 feet [.9-1.2 meters]) that extends 8 to 10 yards (7-9 meters) from the wall and then gradually drops to a depth of at least 8 feet (2.4 meters).

The aquatic classes at West Point are taught in three separate natatoriums located within the Arvin Cadet Physical Development Center. Crandall Pool, which is a six-lane, 50-meter facility, is divided into two 25-yard pools by a submergible bulkhead. The pool also includes two 1-meter diving boards, two 3-meter diving boards, and a 6 1/2-meter and a 10-meter tower facility. The depth in Crandall Pool runs from 8 to 18 feet (2.4-5.5 meters).

The Intramural Pool includes a 25-yard dimension accommodating an 11-lane arrangement with a constant depth of 6 feet 7 inches (2 meters). This facility can also convert to an 11-lane meter-oriented venue. The Combat Water Survival Swim Laboratory houses a 25-yard six-lane pool with a depth range of 4 feet (1.2 meters) to 8 feet 4 inches (2.5 meters). In addition to its traditional design, this facility also houses theater-specific conditional enhancements, including wave production, simulated lightning, falling rain, and surface fog. Although most readers will not have as large a pool complex to operate in, almost every skill taught at the U.S. Military Academy (USMA) can be adapted and taught in a hotel-size pool.

Equipment

While the equipment requirements for swimming as a fitness or recreational activity are minimal, survival skill progressions require additional equipment. Students learn to "swim heavy" wearing battle fatigues and boots, often carrying a rifle and wearing a weighted vest to simulate field conditions. Rucksacks and Kevlar helmets are standard, and skill units often culminate with cumulative conditioning segments utilizing much of this gear. Exposure to swimming while wearing pants, shirts, and shoes is a critical and often neglected component in many instructional curriculums and is key in having a student come to understand the implications of successfully surviving an unexpected or accidental submersion.

Additional training opportunities expose students to emergency water safety options, which in turn utilize such standard safety equipment as reaching poles, shepherd's crooks, ring buoys, rescue tubes, and spinal backboards for establishing a hierarchy of response in managing a potential water irregularity.

Risk Management

An inherent aspect of any well-organized physical activity centers on managing and controlling the element of risk associated with participation. With regard to swimming, the very nature of the environment complicates this issue significantly.

Two fundamental issues are associated with managing risk at USMA:

1. Educating the user. As part of first-day orientation, students get a comprehensive tour of Crandall Pool and are instructed on specific responsibilities in the event of an in-class emergency. Briefing procedures center on danger areas and logistical coordination, as often a number of activities are programmed for the facility simultaneously. Managing an emergency is a twofold challenge that will inevitably involve the user, so education is key for comprehensive prevention and accident scene management.

2. Identifying, minimizing, or eliminating risk. The first step in creating a risk management program or in analyzing an existing one is to identify all areas of exposure to risk. Every facility has some form of inherent risk, some of which is created by design or program implications. What appears to be feasible during facility design in terms of code compliance and acceptable industry standards does not always equate to an accident-free environment. Along with a longitudinal chart designed to track facility irregularities, daily safety checks are an integral part of any risk management system. Usage demands and programming change the complexion of an aquatic environment dramatically. Survival applications can be particularly challenging in light of heavy-equipment usage (load-carrying belt, weapon) and the aspect of swimming fully clothed, which is very different from normal recreational swimming.

While eliminating risk is next to impossible, risk can be minimized through good emergency action planning, comprehensive surveillance systems, and sound progressive teaching practice (see table 5.1). To that end, a sound risk identification and reduc-

Table 5.1   Minimizing Risks in Swimming

Safety devices and procedures	Risk reduction strategies
Shepherd's crook, rescue tube	• Easy accessibility on deck. • Basic extension/reach instruction. • Using proper placement, below victim, and raising gently under shoulder or leg. • Reinforce importance of rescuer stabilization throughout.
Rescue tube, buoy	• Easy accessibility on deck/easy access. • Reach/extension/contact. • Swim and extend to allow for flotation and support. • Reinforce the importance of noncontact throughout.
Entries	• Discuss entry protocol for instruction. • No dive entries permitted at any depth. • Entry only after instructor has given instructions. • Acknowledge depth at entry point. • Reinforce importance of exploring pool depth before entering at all times.
Emergency action planning	• Orient swimmers to the inherent dangers of the facility and their specific role in the event of an emergency. • Discuss site-specific emergency action plan and identify external contact (telephone) locations.

tion strategy template should be included with any course syllabus or general orientation.

Course Overview

All freshmen, or plebes, are given a swim test within the first week of arriving at West Point in the summer. This consists of a 150-yard swim, which is timed. Students who cannot complete the 150 yards have their distance recorded, and anyone who identifies him- or herself as a nonswimmer is evaluated for overall ability and comfort level in the water. All freshmen are then categorized and assigned to classes of approximately 8 to 12 participants of similar ability based on testing data.

U.S. Military Academy instructional classes are segmented into five groups: Advanced, High Intermediate, Low Intermediate, Elementary, and a Foundations course for the absolute nonswimmer. Each course consists of 19 lessons that last 45 minutes (see table 5.2). Students who take the Foundations course move into the Elementary course immediately upon successful completion of the Foundations course. Thus the nonswimmers have 38 lessons rather than the standard 19 lessons for the other aquatic offerings.

The Aquatic Foundations course is an introductory swimming exploration program designed to prepare nonswimmers for success in the Elementary course. The program is arranged sequentially to help students acquire in-water experiences over 19 lessons and gradually refine the motor skills needed to be comfortable, effective, and safe in the water environment.

The Elementary, Low, High, and Advanced courses are designed to develop aquatic proficiency in two areas: basic surface locomotion and combat and survival swim application. Emphasis in all levels is on the military applications of swimming and survival skills, including breath control, buoyancy positions, stroke skills, and swimming endurance. Grading is primarily based on criterion-referenced scales in all these domains.

Each level of instruction comprises at least eight lessons aimed at improving students' basic swimming ability in the elementary backstroke, front crawl (freestyle), breaststroke, and sidestroke. The goal is to have the student swim each stroke 150 yards demonstrating biomechanical efficiency. Every stroke is taught from the point of balance in the horizontal position, with the mechanics of the stroke being taught through a set of progressive lead-up drills.

Table 5.2   Overview of Swimming Lessons

Lesson	Topic	Skills
1	Initial course briefing Classification test (not for record) Teach:	Orientation 5-minute swim • Gutter bobs • Vertical exhalation • Rhythmic bob (RB) • Sculling and finning
2	Review and practice: Teach: Conditioning:	Previous skills • Treading water • Buoyancy intro Bob and travel
3	Review and practice: Teach: Test: Conditioning:	Previous skills • Survival floating • Elementary back Tread water Skill iterations
4	Review and practice: Teach: Test: Conditioning:	Previous skills Front crawl, part 1 Elementary backstroke Skill iterations
5	Review and practice: Teach: Conditioning:	Previous skills Front crawl, part 2 Front crawl balance and breathing drills
6	Review and practice: Teach: Teach, practice, test:	Previous skills Breaststroke Front crawl
7	Review and practice: Test: Teach, practice:	Previous skills Breaststroke • Sidestroke • Underwater swimming
8	Review and practice: Teach, practice, test: Conditioning:	Previous skills • Sidestroke • Intro to BDUs Skill iterations
9	Review and practice: Teach:	• Previous skills • Stroke continuance (if needed) Equipment removal
10	Review and practice: Teach, practice: Conditioning:	Previous skills • Equipment removal options • Bob and travel with equipment Skill iterations

Lesson	Topic	Skills
11	Review and practice: Practice, test: Conditioning:	Previous skills • Bob and travel with equipment • Equipment removal Skill iterations
12	Review and practice: Teach, practice: Conditioning:	• Previous skills • Wet carry • Clothing inflation Skill iterations
13	Review and practice: Practice: Conditioning:	Previous skills Clothing inflation 5-min BDU swim
14	Review and practice: Teach, practice: Test: Conditioning:	Previous skills • 1-meter entry • High-level entry 1-meter entry Skill iterations
15	Review and practice: Test: Conditioning:	Previous skills High-level entry Skill iterations
16	Review and practice: Teach, practice:	Previous skills Survival problem
17	Review and practice: Test: Conditioning:	Previous skills Survival problem Skill iterations
18	Review and practice: Test: Teach, practice:	Previous skills 10-min swim Tactical swim training
19	Survival swimming: Teach, practice: Additional training opportunities:	Personal water safety • Lifesaving protocols • Rescue and response hierarchy • Advanced tactical training • Rucksack and Kevlar • Mask, snorkel, and fin usage

In addition to receiving basic instruction, students develop breath control and overall comfort in the water while mastering such skills as treading water, supine and prone flotation, and underwater swimming. Attention is also paid to understanding various body buoyancy postures and how to remain calm while performing subsurface.

After students complete the basic stroke module, 10 lessons focus on survival and tactical swimming, through which they learn military-specific survival applications. This involves swimming fully clothed in battle dress uniform (BDU) with operational gear such as a weapon, load-carrying equipment vest, and Kevlar helmet.

SAMPLE LESSON PLANS

LESSON 14

Equipment

- BDUs, boots, load-carrying equipment (LCE), rifle
- Safety lines, spine board, rescue tube
- Standard operating procedure (SOP) safety equipment

Activity	Time (min)
1. Warm-up (BDUs/boots) • Appropriate for skill level • Include: giant stride entry, sidestroke, breaststroke, and sidestroke with hand on hip	5
2. Skill test • 1-meter entry and swim: choice of either sidestroke with weapon at hip or breaststroke with weapon slung over arm and head	15
3. Review/Practice • High-level entry • One practice high-level entry from pool side • One practice high-level entry from 3-meter diving board	15
4. Conditioning • 3- to 5-minute continuous swim without BDUs and boots in preparation for 10-minute swim—choose appropriate distance • Four by 25/50 intervals with a set given rest interval	10
5. Next lesson • Tower entry (6.5-meter) skill test • Optional 10-meter entry • Retest any survival skill	

LESSON 15

Equipment

- BDUs
- Backboard, rescue tube
- SOP safety equipment

Activity	Time (min)
1. Warm-up • Rhythmic bobs • Sidestroke • Breaststroke	5
2. Review • High-level entry from side; if necessary also from 3-meter board	5
3. Skill test • High-level entry (6.5 meter) and underwater swim • Optional high-level entry from 10-meter platform	15
4. Conditioning • Up to four by 25 swims with BDUs and boots with short rest in preparation for survival problem; may include rifle for higher levels • Strip swim—remove a piece of clothing after each length (boots, BDU pants, BDU top); goal to not touch wall throughout swim	20
5. Next lesson • Introduction to survival problem	

LESSON 19

Equipment

- Stopwatch
- BDUs, boots, LCE, weapon, rucksack
- Ring buoy, rescue tube, shepherd's crook

Activity	Time (min)
1. Warm-up: partner water wrestling	5
2. Demonstrate, teach, practice: • Distress vs. drowning • Reaching assist with shepherd's crook, military implications • Throwing assist with ring buoy, military implications • Contact priorities—rear vs. front vs. submerged • Active assist options: reach, throw, row, go and tow • Passive towing options: wrist, collar, rucksack	15
3. Skill segments—circuit • Active rescue (reach, throw, go and tow) • Passive front surface rescue (wrist/collar tow) • Submerged (equipment release, collar tow)	15
4. Warm-down: drown-proofing (hands/feet tied)	10

Skills and Techniques

The skills and techniques that follow are examples of activities that can be taught during a class period. A normal class sequence includes (1) accountability of the students, (2) brief overview of class activities, (3) demonstration, (4) warm-up, (5) practicing new skill or skills, (6) assessment and feedback, (7) more practice, (8) lesson closure and dismissal. As with any movement course, the key is time on task. Out-of-water explanation of activities must be kept to a minimum. Additionally, it is important to be prepared to have additional skills for those students who become proficient in a movement quickly.

Water Acclimatization and Breath Control

Some students have never had the opportunity to swim, so submerging their face underwater can be a frightening experience. The introduction of the gutter bob and vertical exhalation allows students to become more and more comfortable in a water environment. Through the use of various progressions they will let go of the wall and eventually float.

Gutter Bob

DESCRIPTION

The gutter bob is a basic submersion technique, utilizing the gutter as a base of support for descending and ascending continuously, with the intent of developing a relaxed breathing pattern and a degree of comfort underwater.

TEACHING CUES

- Exhale through the nose with the head above the water and eyes remaining open.
- Blow bubbles through the mouth and nose at surface level while humming.
- Blow through the mouth and nose with face slightly submerged.
- Hold on to the gutter with both hands utilizing a loose grip.
- Take a deep breath through the mouth.
- Slowly submerge, exhaling through the mouth and nose until the arms are fully extended.
- Slowly pull up on the gutter until the head is above the surface, all the while continuing to exhale.
- Repeat this skill continuously three to five times as part of the daily warm-up.

SUGGESTED LEARNING ACTIVITIES

- Emphasize slow and proper movement with chest next to the wall.
- Have students focus on slow continuous exhalation throughout the movement.
- Have students try to expend all air during one execution before they reach the surface.
- Allow students to observe each other from the deck during skill execution while you give constructive feedback.
- Provide explanation of open eyes as a way to develop and maintain awareness and confidence during submersion.
- Tell students who inhale water when submerged to exhale through their nose.

Vertical Exhalation

DESCRIPTION

The vertical exhalation, an extension of the gutter bob, allows students to develop confidence in their ability to continuously exhale in a position away from the wall while at the bottom of the pool. Students also develop an understanding of how to use the bottom to return to the surface without attempting to swim. Students follow this sequence:

- Grasp the gutter and descend next to the wall while exhaling continuously through the mouth and nose. Eyes should be kept open, just as in the gutter bob.
- When the arms reach full extension, release the gutter and continue the descent until the feet touch the bottom.
- Allow the fingertips to feel the wall while descending.
- When the feet touch the bottom, go into a crouch position.
- Position the hands against the wall and push the body back away from the wall while still in the crouch position.
- The crouch position is executed as follows: one knee up and one knee down with arms and hands extended either straight up or out at a 45-degree angle.
- From this position, away from the wall, look up at the gutter, extend the arms toward the gutter, hands together, fingers extended and joined, and pause for 1 to 3 seconds.
- Push off the bottom with enough power to glide to the gutter.
- Pull up on the gutter enough to get the head above the surface and breathe.

SUGGESTED LEARNING ACTIVITIES

- Emphasize the importance of slow and steady improvement.
- This is not a race for time but rather calls for strict adherence to technique.
- Ensure that students adhere to the gutter bob position going into the vertical exhalation.
- Make sure the students do not automatically let go of the gutter and descend out away from the wall at the start.
- Remind students that it is very important to keep the eyes open in order to maintain orientation in the water.
- Remind students that their hands are the rudders of their bodies. Where they point their hands is the direction their body will travel in.

Rhythmic Bob

DESCRIPTION

This breath control drill is a stationary, continuous, vertical movement up and down in the water. It allows students to get away from the wall and survive with use of the pool bottom (to push them to the surface to breathe), their arms (to push them up and down), and gravity (to pull them down).

TEACHING CUES

- Move students 3 to 4 feet (.9-1.2 meters) away from the wall. Have them begin from the "position of attention."
- Let gravity initiate the descent. Extend the arms out and up from the sides of the body and begin to press against the water to help with descent. The palms of the hands should be out and up, with the fingers extended and joined.
- As in all other breath control drills, the exhalation is continuous.
- Once on the bottom of the pool, slowly get into a crouch position.
- Position the hands over the head in the glide position (hands overlapping) and push back to the surface until the fingertips break the surface.
- When the fingertips break the surface, the arms pull outward in a circular pattern down to the sides (side-straddle hop motion).
- When the head breaks the surface, inhale and begin the upward and outward extension of the arms to the overhead position.
- Students should repeat continuously from the second step on until all are comfortable with the skill.

SUGGESTED LEARNING ACTIVITIES

- Instruct students to execute a full range of motion with the arms going up and going down.
- Do not emphasize "flutter kicking" or "dog paddling" toward the surface.
- Have students use proper form as a very important lead-in to executing this skill with equipment during the survival phase.
- Allow students to practice the skill on the deck before getting into the water to develop the proper motor pattern.

Sculling and Finning

DESCRIPTION

Sculling and finning are rudimentary arm-hand movements designed to reinforce basic water displacement and lift in both the horizontal and vertical positions. Sculling provides a constant forward movement that is performed with figure-eight arm-hand motions. Finning is a limited-motion arm-hand displacement technique that also reinforces "still-water" movement. Unlike sculling, which is completely positive in terms of application, finning is based on a positive–negative formula and is often used as a lead-up training tool for basic locomotion.

TEACHING CUES

- Introduce both techniques in the supine position with an emphasis on center of gravity placement.
- Emphasize the concept of "pressing," in which the arm-hand is resistive through a positive range of motion.
- Thumbs are always high; wrist is rotated and presents an angled surface, like that of an airplane wing, which provides lifting power as the hand is drawn to the side and parallel to the surface.

- Movement of the hands away from the hips begins while the wrist is being rotated at the thigh.

SUGGESTED LEARNING ACTIVITIES

- Remind students to keep hands engaged beneath the surface of the water at all times.
- Emphasize lateral arm-hand movements rather than down and up movements.
- Teach a smaller displacement radius position for movement and efficiency.
- Remind students that the "paddle" in swimming uses both the hand and the forearm, so the entire lever system (wrist, elbow, shoulder) is always engaged.

Buoyancy and Basic Displacement

While success in the water is based on any number of factors, generic elements of buoyancy and basic displacement are important for specific skill acquisition.

Prone Float

DESCRIPTION

With the prone float, swimmers lie on their front side, with their face near the water's surface and arms extended out in front slightly wider than the shoulders, in a "superman-like" body position (see figure 5.1). The prone float helps students become comfortable in a position that involves holding their breath. Understanding the principles of the prone position will enable students to learn swimming strokes from this position.

TEACHING CUES

- In chest-deep water, students flex their knees until their shoulders are submerged. They extend their arms on the surface, take a deep breath, place their face in the water, lean forward, and gently push toes off the bottom. If a student's normal floating position is near vertical, his or her toes will return to rest on the bottom. It is important for these students to press on the water with their chest (lungs) in order to keep the legs up.

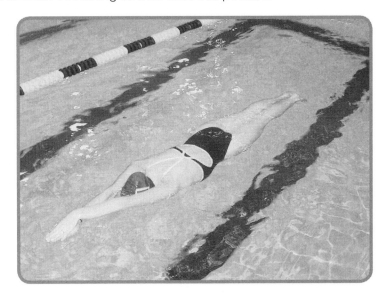

FIGURE 5.1 **Prone floating position.**

- In deeper water, students hold on to the side of the pool, take a deep breath, put their face in the water, and extend the body to a superman-like position in the water and release from the wall, all the while trying to maintain a horizontal body position at or near the surface.

SUGGESTED LEARNING ACTIVITIES

- To help students keep the nose from filling with water, have them lift the chin just slightly and gently blow some air through the nose. Since breath holding assists in floating, they should not forcibly exhale.
- Have students, in the superman position, gently push downward with the chest (lungs). Referred to as "pressing the buoy," this helps to keep the legs at or closer to the surface.
- For students who are still unable to maintain position at or near the surface, suggest that they utilize a gentle sculling action with the hands and light flutter kicking.

Supine Float

DESCRIPTION

The supine float is a float on the back with the head back and arms stretched overhead with the lungs full of air (see figure 5.2). An understanding of the supine position enables students to learn swimming strokes on their backs with an effective streamlined body position.

TEACHING CUES

- Take a deep breath, lay the head back, and bend the knees slightly, holding arms out from the shoulders and relaxed.
- Do not push off the bottom, but let the feet rise up to the floating position.
- Position the head to find body balance position.
- Press the navel to the surface of the water.

SUGGESTED LEARNING ACTIVITIES

- Have students fill their lungs to help them float. Have them breathe in and out through their mouths every few seconds.
- If students' natural floating position is diagonal or vertical, have them float more horizontally by moving their arms in the water above their head and straightening their knees.
- If students cannot float without motion, have them do sculling motions with the hands and gentle flutter kicks to help them maintain their position with minimal effort.

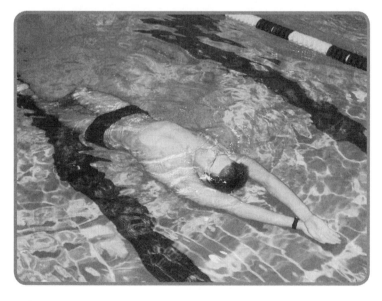

FIGURE 5.2   Supine floating position.

Survival Floating

DESCRIPTION

Survival floating allows a person to minimize energy expenditure and facilitates a stationary resting position in deep water. The student floats facedown in the water near the surface with the body, arms, and legs relaxed. The arms and legs hang in a "jellyfish-like" position with the back up near the surface (see figure 5.3).

TEACHING CUES

- Take a full inhalation and hold it. Assume a jellyfish floating position with arms extended to the front and relaxed.
- Turn the head to the side, keeping one ear in the water and eyes open. Forcefully exhale, then immediately inhale deeply.
- After each breath exchange, resume the jellyfish float position.
- The upper back should be exposed to air. The body position is similar to what it would look like if one were lying over the top of a barrel.

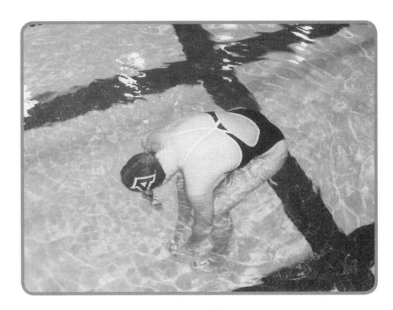

FIGURE 5.3 Survival floating position.

SUGGESTED LEARNING ACTIVITIES

- In the jellyfish floating position, the legs should be slightly tucked up under the buttocks.
- Students can use a sculling motion to help with breath exchange. They should continue the sculling motion while the head is rotated to breathe.
- A split second before rotating for breath exchange, swimmers begin exhaling in the water. They continue exhalation as the head rotates, then finish exhaling. Inhaling is the only task that must be done with the face out of the water. (This technique will limit the amount of time students spend with their head out of water.)
- Students who constantly sink to the bottom of the pool because of their buoyancy may utilize one or more light sculling or rotary kicking motions (or both) to stay at or near the surface.
- Head should be slightly under water with the arms extended down and relaxed.
- Utilize a swim egg for any student having difficulty.

Front Surface Support (Treading Water)

DESCRIPTION

Treading water consists of maintaining a stationary upright body position in the water with one's head above the water's surface.

TEACHING CUES

- Stay nearly vertical with the upper body bent slightly forward at the waist.
- Make continuous broad, flat, sculling movements with the hands a few inches below the surface of the water in front of and to the sides of the body.
- Use the scissors, breaststroke, or "eggbeater" kick along with sculling movements of the hands, producing just enough thrust to keep the head above water.

SUGGESTED LEARNING ACTIVITIES

- Have students keep their head as low in the water as possible.
- Have them move the arms and upper body in a slow, coordinated, and relaxed manner, keeping the body vertical and the head above the surface.
- Have students, keeping elbows slightly bent, move their arms using the shoulders to reduce fatigue and energy expenditure.
- The movements of the hands and leg kicks should be coordinated in order to enhance the position.
- A swim egg can be used for any student having difficulty.

Basic Stroke Mechanics

In most swimming instruction, stroke acquisition has focused primarily on the enjoyment of swimming as a means of recreation, fitness, or both, with additional implications for both personal safety and survival. Four fundamental strokes are central to the survival curriculum at USMA. These are (in order of delivery progression) the elementary backstroke, front crawl, breaststroke, and sidestroke.

Elementary Backstroke

DESCRIPTION

The elementary backstroke is one of the simplest forms of swimming. It is primarily a restful stroke that is useful for many survival and lifesaving scenarios. Muscle groups are not strenuously employed, but rather coordinated to enhance efficiency. This stroke also allows the swimmer to breathe freely with the face out of the water. Therefore, the elementary backstroke is a good stroke for swimmers to use while they are trying to recover during their endurance swims yet still make forward progress. This could be called "active rest." Since this stroke can be modified (done with one or no arm pulls), it is also ideally suited for the towing and rescue techniques employed by lifeguards.

The elementary backstroke is primarily taught at USMA to afford the swimmer an effective survival stroke. It is a symmetrical stroke that uses coordinated movements of large muscle groups to generate propulsion. It also takes advantage of the principles of inertia, momentum, and balance, as the students need to learn to "GLIDE" between strokes.

The stroke is done from the supine position with the arms at the side in the position of attention, with legs extended. Students should try to keep the body in the horizontal plane with the back fairly straight, but the legs may drop slightly lower to perform the kick. The arms and legs are symmetrical, and their movements are coordinated so that they do not counteract each other but rather enhance the propulsive force in the desired position. The arms and legs move as if connected by a string.

Generally, as the arms extend along the body line, the legs are drawn toward the buttocks. Similarly, as the arms spread into the propulsive phase, the legs separate in order to kick. Finally, the propulsive movements of the arms and legs occur simultaneously and propel the student into a supine glide position.

TEACHING CUES

The two hardest skills to acquire in the elementary backstroke are the kick and the coordinated timing of the whole stroke. However, since the movements of the legs and arms are linked, if the kick is wrong it will be harder to coordinate the whole stroke. Therefore, mastery of the kick is essential for achieving efficiency.

Kick

- The kick utilized in the elementary backstroke is known as the "whip kick." From the supine position and with the legs straight and the toes pointed, the kick is started in the recovery phase as the swimmer bends the knees and draws in both legs toward the buttocks. As the feet get closer toward the buttocks, the legs separate and the feet are dorsiflexed. It is important that the knees remain inside the ankles as they separate and that the feet rotate outward (dorsiflex) as they prepare for the propulsive phase of the kick. The knees should also remain beneath the surface and should be at least as wide as the hips. At this point, all the student has done is to set the kick up for the propulsive phase (this is similar to drawing back on a slingshot before firing). Once the student has set up all the potential energy for the kick, he or she converts it to power by simultaneously "whipping" the legs around in a circular motion until the feet come together again with the toes pointed.

- Students with poor flexibility might have difficulty with the whip-style kick and might have more success with a "frog-style" kick. In the frog kick the knees do not remain inside the ankles. Instead the knees lead the way, whereas in the whip, the feet lead the way. However, the frog-style kick is less efficient. Whip kicks should follow this sequence:

  - Recover legs by bending the knees and separating them slightly. (RECOVER)
  - Draw feet downward first, then toward buttocks. (RECOVER; feet should remain outside the knees)
  - Separate knees to at least as wide as the hips or wider. (OPEN)
  - Knees stay inward as the feet dorsiflex and rotate outward. (OPEN)
  - Keep head, back, hips, and thighs in a relatively straight line.
  - Feet press against the water in a circular motion and whip together. (CLOSE)
  - The speed of the kick should increase throughout the propulsive action. (CLOSE)

  - This kick can be taught by having students first learn the movements corresponding to the command sequence ("RECOVER"–"OPEN"–"CLOSE") while they hold on to the wall from the supine rack-out position. Once the movements correspond, students can use the kick to propel themselves in the water. If students have difficulty moving in the water via this kick, try having them hold on to a kickboard in order to facilitate a greater degree of leg specificity.

Arms

The arms and legs should be linked and their movements coordinated in order to assist each other. The arm movements begin with the recovery, like the legs, and are bent at the elbow as the hands are drawn up the side toward the shoulders, all while remaining beneath the surface. The thumb should run along the inside of the body until the hand reaches the shoulders with the palm facing downward. Once the hand is at the shoulders, it may continue to extend and reach over the shoulders or head. This is an individual preference, and the instructor should encourage students to figure out what works best for them. The important point is for the arms to remain linked to the kick. The arms at their highest point trigger the propulsive phase by pushing and accelerating the water with the palm of the hand in the direction of the desired movement. This is a symmetrical stroke, and the arms will complete the following actions:

* Arms recover with bent elbows, and hands slide upward along the body. (RECOVER)
* Arms extend up and outward over shoulders. (RECOVER)
* Arms spread wide, and the hands rotate so that the fingers point outward and the palms face toward the feet. (OPEN)
* Arms should be bent to provide the best leverage for the pull.
* Hands sweep toward the feet, keeping pressure on the palms in order to generate propulsive force. For best results, the arm pull should be accelerated. (CLOSE)
* Continue the arm pull until both hands are at the side. (Tell students to imagine throwing a tennis ball with each hand toward their feet.)

TIMING AND BREATHING

The most critical component in learning the elementary backstroke is the coordinated movements or the timing of the stroke. The stroke is symmetrical, and the arms and legs move at the same time. Breathing is done at will; however, it is best to instruct students to use a rhythmic-like pattern to prevent hyperventilation. Have the students inhale during the recovery phase and exhale during the propulsive phase. To begin this exercise, students should push off the wall and rotate into a streamlined position on their back. Next they get into the supine position of attention. Then, the timing of the stroke is as follows:

* Arms and legs recover almost simultaneously, arms first, and the legs lag slightly. (Swimmer would inhale during recovery.)
* Arms extend or spread, and legs spread to prepare for the propulsive phase.
* Arms and legs begin and end the propulsive phase together by accelerating the movements back to the supine position of attention. (Swimmer would exhale during propulsion.)
* Swimmer glides as far as possible before taking next stroke, does not stop.

SUGGESTED LEARNING ACTIVITIES

- Inertial forces and momentum are used to enhance performance after the propulsive phase—"GLIDE." To enforce this, have students count to a set number between strokes.
- Have students practicing the kick hold the kickboard in front of them or "hug" the board. They should not place it underneath their head.
- Have students master the kick first and then move to whole-stroke coordination.
- Have students keep their chin up with the head resting back on the water, as if they were putting their head on a pillow.
- The head, chest-back, and hips are kept connected as a unit. The head can submerge as long as the rest of the body submerges with it evenly. Students will need to exhale if the head is submerged.
- Have students exhale on the power phase and inhale during the recovery.
- Students may find learning the timing easier on land. Have them squat as they simulate the kick and bring the arms over their shoulders during recovery, then bring arms back to the side as they simulate the power phase.
- Have students keep their eyes open in order to stay aware of what is around them. Use markers along the ceiling to keep them swimming straight. Also, identify backstroke flags that can provide guidance.
- For best results the legs should lag behind the arms just slightly. The recovery of the legs begins once the arms are at about shoulder height.
- Have students keep an even pressure on the back of the head and the center of the shoulder blades to assist with body position.
- For swimmers who struggle to stay near the surface, have them inhale after the power phase of the stroke to assist with body buoyancy during the glide phase.
- Use a swim egg for any student who cannot maintain the body in the supine position. Once they have mastered the movements and timing, remove the egg.

Front Crawl (Freestyle)

DESCRIPTION

The front crawl, commonly referred to as the freestyle, is the fastest swimming stroke. This is the stroke most people think of as swimming in its purest form and the one most people want to learn and perfect first. The origins of freestyle lie with the sidestroke, and it is important to stress that the body rolls as a unit onto its side in order to achieve the most efficient "active streamlined" position for the front crawl. The most effective freestyle swimmers try to spend as much time as possible near their side in order to "slip" through the water.

The better freestyle swimmers are not necessarily the stronger or better-conditioned students but rather the ones who have the best body position in the water (body balance). They therefore swim through the water with less resistance.

The front crawl starts in the prone position, and the body rotates from side to side as the swimmer pulls the right and then the left arm (one arm cycle) and uses a flutter kick

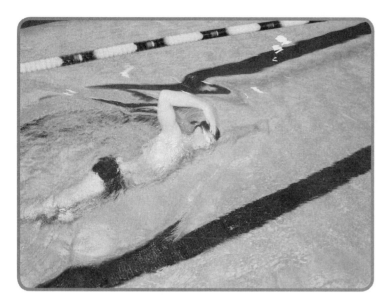

FIGURE 5.4   Front crawl, or freestyle, position.

(see figure 5.4). It is the arm pull that provides the majority of the propulsive forces. However, it is what the body does between arm pulls that makes it less resistive to the water, allowing it to travel at a greater distance per arm pull. The kick provides little forward propulsion but aids in creating the best possible body position in the water. Research has shown that the fastest swimmers in the world take fewer strokes compared to their competitors. Getting swimmers to realize that good freestyle swimming is not a product of pounding their arms and churning their legs, but rather of staying horizontal in the water as long as possible between strokes, is the key to their perfecting this movement.

TEACHING CUES

- Body position is the most critical component of efficient freestyle swimming, and the element that influences the body position the most is the position of the head. The head should allow the water to ride around the hairline, depending on the individual's buoyancy. Students with little buoyancy or with a poor body position may have to lower their head a little in order to raise the hips and get into a straight line in the horizontal plane. From the instructor's point of view, only the top of the student's head ("head is hidden") and the buttocks should be seen while he or she is in the prone position. The eyes should focus on the bottom of the pool, and students should use peripheral vision to look forward. It is important for the swimmer to stay connected as a unit (hips-shoulders) and roll the body in order to breathe. Lifting the head will create poor body position horizontally and laterally.

- The crawl stroke employs the flutter kick. The flutter kick emanates from the hips and releases at the feet, much like the crack of a whip. The kick is a pendulum-like action, from the hips through the legs with the feet pointed (plantarflexed) at the end. The kick should be about 6 to 12 inches (15-30 centimeters) in depth and should barely break the surface, thus creating the appearance of boiling water. The kick can be taught using many different scenarios depending on the student's ability level. It can be taught from the wall or on a kickboard. Perhaps the most effective way to teach it is from the prone position, with the students' hands at their sides so that they experience the proper body position. Have the students roll their bodies in order to breathe. Whatever the method, the following are characteristics of a correct kick:

  - The kick moves up and down the horizontal plane, starting from the hips and ending at the feet.
  - The kick is about 6 to 12 inches in depth, creating "boiling water" at the surface.

- The feet plantarflex ("point the toes") at the end of the kick.
- The two legs kick alternately.
- The knees may bend slightly to create greater flexibility on the downbeat.
- The legs straighten toward the surface during recovery or the upbeat.
- The ankles are kept loose, not locked. The force comes from pressure on the top of the foot.

- People naturally want to focus most on the arm stroke. Most individuals have high stroke rates. The key is to get students to slow down their stroke rate in order to increase stroke length.

- The arms should be viewed as a simple extension of the body, and the most important thing the arm does is to lengthen the body. To help students achieve this, make sure they wait for the recovering arm to get in front of the head before the opposite arm begins its pull. This is referred to as front quadrant swimming (FQS) and is a key component to efficient freestyle. The simplest form of the arm pull is to just pull back when the hips and shoulders rotate toward that particular side. The arm pull needs to stay connected with the hips and shoulders, acting as a unit to create power through the kinetic chain. The phrase "swing and turn" can help students with the recovery phase of the stroke. Freestyle is an asymmetrical stroke, and the arm pull will divide the body down the midline. Each arm pattern has the following components:

  - Hands sweep downward and outward just outside the shoulder.
  - Hands pull back toward the feet and slightly up toward the midline.
  - The elbow bends 90 degrees and the hand does not cross the midline.
  - The hand exits the water little finger first, and the elbow comes high out of water.
  - The arm recovers forward and over the shoulder and ends up relaxed with the elbow higher than the hand.
  - The hand leads the elbow after passing the shoulder.
  - The hand enters the water fingertips first, aligned in front of the shoulder, and the arm extends forward.
  - The arm extends fully in front of shoulder, and the body rotates onto the same side.

TIMING AND BREATHING

The stroke starts out in the prone position and uses body roll like a log (hip-shoulders-arms as a unit) to generate inertial forces and propulsion. The arms are viewed merely as a connecting point to the water through the kinetic chain. Breathing occurs, when required, during the body roll, and the swimmer's hands will be opposite one another (in a sidestroke-like position) to enable inhalation. Before inhaling and before the face leaves the water, the student exhales. If this is done properly, bubbles will appear in the water as the head-body begins to pivot. The kick is done as required to lend support to proper body position, but should not inhibit the body roll. Actually, the kick should be part of the body roll, and at times the student may flutter kick in the sideline position. The sideline position refers to balance progression used in teaching both the freestyle and sidestroke. A rhythmic breathing pattern is best. Ideally, the student should be able to breathe on both sides and should take an equal number of breaths on the two sides. Called bilateral breathing, this is a breathing pattern that is done once every three arm pulls, or twice to the left every two arm cycles and twice to the right every two arm cycles. Envision a barbecue skewer down the center of the body, with symmetrical and equal execution on both sides. Performance points are as follows:

- The head-body turns to the side as a unit and stays connected to the kinetic chain.
- The swimmer remains as long as possible on the side while making forward progress.
- The swimmer exhales to breathe just before turning and inhales once on the side.
- The swimmer rotates back toward the middle as the hand recovers, and does not pull the rest arm until the recovery hand passes in front of the head (FQS).
- The face should be down before the hand enters, fingertips first.
- Bilateral breathing improves balance and body roll, but may be too advanced for some. Students should begin with dominant-side breathing and progress to a bilateral pattern once the rhythmic breathing process is comfortable.

SUGGESTED LEARNING ACTIVITIES

- Emphasize proper head position ("head hidden") since this determines correct body position. Only the top part of the crown of the head should be above the water.
- Remind students that it is how far they travel on each stroke that is important, not how fast they stroke.
- Have students roll the body as a unit (legs-hips-shoulders-head-arms) to stay connected to the kinetic chain.
- Have them practice flutter kicking in the prone or side-lying position with the hands at the side or in front. A good drill is to have the students start kicking in the prone position, both hands in front, count to 3 seconds, then stroke to one side in a sidestroke-like position. They continue to flutter kick and count for 3 seconds, then recover the arm and rotate the body back to prone position; do the same for the other side; and keep repeating. This is called the "three-count prone, slide and glide on the side." As the students' skills advance, swimmers will be able to skip the prone position and switch from one side to the next in unison about every 3 seconds. This is referred to as "six kicks on each side"—taking about six flutter kicks on each side before switching to the other side. This drill teaches balance and how to move the body as a unit throughout the stroke. Be creative and use variations of these drills to improve students' crawl stroke.
- Have students wait until their recovery hand passes by their shoulder before they start the next arm stroke (FQS). Emphasize this in the preceding drill as well.
- Have students practice bilateral breathing. (Some may not be able to master this in the time allotted; it may be preferable for them to choose a favorite side in order to continue to practice rhythmic breathing.)
- Beginners may require a lot of time to develop a smooth transition of rhythmic breathing. Sometimes it helps to have them walk through the water or hang on to the wall or a kickboard in order to practice rhythmic breathing while coordinating the movement with the arms and body.

- For proper arm recovery, have the students imagine that they are taking their hand out of their pant pocket and bringing it out of the water little finger first. Then have them practice a movement similar to zipping up a zipper (this is done along the shoulder) and extend their fingertips first in front of the shoulders.

- When practicing kicking, emphasize loose ankles with a supple kick that gives the appearance of water boiling at the surface.

- Look for good mechanical advantage points during the arm pull, for example a 120-degree elbow bend during the power phase of the stroke.

- Use a swim egg for any student having difficulty keeping the body in the prone position. Once the movements and timing are mastered, remove the egg.

Breaststroke

DESCRIPTION

The breaststroke is the oldest documented swimming stroke. It is well suited for open-water swimming, as swimmers can look up on every breath to check their direction. This stroke is the slowest of the four competitive strokes and is also a survival stroke. It is primarily a restful stroke that uses the coordinated movements of large muscle groups in the legs to make forward progress. Effort is reduced as gliding makes use of momentum between strokes. At USMA, the focus is on an efficient and restful style of swimming breaststroke.

The breaststroke gets most of its propulsive force from the whip kick. The timing of the kick and the placing of the body into a streamlined position between kicks are critical for success. The arm pulls have a symmetrical sculling pattern, which translates to lateral sweeping hand action (see figure 5.5). There is really no front-to-back component to the arm pull. It is important for students to learn how to streamline the arms and legs equally during the recovery phase so that these components do not counteract each other. Therefore, the timing of the PULL–BREATHE–KICK–GLIDE becomes one of the most difficult yet important tasks the student faces in mastering this stroke.

TEACHING CUES

As with all of the strokes taught thus far, body position and coordinated timing are key to successful performance. The kick, however, plays an even greater role in the breaststroke because students rely heavily on it for their forward movement. Without a propulsive breaststroke kick, the stroke will be relatively ineffective. With this in mind, the instructor introduces the stroke by first teaching the kick.

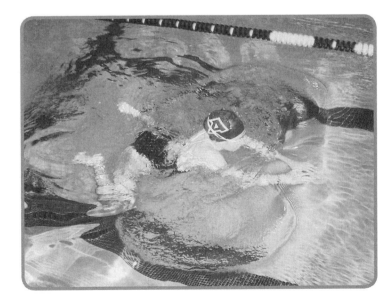

FIGURE 5.5   **Breaststroke.**

Kick

- The breaststroke uses the whip kick. The kick is done in the prone position and becomes much more powerful because of the advantageous mechanical position for the quadriceps. It should not take too long for students to master this kick since they have already learned the whip kick in the elementary backstroke. There are only slight variations between the two. From the prone position with the legs straight and the toes pointed, the swimmer starts the kick in the recovery phase by bending and dropping the knees, then drawing both heels toward the buttocks. It is important to keep the legs within the slipstream or active streamlined position of the body during recovery.

- Keeping the legs within the slipstream of the body will reduce any forward resistance during the recovery of the kick. As the feet get close to the buttocks, the hips drop slightly, the legs separate, and the feet dorsiflex. The only body part from the waist down that should go outside the slipstream is the feet when they dorsiflex and get ready to apply force. Students can accomplish all this with the aid of reminders to keep their knees inside their feet during the recovery. Once the feet are recovered, swimmers are ready to apply force. They do so by keeping pressure on the balls of their feet, which simultaneously whip in a circular motion until the feet come back together with the toes pointed.

- Students who cannot master the whip kick can use a frog-style kick, but it is less efficient. The main difference is that the frog kick breaks the slipstream of the body because the knees flex outward. Also, the frog kick employs more of a squeezing action as opposed to a whipping action. Whip kicks exhibit the following movements and positions.

- A way to teach the kick is to have students first learn the movements corresponding to the command sequence "RECOVER"–"OPEN"–"CLOSE" while they hold on to the wall from the prone position. Once the students can match the movements to these commands, they are ready for application while moving in the water. Use of a kickboard isolates the kick for further refinement. A more advanced method is to have students kick in the prone position with hands at the sides.

Arms

The arms perform more of a sweeping than a pulling action. The arms can create an efficient streamlined body position to allow the kick to provide as much propulsive force as possible. The arm pull pattern is symmetrical and is initiated with the hands out in front of the head (from a streamlined position). The hands start with a scull or sweep out beyond the shoulders. The elbows get wider than the shoulders, and the hands are wider than the elbows. Then, as the elbows bend, the hands drop and sweep in front of the shoulders. They should come together approximately under the chin. "Sweep out–sweep in–keep your hands under the chin" is a rhyme the students can use to help them perform a sound arm pull pattern. Once the hands are together in a praying position under the chin, they shoot forward to the starting point. The important concept is that once the stroke starts, there is no delay to the starting point out in front of the head. Also, there is a gradual acceleration of the arm pull pattern. That is, as the hands sweep out, they slowly feel for the water. As the hands grab and sweep in, they should accelerate and use lifting principles to generate force. The students want to slip the hands forward at this point and get their bodies into a streamlined position to take advantage of the kick. The arm pull pattern from the instructor's point of view is a circular pattern formed by the following movements:

- From the prone streamlined position, the palms turn out and the hands sweep out.
- The hands gradually sweep out until the elbows are beyond the shoulders and the hands are wider than the elbows.
- The hands grab the water in a circular motion and drop down slightly to prepare to sweep in. Palms will face somewhat inward at the end of this motion.
- The hands accelerate as they sweep in toward the midline.
- The hands are brought together under the chin, with elbows drawn inward much as in a praying position. The most common mistake is for the student to pull back too far.
- The swimmer continues to move the hands fast and slip them forward to the starting point, dropping the head for an effective glide position.

TIMING AND BREATHING

- The timing for the breaststroke is PULL–BREATHE–KICK–GLIDE. These are not four distinctive movements, but rather a continuous flow in which the movements "connect" or overlap each other. The timing is simply the order in which the movements are initiated. The stroke starts out in the prone streamlined glide position and begins with the hands sweeping out. Once the hands are in the position to sweep in, as already described, and before the completion of the sweep, the head will naturally rise. As the hands continue to sweep inward, they create a natural lifting force, part of which is used for forward motion and part of which is used to raise the body. It is at this point that students should lift their head in order to begin inhalation. It is also right after this point that they should begin recovery of the legs to start the whip kicking cycle.
- A snapshot taken at this point would show the swimmer with the head and shoulders up out of the water, hands together near the chest, and feet recovered near the buttocks. As the hands slip forward, the head should follow the hands forward beneath the surface, and the water should roll over the head. There are always less resistive forces beneath the surface. As the arms and hands continue to stretch forward toward an active streamlined position, the kick will move into its propulsive phase. The finish of the kick should occur after the arms reach full extension. At this point comes the most enjoyable part of the stroke, the glide. Have the students continue to move forward using principles of momentum and wait for the next stroke cycle. The timing and breathing of the breaststroke occur in the following sequence:
  - Arm stroke begins sweeping out. (PULL)
  - Arms sweep in as swimmer exhales in water. (PULL)
  - The head lifts up in order for swimmer to inhale. (BREATHE)
  - The legs begin to recover to prepare for kick. (KICK)
  - The arms recover, the face returns to the water, and the propulsive phase of the kick begins. (KICK)
  - The arms go to full extension, the body is streamlined, and the kick finishes. (KICK)
  - Swimmer uses the principles of inertia and momentum to glide. (GLIDE)

SUGGESTED LEARNING ACTIVITIES

- Make sure students understand what dorsiflexion is and when their feet dorsiflex in this stroke. Without dorsiflexion, the kick is relatively ineffective.
- For students who pull too far back, have them lie over a lane line on their armpits and pull. The lane line will prevent them from pulling back too far. They can also do this by lying on the deck and utilizing the wall in the same fashion.
- Have students exhale in the water right before they lift their head out.
- Have students count to a set number between strokes to help them emphasize a prolonged glide position.
- Have students do a one-pull–two-kick drill to teach them how to glide between strokes. For every arm pull executed, the swimmer takes two kicks. On the second kick, they focus on a streamlined body position. For those who struggle with the arm pull, reverse the drill to a two-pull–one-kick stroke.
- Use dryland practice for any part of the stroke—kick, arm pull, and timing. Use the deck or starting platforms and have students stand up or stand bent at the waist. Be creative in teaching the different mechanisms of this stroke.
- Prone kick drills: Have students in the prone position, with hands at their sides, perform a whip kick.
- Use a swim egg for any student who is having difficulty keeping the body in the prone position. Once the movements and timing are mastered, remove the egg.

Sidestroke

DESCRIPTION

The sidestroke is a pure resting stroke that employs elements of rest and propulsion (see figure 5.6). Interestingly, its evolution is traced back to the 19th century, and it developed because swimmers wanted more speed than they attained in the more commonly performed stroke of the time, which was the breaststroke.

- The sidestroke is a very effective resting stroke, with exceptional suitability and adaptability for endurance swims with minimum energy cost. It is also a stroke of choice for towing and carrying.
- Students recognize the ease of this stroke right away because it allows them to keep their face out of the water in order to breathe freely, thereby reducing anxieties associated with submersion. Since this stroke minimizes drag, it requires less

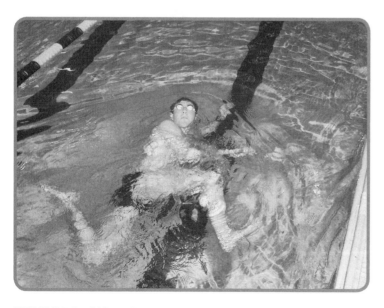

FIGURE 5.6 Sidestroke.

energy, and swimmers can use it for longer distances without tiring. An efficient, powerful, and well-coordinated sidestroke is absolutely essential in rounding out a swimmer's in-water repertoire.

TEACHING CUES

It is essential that students learn to master either the scissors or the inverted-scissors kick early in the development of the stroke. Without a propulsive kick, the sidestroke is relatively ineffective. In addition, learning the kick first enables the student to master the coordination of the entire stroke later on. Therefore, it is the instructor's first priority to get the student to achieve an efficient scissors or inverted-scissors kick.

Kick

- The scissors or inverted-scissors kick is best taught initially from the rack-out position. Once students understand the correct movements, they can use a kickboard for in-water iterations. The whole-stroke method may also be employed at this point for more advanced students. The sequence of the scissors kick is as follows:
    - Hips and knees flex to begin recovery of legs. (HEEL)
    - Heels are drawn toward buttocks together. (HEEL)
    - The swimmer dorsiflexes the top foot, and the top leg extends forward. Imagine the top leg kicking a door down. (FLEX)
    - The swimmer plantarflexes the bottom foot, and the bottom leg continues to flex toward the buttocks. (FLEX)
    - Simultaneously, the top leg presses backward and the bottom leg kicks forward. (TOE)
    - Legs straighten to sideline glide position, with toes pointed. (TOE)
- The commands "HEEL"–"FLEX"–"TOE" correspond to the anatomical positions described. Having students repeat these commands while performing the kick will help them remember the sequencing as well as the correct anatomical positions for the kick. The inverted-scissors kick is accomplished by reversing the top and bottom leg ("flex" position). Both kicks, the scissors and the inverted scissors, are acceptable to use with the sidestroke.

Arms

In the sidestroke, it is important to identify the lead and trail arms. The lead arm is on the same side the individual is swimming on to execute the stroke. It points or leads the way. The trail arm is the arm at the individual's side, hand at thigh, and it lags or trails behind the stroke. Details of the proper execution of the arm movements are as follows:

LEAD ARM

- The hand sweeps *slightly* downward and back toward the chin. (PULL)
- The wrist is flexed down and elbows are bent, and the shoulder rotates. (PULL)
- The hand pulls back to the shoulder so that it is under the chin. (PULL)
- Recovery is made in the water as the hand moves forward and "slips" past the lower ear (the ear that is in the water).

TRAIL ARM

- The forearm recovers along the side, and the hand slips forward toward the chin.

- The hand meets and overlaps near the chin.
- The hand sweeps downward and backward (close to body) toward the feet. (PUSH)
- The hand continues a sweeping motion until it reaches the thigh. (PUSH)
- The lead arm does more of a PULL, and the trail arm does more of a PUSH. More force comes from the push than from the pull.

TIMING AND BREATHING

- The starting point for the stroke is the prone streamlined glide position. Students rotate onto one of their sides by sweeping back with the trail arm in order to begin. Once they are on their side, the lead arm should be forward, with the head resting on the shoulder and the trail arm back. This is referred to as the sideline glide position, from which all coordination of the stroke starts. The sideline glide position is the most effective active streamlined position throughout the stroke. The timing of the stroke always begins with the lead arm pull. The sequencing is as follows:
  - From a side glide position, the lead arm sweeps back, and trail arm and legs recover.
  - The lead arm begins recovery, the trail arm sweeps toward the feet, and the legs begin the kick.
  - The lead arm reaches full extension, the trail arm finishes at the side, and the legs finish the kick.
  - Arms and legs extend to the sideline glide position; students should remember to use momentum at this point. (GLIDE)
- Even though the swimmer can breathe at will, a controlled rhythmic breathing pattern is recommended. Have students inhale on the lead arm pull and exhale as they finish the kick and reach the sideline glide position.

SUGGESTED LEARNING ACTIVITIES

- Emphasize correct body position—one that is balanced along the horizontal plane.
- Let the students learn the stroke on their side of choice. They will usually have a dominant side that is easier for them to learn on and should be encouraged to experiment and find that side. Students can experiment with this when they learn the kick in the rack-out position. Have them practice on each side while hanging on to the wall. Instruct them to discover which side (if either) feels more natural.
- Explain that the scissors kick is so named because it opens and closes much like a pair of scissors.
- Drills on land may help with the kick and with coordinating the timing of the stroke.
- When students use a kickboard to practice their kicks, they can hold on to the kickboard and place it underneath their head with the lead arm beneath the board. They can also hold on to the board with the lead arm on top of the board and the head on resting on the shoulder.
- Emphasize the principle of inertia and the use of momentum—"GLIDE"—between strokes. To reinforce this principle, have students count to a set number before taking their next stroke.

- While holding on to a kickboard with the lead arm, students can practice the kick and the trail arm push sequence.
- Use a swim egg for any student having difficulty keeping the body in the sideline position. Once the movements and timing are mastered, remove the egg.

Underwater Swimming

DESCRIPTION

The underwater swim is an important breath control exercise intended to get the swimmer moving by applying propulsive force below the surface. This normally applies when a swimmer needs to go under obstacles or avoid observation in the water. This is the most advanced breath control exercise taught in the swimming curriculum at USMA.

TEACHING CUES

Students begin the underwater swim at the pool's edge. They take several quick deep breaths (holding on to the last breath) and duck under the surface. Students then push off the wall and swim, using both arm pulls (as in the breaststroke) and leg kicks (either whip or flutter), under the water as far as possible.

SAFETY TIPS

- Remind students to exhale slightly at least two times during the execution of this drill in order to avoid shallow-water blackout.
- Discuss the implications of hyperventilation as it relates to underwater swimming.

Kick

The flutter kick, breaststroke kick, and scissors kick (or some combination of these) may be used for underwater swim segments.

Arms

The breaststroke or a modified breaststroke pull is used for the underwater swim.

SUGGESTED LEARNING ACTIVITIES

- Remind students to take a deep breath prior to starting the swim.
- Emphasize using both an arm pull and a leg kick.
- Emphasize exhalations during execution of this drill.
- Remind students not to break the water's surface until completion of this drill.
- Have students keep their eyes focused downward to avoid drifting to the surface during the swim.

Survival Swimming

The following activities focus on the survival portion of the aquatics program. Various ways of entering the water with full equipment and without sinking are introduced, as well as the bob and travel, which can be used as an effective method of moving through the water with equipment. Equipment removal and subsequent clothing inflation are also presented as an alternative when it is impossible to get to land safely.

Stride Entry

DESCRIPTION

Stride entry is performed facing forward as the student steps off the side of the pool (see figure 5.7). The goal is to keep the head above water on entry. This is generally considered a lifeguarding technique and is executed so that the rescuer can keep focused on the victim while entering the water.

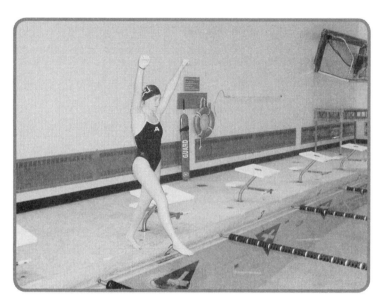

FIGURE 5.7 Stride entry.

TEACHING CUES

- Stand on the edge of the pool deck facing the water with both arms extended out to the side.
- Step off with a big stride, keeping the legs apart until the feet touch the water. Lean the torso slightly forward. Arms sweep together until the hands meet. At the same time the legs squeeze the water in a scissors action to prevent the body from sinking.
- Transition into a swimming stroke upon completion of the entry.
- The following is the command sequence in order of progression:
  - "Toes on the edge"
  - "Step off"

SUGGESTED LEARNING ACTIVITIES

- Have students "hug" the water in order to help with the arm motion.
- Emphasize timing so that the scissors action of the legs and the sweeping action of the arms squeeze water to keep the body at the surface.

Rear Entry

DESCRIPTION

The rear entry technique is used for safe entry from a height of no more than 3 to 4 feet (.9-1.2 meters) above the water's surface, since it produces an element of disorientation. Students enter the water rear first. After entry, they must completely exhale through the nose. This breathing technique allows the body to descend to the bottom. Once on the bottom, the student goes to a one-knee-up and one-knee-down position, with the arms fully extended and pointing up toward the direction of travel. Rear entry swimming exercises are done at USMA only when the cadets are wearing their battle dress uniforms (BDUs). Rear entry is used to initiate the performance of the following survival skills: equipment removal and recovery, bob and travel, clothing inflation, and the tackling of survival problems.

TEACHING CUES

- Turn the back to the water and place the heels of the boots over the edge of the deck.
- Tuck the chin.
- Clasp hands, extend arms to the front, and bend at the hip. This is the hookup position without equipment.
- Flex the knees.
- Take a breath.
- Sit down into the water in a "V" position with the buttocks entering first.
- Exhale completely through the nose and mouth and descend to the bottom.
- Recovery to the gutter should be relaxed and under control through use of a fingertip lead.
- The following is the command sequence in order of progression:
  - "Heels over the edge."
  - "Hook up." (Hands are extended to the front and clasped, and the swimmer bends forward at the hip.)
  - "Tuck the chin."
  - "Hit it."

SUGGESTED LEARNING ACTIVITIES

- As an instructor you can control the entry by holding a swimmer's clasped hands. Release the hands as the swimmer's body extends over the edge.
- The swimmer keeps the body in a tight "V" to facilitate movement to the bottom.

Equipment Removal and Recovery

DESCRIPTION

The skill of equipment removal and recovery is used to enhance poise, composure, and breath control during the execution of a task. This skill is also required at the U.S. Army Ranger school. To execute it correctly, students at the Ranger school perform a rear entry with LCE and a rifle. On the way down, they remove the rifle, bob to the surface, and take a breath. They then return to the bottom and remove their load-carrying equipment, then perform five rhythmical bobs in succession. Load-carrying equipment (LCE) is the harness that fits around the waist and over the shoulders and the applicable military gear (canteen, ammunition pouches, etc.) that is attached. After the last bob, they retrieve the equipment one piece at a time (rifle first, then the LCE) by using the bob and travel to and from the side of the pool.

TEACHING CUES

- Before having the students execute a rear entry and LCE removal, have them practice blind belt buckle release on the deck—closing their eyes, finding the buckle by feeling for it, and then unhooking it. Practice this technique several times.

- Execute a rear entry with the LCE only.
- Exhale through the mouth and nose while descending to the bottom of the pool, and remove the LCE.
- Perform five rhythmic bobs in succession and recover to the gutter.
- Recover the LCE. Move feetfirst to and from the equipment. Do not swim with the LCE. When retrieving the LCE the swimmer will sling it on one shoulder. Once the suspender is slung over a shoulder, the swimmer bobs and travels to the side.
- Perform the three preceding steps with the rifle.
- To hook up with the rifle, one hand grasps the butt where the sling is attached, and the other hand grasps the sling higher up on the chest. Trace the sling of the rifle with the thumb from top to bottom to ensure that it is not tangled. The weapon is then pulled snug to the back.
- Recover the rifle. Move feetfirst to the rifle. Sling the rifle on one shoulder. Do not hand carry the weapon from the bottom. Once the rifle is slung over a shoulder, perform a bob and travel to a position of safety.
- Practice these steps together, with the LCE and the rifle at the same time, and then execute the skill test.
- For the skill test, students perform a rear entry first—removing rifle, execute one rhythmic bob, then remove the LCE, execute five rhythmic bobs, and immediately recover the rifle and LCE separately.

SUGGESTED LEARNING ACTIVITIES

- This skill is designed to test composure under duress, breath control, and underwater movement. Emphasize relaxing and going slowly and methodically through each of the steps.
- When removing the equipment, the student should drop both the weapon and the LCE an arm's length away to prevent entanglement.

Bob and Travel

DESCRIPTION

The bob and travel stroke is generally used in a water depth of no more than 10 feet (3 meters). The bob and travel allows a person to make it to a position of safety while carrying equipment, regardless of swimming ability. This skill can be very useful if people fall from a watercraft, are forced to disembark suddenly, or unexpectedly find themselves in deep water.

TEACHING CUES

- Begin in the water at the side of the pool. Let go of the gutter, and exhale down to the bottom of the pool in the direction of travel.
- Go to the one-knee-up and one-knee-down position with the hands side by side and the thumbs interlocked, arms fully extended and pointing upward toward the surface at a 45-degree angle in the direction of travel. Keep eyes open.
- Push up vigorously with the legs at a 45-degree angle, arms streamlined, and break the surface of the water with the fingertips; then, with the arms still fully extended, thrust the arms downward to the hips.

- Bring the knees up to the chest and then execute a modified rhythmic bob traveling forward and keeping the legs slightly in front of the hips. Take only one breath at the surface and keep eyes open.

SUGGESTED LEARNING ACTIVITIES

- Have students simulate the motion on the pool deck using a number sequence.
- Emphasize "clapping the hands" at the beginning of the descent to the bottom of the pool in order to produce enough force to push the body down to the bottom.
- Have students who are landing on their backs or rear ends keep their feet directly below their hips when going to the bottom.
- Remind students to keep feet together on the descent.
- Students may want to make forward progress on the descent as well.

Clothing Inflation

DESCRIPTION

Clothing inflation is a water survival skill that can keep a person afloat for extended periods of time. Students execute a rear entry, remove their boots and BDU trousers in the water, and then inflate the trousers so that the trousers fully support them at the surface.

TEACHING CUES

- Execute a rear entry.
- Assume a good drown-proofing position, remove the boots, and let them fall to the bottom of the pool.
- Remove the trousers and ensure that both legs are either right side out or inside out.
- Tie an overhand knot near the end of each trouser leg, or tie the trouser legs together using an overhand knot.
- Position the trousers in front of the body as if to put them on, with the zipper facing forward. Grasp the waistband equidistant from front to back.
- Circle the arms overhead, bringing the trousers to a position behind the neck. "Pop" the trousers open, making the waist as wide as possible.
- Extend the arms straight up, keeping the waist of the trousers as wide as possible, while performing a vigorous kick to allow the extended arms and trousers to be positioned up and out of the water.
- Bring the trousers straight down with the waist pointed downward, capturing as much air as possible to inflate the trousers.
- Keep the waist of the trousers pointed down and pinch off the waist to prevent any air from escaping.
- If an overhand knot was tied at the end of each leg, students put both shoulders over the inflated pants so that the pants provide support under the armpits. If the trouser legs were tied together with one knot, students put their head in between

the trouser legs with the knot behind the neck. With both methods they should keep the waistband pinched off and facing the bottom of the pool.

- Cross the legs and relax in a position fully supported by the inflated trousers.

SUGGESTED LEARNING ACTIVITIES

- Demonstrate the overhand knot at the end of the trouser legs by tying the trouser legs together on the deck. Have the students practice this with their eyes open and then with their eyes closed.
- Have students feel their way from the end of the trouser leg to the reinforced knee and make the overhead knot at this point.
- On the pool deck, have students practice circling the trousers behind the head, extending the arms upward, and thrusting the trousers straight down, keeping the waist opening wide.
- Have students circle the trousers behind their head. Once the trousers are extended over the head, have the students step off of the pool deck and thrust the trousers downward, capturing as much air as possible. Pinch off the waist to prevent any air from escaping, put both arms over the inflated legs with support under the armpits, then cross legs and relax.
- Have students practice just the inflationary aspects in the water as well.
- Students can add air to the trousers by splashing water in a downward "J" stroke toward the opening in the trousers at any time to supplement or add buoyancy.
- Students can also add air to the trousers by going underwater and exhaling air into the trouser opening.

One-Meter Wet Carry

DESCRIPTION

In this carry, students execute a stride entry into the water facing forward and keeping the body at or near the surface of the water. Holding the weapon at high port arms, they slap the weapon on the surface and lean forward, attempting to keep the head above the water. From the stride entry, they transition into a swimming stroke and swim 25 yards with the weapon cross-slung.

TEACHING CUES

- Button the top button of the BDU and roll the collar inward to facilitate buoyancy by catching air in the shirt during entry.
- Step up to the edge of the pool deck. Hold the weapon at port arms, with the trail hand of the sidestroke grasping the hand guard under the sling.
- On command, raise the weapon over the head to high port arms.
- Step off using a stride entry and slap the weapon on the surface.
- Command sequence:
  - "Toes over the edge."
  - "High port arms."
  - "Step off."

- Cross-sling the weapon on entry and utilize choice of stroke to swim 25 yards, emphasizing a strong kick.

SUGGESTED LEARNING ACTIVITIES

- Have students lean the torso slightly forward on entry to facilitate staying at the surface.
- Timing is critical for bringing the legs together and slapping the weapon on the surface.
- Have students button the top button of their BDU and roll the collar inward. Emphasize laying the head down in the water, using a strong kick, and not relying on the glide.
- Remind students to transition quickly from the stride entry to the sidestroke or breaststroke to minimize sinking. They use momentum from the entry to initiate forward momentum.
- Remind them to keep the weapon under control and swim streamlined through the water.

High-Level Entry

DESCRIPTION

The purpose of the high-level entry is to help students overcome fear of heights and remain calm and focused in a stressful situation. At West Point, this exercise is done only in Crandall Pool. It is first done from the 3-meter diving board to build confidence. Students then step off the 6 1/2-meter tower in the hookup position, first for practice to ensure proper entry positioning. On the second attempt, students swim underwater to the opposite side of the pool for record.

TEACHING CUES

- Perform the hookup position by placing the thumb and pinkie fingers of one hand on the cheekbones and the other three fingers across the forehead, creating a cage across the face. This air pocket will help to prevent injury to the face. With the other hand, grasp the elbow and hold it in close to the body.
- Look out at the horizon (top row of orange chairs in the seating area of the pool).
- Bring the rear leg inward after stepping off the edge, so that the legs are crossed.
- The following is the command sequence in order of progression:
  - "Step up."
  - "Hook up."
  - "Look up."
  - "Step off."
- On the record attempt only, swim underwater to the opposite side of the pool, or as far as possible. Make three exhalations underwater to prevent shallow-water blackout.

SUGGESTED LEARNING ACTIVITIES

- Instructor goes off tower as a demonstration.
- Students react to the commands.
- Students who balk should not be allowed to remain at the edge of the tower. Have them step away, and then start the command sequence again.

Survival Problem

DESCRIPTION

The survival problem is the ultimate water survival challenge. Once students can pass this segment, they are well on their way to safely handling almost any water situation they may encounter within typical Army standards. The survival problem consists of a combination of equipment removal, swimming for 25 yards, and clothing inflation. The three skills are performed in succession with no rest.

TEACHING CUES

- Perform equipment removal (no recovery). Have students who are not testing recover equipment and then get themselves prepared to test. Make sure they perform one rhythmic bob between removing the weapon and LCE.
- Swim 25 yards.
- Inflate clothing.

SUGGESTED LEARNING ACTIVITIES

- A survival stroke is less tiring than the front crawl and is not significantly slower over the 25 yards. Students should use the stroke that they are strongest in and most comfortable with to minimize exhaustion.
- Emphasize inflating on the first attempt.
- Students should push off in a 45-degree angle in the direction of swim after removal of LCE.

Adapting This Course for Your School

Having access to a pool allows you the opportunity to teach swimming and water safety to students— an activity that can truly save lives! Whatever the age of your students, elementary, middle school, high school, or college, you may have all ability groups from nonswimmer to advanced. The following section will give you some ideas on ways to adapt what we do at West Point for your unique setting.

Understanding the Learning Process

When one thinks of swimming, the idea of locomotion immediately comes to mind. However, swimming in a general sense is more aligned with water displacement, which is required to keep our bodies afloat and breathing. One need not be "moving" through the water to experience this process.

Acquiring swimming skills is a longitudinal process that entails elements of specificity (exposure), instruction, and facilitation. Of the three, perhaps the most integral element relies on the specificity of time spent in the water, as it is truly through the process of experimentation that the learner acquires the necessary skills to be successful. While teaching, guidance, and effective supervision remain key elements within the learning environment, master teachers strive to teach less and thereby create an "unstructured–structured" environment where learners explore at a pace relative to their individual needs. Perhaps the best way to describe this process is through reference to Kolb's Learning Theory. Kolb's Learning Theory (Kolb, 1984) is based on John Dewey's emphasis on the need for learning to be grounded in experience. Kolb defines learning as a four-stage "window" that the learner (as well as the teacher!) carefully navigates during the instructional process. Four concepts that make all the difference in terms of skill acquisition are observation, reflection, experimentation, and implementation.

Many years ago one of the authors saw a documentary piece with former baseball great Pete Rose, who was being interviewed after breaking Ty Cobb's base hit record. One of the reporters asked, "Hey Pete, can you explain how you became such a great hitter?" Rose replied, "Sure, I practiced my tail off." The reporter, dissatisfied with the answer, questioned again, "No, I meant what's the science behind hitting that ball?" Rose thought about it for a moment and said, "Hey, I see it, I swing at it, and it just meets my bat in a sweet spot that's been very good to me!"

Does this sound familiar? Surely you remember your own initial swimming experiences: the gothic YMCA pool, the beautiful mountain lake at camp, or even the distinct smell of the backyard pool cover when it was removed in the morning. You clearly remember events surrounding your pursuit of swimming prowess, but it can be challenging to describe the process through which you came to take those first few strokes so successfully.

Observation   Often the stimulus that facilitates the learning process begins with watching others "doing" the activity. Let's apply this to a land-based activity for a parallel illustration. Think of the baby who goes from crawling to walking. Don't be fooled! Countless hours have been spent watching all those "big people" wandering about effortlessly on their own two feet; and the realization, be it conscious or unconscious, after all this watching is to think, "Why not me?"

It is the observation of performance that initially draws us in. It is the very act of "watching" that attracts us. While peers, parents, and perceptions are important, seeing someone perform the action is often the true igniter.

Reflection   True reflection on what you "observed," be it someone swimming or an instructor demonstrating a technique, will pave the road to success. Often, this process occurs both before and after immersion, so don't be alarmed when you find yourself thinking about streamlining as you lie in bed at night counting sheep. Your ability to think about things and envision how you look as a performer goes a long way toward your becoming a more effective and successful learner!

Experimentation   You've now made it to that all-important third tier of learning. Be patient, because you'll be spending a lot of time here. Even great swimmers revisit experimentation during training sessions. It has been estimated that world-class swimmers, those we see wearing Olympic hardware, spend upward of 60 percent of their training time learning how to become more streamlined and less resistive as performers.

Great swimmers are still learning how to "carry" their head more efficiently, extend their reach, punctuate a pull lever—this after years and years of countless hours of water time. Do not get frustrated—true learning here will be fast, then slow, then fast, then slow.

You will often want more than you are ready for, and sometimes less than you're actually capable of achieving. Consistency will come; but as an all-important axiom of motor learning has it, if you want to be good, you've got to do it, and if you want to get better, you have to repeat it.

As a quick side note, this tier is particularly challenging for instructors as well, in that they often try to fine-tune learners before the larger battles of comfort and basic displacement have been experienced and understood.

What is the bottom line to this tier? A sound instructional program centers on a mode of facilitation rather than a rigid, structured learning template. In a perfect world, novice learning centers on specific body positioning (prone, supine, and vertical) as opposed to stringent stroke application. Learning how to scull or fin effectively is a wonderful way to master "still water" movement, to get that pesky center of gravity elevated and moving.

Learning to swim and learning how to do algebra are more alike than you would guess. Both have a strong dependence on the acquisition of basic formulas. Miss these, and you miss a lot. Get a learner buoyant and moving as soon as possible, and the technical aspects will soon begin to flow effortlessly.

Implementation   If all goes well through the first three windows, making your newfound skill work for you as a swimmer is a little closer to becoming a reality. Students should be careful, however, as "implementation" and "mastery" have two very distinct definitions. The process of implementing a skill or a technique in this instance implies utilizing a movement or skill set (or both) to successfully perform some degree of water locomotion with less drag and resistance. More importantly, however, it is now achieved unconsciously because of all the conscious drill work performed within the experimentation phase.

Skill refinement and implementation take time; and learning how to "plug in" a new skill, particularly a skill related to motor performance, is always in progress.

Establishing a Safe Water Environment

As with any skill development process, there is a psychological as well as a physiological aspect to developing watermanship skills, and this process is especially important for children. The term watermanship refers to an overall comfort within water, in varying postures, along with a baseline ability to swim comfortably at both the surface and the subsurface.

Each year in the United States, about 4,000 people die from drowning (National Center for Health Statistics, 2000). Drowning was a leading cause of unintentional injury death among all ages in 1998 and was the second leading cause of unintentional injury death among children ages 1 to 14 in that same year (National Center for Health Statistics, 2000). About 60 percent of drowning deaths among children occur in swimming pools (Dietz & Baker, 1974).

What can you do to drown-proof a child? The first line of defense is recognizing that there is no such thing as drown-proofing. Even the most skilled swimmers can drown, so ability level in and of itself is not a deterrent.

Children must be taught to recognize and analyze dangerous situations in and around the water environment *before* they begin to swim. Too often we teach from a reactive rather than a proactive point of view. Children need to understand that skill development is an evolving process with numerous limitations that are often complicated by a number of factors, with water conditions being the most notable of these.

A water park is very different from a wading pool; a river current doesn't parallel that found in a pond, and an ocean's fury can change quite

dramatically in a very short period of time. Watch people who spend their lives in and around water, and you will see two very interesting things when they go to a new place to swim:

1. They always talk to aquatic supervisors or lifeguards about site-specific conditions that may differ from conditions they are accustomed to.
2. They take the time to study the facility or environment before entering the water. Surfers often stand at water's edge for 10 to 15 minutes watching how waves break and how the surface water flows. This observation period assists in their safe performance once they have entered the water.

Of course, enrolling children in an accredited swimming course taught by a licensed or certified professional is a tremendously helpful beginning and certainly should not be discounted as an effective method toward becoming a safer and more efficient swimmer. But always understand that completion of a course does not guarantee competency in terms of safety and survivability. Water acclimatization and skill acquisition are both dependent on lifelong experiential episodes.

Teaching Swimming at the High School and College Level

Historically, most courses at the college or university level have been geared either toward a traditional learn-to-swim format or toward enabling students to become better swimmers at an intermediate or advanced level. In recent years, a peripheral interest has developed in aquatic fitness activities (water aerobics, water exercise, etc). Interestingly, water survivability is very infrequently offered as a stand-alone course; instead, survival skills and techniques are often utilized as filler options within curricular programs.

As recreational activities in and around the water continue to gain popularity, perhaps more consideration should be given to a stand-alone survival module that addresses situations and scenarios not dealt with in a basic instructional segment. The following three themes can easily be adapted and utilized as discrete instructional units or as supplemental programming options for any traditional swimming curriculum.

Swimming to Survive

OBJECTIVE

To teach students how to recognize a water emergency, understand stroke priorities when faced with fatigue, and explore various body postures in establishing buoyancy

LESSON SEGMENTS

1. Distress versus drowning: a definition
2. Resting stroke options
3. Buoyancy, balance, and drown-proofing

PROCEDURE

1. Describe characteristics of active and passive victims and have students demonstrate postures generic to each.
2. Students perform four basic resting stroke variations: elementary backstroke, sidestroke, breaststroke, and modified front crawl (survival option with underwater recovery).
3. Students experiment with three basic buoyancy postures—prone, supine, and vertical—as well as the "jellyfish" drown-proofing position.

EVALUATION

1. Students demonstrate three characteristics of an active victim and three characteristics of a passive victim, and have assigned partners identify behaviors accordingly.
2. Students perform a 200-yard survival swim, utilizing different resting strokes at 25-yard intervals.
3. Students drown-proof for 2 minutes with arms and legs tied, with proper safety measures utilizing an in-water partner spotter.

Basic Water Safety Principles

OBJECTIVE

To teach students how to recognize an emergency, prioritize a response mechanism, and maintain a position of safety throughout

LESSON SEGMENTS

1. How can I help?—reach, throw, row, tow
2. Spinal injury recognition and immobilization
3. Defenses, releases, and escapes

PROCEDURE

1. Define priority usage of rescue equipment and explain how each type is used safely.

2. Identify the condition of spinal injury as it relates to water, and practice victim immobilization procedures.

3. Demonstrate in-water defense mechanisms and how to safely escape or parry a victim's grasp during an in-water contact scenario.

EVALUATION

1. Students must successfully provide assistance in a simulated victim submersion sequence, utilizing at least two different rescue strategies.

2. Students must successfully activate a mock emergency action plan and identify and immobilize a suspected spinal cord–injured victim in shallow water.

3. Students must successfully defend, escape, or parry, singly or in combination, either a front head hold or a rear head hold grip, employing techniques specifically designed for in-water application.

Open-Water Considerations

OBJECTIVE

To teach students condition-specific techniques for open-water or surf survival and safe recreational small craft operation

LESSON SEGMENTS

1. Waves, currents, and moving water

2. Small craft safety and usage of personal flotation devices

3. Clothing inflation options

PROCEDURE

1. Discuss characteristics of moving water and tidal conditions and how they differ from those in still-water survival situations. A wave pool facility is desirable.

2. Demonstrate canoe and personal flotation device usage before and after controlled swamping.

3. Practice disrobing and clothing inflation options utilizing both shirt and pant options.

EVALUATION

1. Students simulate a 25-yard diagonal open-water swimming pattern, utilizing resting stroke of choice and proper sighting technique.

2. Students demonstrate proper canoe-trimming technique, perform controlled swamp, and properly apply personal flotation device after submersion.

3. Students demonstrate a proper disrobing and inflation progression for both shirt and pants while blindfolded. For successful completion, a 60-second flotation interval is required for each.

Teaching Swimming at the Elementary and Middle School Level

Teaching children to swim has traditionally been looked on as a structured 10- to 14-day process revolving around the start of the summer season. Rarely do you find swimming instructional programs at the elementary school level. Lifeguard supervision, specialized instructional certification, and the limitations of facility space are the main barriers to the implementation of this curriculum at many elementary schools.

The most interesting aspect of any introductory program is that in many cases, parents or caregivers leave the process feeling that very little has been accomplished. More alarmingly, there is often the false assumption that finishing a course automatically translates into a fully water-safe child, and this is simply not true. Swimming must be viewed as a lifelong skill, and success in terms of survival aspects should be viewed as more positional than related to stroke and technique completion.

Within the Foundations program at USMA, the instructional focus first and foremost is on developing comfort and basic locomotion in relation to varying in-water posture positions as opposed to the specific stroke development paradigm used in most traditional programming venues. Developmental research seems to support this concept, showing that skill acquisition in many areas, including both the cognitive and social domains, depends on essential prerequisite readiness skills and durational elements for any type of long-term success (Langendorfer, 1994).

The Foundations course revolves around a concept of positional exposure that is based on three fundamental in-water postures: the prone, supine, and vertical positions. Students progress through a 15-lesson course with small positional modules, each involving three progressive benchmarks associated with specific body positioning.

Course adaptation to the Elementary level of instruction at West Point has been outstanding in that students are more positioned for success after having had the opportunity to develop more baseline readiness. While implementing a unit based solely on readiness and exploration may prove difficult within the structure and confines of a larger public school curriculum, any degree of water readiness or exploration is a highly suggested first step within any sound learn-to-swim curriculum.

USMA AQUATIC FOUNDATIONS CURRICULUM (SAMPLE)

COURSE CONTENT

    I. Basic hydrodynamics module—vertical position module

    II. Supine position module

    III. Prone position module

    IV. Stroke and survival position module

LESSON 1: BASIC HYDRODYNAMICS—VERTICAL POSITION MODULE

- Introduction, administration, emergency action plan
- Entries: ease-in, stride jump
- Bobbing mechanism
- Buoyancy mechanism
- Breathing mechanism
- Displacement mechanism
- Combined skills: bobbing, breathing

Performance Benchmarks

- Benchmark A: ease-in, bob
- Benchmark B: ease-in, bob, displace (:10)
- Benchmark C: stride jump, bob, displace (:15), buoyancy (vertical, supine)

LESSON 2: VERTICAL POSITION REVIEW

- Drown-proofing, survival displacement
- Treading options
- Basic locomotion
- Combined skills: treading, breathing

Performance Benchmarks

- Benchmark A: stride jump, drown-proof (:15)
- Benchmark B: stride jump, tread, drown-proof (:20)
- Benchmark C: stride jump, tread, drown-proof (:15), survival swim 10 yards (9 meters)

LESSON 3: SUPINE POSITION MODULE (WITH FINS)

- Supine streamlining options with fins
- Supine streamlining with displacement (scull, fin)
- Combined skills: push-off, streamline, displace, streamline

Performance Benchmarks

- Benchmark A: side(s) 10 yards
- Benchmark B: one fin 10 yards
- Benchmark C: no fins 10 yards

LESSON 4: SUPINE POSITION CONTINUED

- Streamline maintenance with effective arm scull action
- Whip kick introduction and drill options
- Combined skills: push-off, streamline, displace, breathe, streamline

Performance Benchmarks

- Benchmark A: elementary backstroke 10 yards
- Benchmark B: elementary backstroke 15 yards (14 meters)
- Benchmark C: elementary backstroke 20 yards (18 meters)

LESSON 5: PRONE POSITION MODULE (WITH FINS)

- Prone streamlining with fins
- Prone streamlining: sweet spot coordination
- Prone streamlining with displacement (scull)
- Combined skills: push-off, streamline, scull

Performance Benchmarks

- Benchmark A: both fins 10 yards
- Benchmark B: one fin 15 yards
- Benchmark C: no fins 20 yards

LESSON 6: PRONE POSITION CONTINUED

- Introduction to front crawl arm options (human stroke, etc.)
- Head, streamline, sweet spot
- Arm action progressions, drill options
- Introduction to breathing mechanism

Performance Benchmarks
- Benchmark A: side(s) 10 yards
- Benchmark B: one fin 15 yards
- Benchmark C: no fins 20 yards

LESSON 7: PRONE AND SUPINE COMBINED MODULE

- Changing positions
- Changing strokes
- Equipment usage
- Stroke review
- Cardiovascular option: kick, scull, swim set

Performance Benchmarks
- Benchmark A: stride jump, streamline, human swim 15 yards
- Benchmark B: stride jump, streamline, front crawl 20 yards
- Benchmark C: stride jump, streamline, front crawl, back scull 25 yards (23 meters)

LESSON 8: STROKE-SPECIFIC APPLICATION AND REFINEMENT

- Review of elementary backstroke
- Review of front crawl
- Introduction to breaststroke progressions

LESSON 9: STROKE-SPECIFIC APPLICATION AND REFINEMENT

- Stroke potpourri
- Introduction to sidestroke progressions

LESSON 10: STROKE-SPECIFIC APPLICATION AND REFINEMENT

- Stroke review, inclusive
- Conditioning circuit

LESSON 11: BASIC SKILLS CHECK-OFF: PART 1

- ☐ Deep water bobbing 5 repetitions
- ☐ Survival float and buoyancy 1 minute
- ☐ Elementary backstroke 20 yards
- ☐ Treading water 3 minutes
- ☐ Stride jump entry, prone level 15 yards

LESSON 12: BASIC SKILLS CHECK-OFF: PART 2

- ☐ Underwater swim 10 yards
- ☐ Front crawl 20 yards
- ☐ Submerged object recovery 8 feet (2.4 meters)

☐ Changing-position swim 20 yards

☐ Stride jump entry, supine level 15 yards

LESSON 13: COMBINED SKILLS MODULE A

Start in deep water, push off into crawl stroke position (10 yards [9 meters]), and turn onto back and continue (10 yards) with a scull and flutter kick. Stop approximately 5 yards (4.5 meters) from the opposite wall and tread water for 15 seconds, level, and swim and kick to opposite wall.

LESSON 14: COMBINED SKILLS MODULE B

Stride jump into deep water, tread water for 15 seconds, level into a crawl stroke (12.5 yards [11 meters]), turn onto back, and continue to opposite wall with a scull and flutter kick.

Key Terms

balance—Float on the surface of the water so that all parts of the body are supported equally.

battle dress uniform (BDU)—Camouflaged trouser and shirt worn by military during field operations.

bob and travel—Method of in-water locomotion, performed by descending and pushing off the bottom to initiate a forward movement. Typically performed in water no deeper than 8 to 10 feet.

dorsiflexion and plantarflexion—Rotation of the foot commonly seen in resting stroke variants. In the normal foot, the reference point for a dorsiflexed or plantarflexed position is a transverse plane that runs through the heel. If the foot is positioned below this transverse plane, it is said to be plantarflexed; above this transverse plane, it is said to be dorsiflexed.

drown-proofing—Also known as survival floating, this technique is performed in a facedown floating position, which is utilized in emergency situations to conserve energy and maximize buoyancy.

eggbeater or rotary kick—A kicking technique used for treading water and personal safety.

finning—A displacement technique that the swimmer utilizes by performing a winging motion with the arms, typically done in a supine position.

freestyle—The most commonly used swimming stroke, also called the front crawl. The fastest of the four competitive strokes.

front quadrant swimming (FQS)—Form of swimming in which the stroking hand is still in front when the recovering arm is about to enter the water. Staying on one's side and keeping an arm outstretched in front of the body ensure a long streamlined position.

giant stride entry—Method of entry performed with the intent of keeping the head above the water's surface.

Typically used at a height no greater than 3 feet above the surface.

high-level entry—Compact jump entry performed off a 6.5-meter platform while wearing BDUs and boots.

Kevlar—Helmet worn by the U.S. Army in combat operations.

load-carrying equipment (LCE)—Harness that fits around the waist and over the shoulders and has applicable military gear (two canteens, two ammunition pouches, etc.) attached.

M-16 rifle/weapon—Standard firing weapon used by the U.S. Army.

rack-out position—Technique used to brace and support the upper body using the pool side or gutter, enabling lower body isolation for kick iterations.

rear entry—Entering the water in a backward crouched body position; this type of entry is disorienting.

sculling—A technique for moving through the water or staying horizontal using only the arms and hands.

sideline kick—The balance progression used in teaching both the freestyle and sidestroke.

starting block—Elevated platform typically used in competitive swimming venues.

streamline—A body position that eliminates drag and resistance during swimming.

survival problem—Connected series of tactical swimming skills designed for evaluation of comprehensive survival competency.

swim egg—Flotation device, typically worn at the center of gravity to increase buoyancy in the lower body quadrant.

tactical—Relating to military operations in a battlefield environment.

wet carry—Surface locomotion or swimming with BDUs, LCE, boots, and M-16 rifle.

References

Dietz, P., & Baker, S. (1974). Drowning: Epidemiology and prevention. *American Journal of Public Health, 64(2),* 303-312.

Kolb, D.A. (1984). *Experiential learning.* Englewood Cliffs, NJ: Prentice-Hall.

Langendorfer, S.J. (1994). *Aquatic readiness: Developing water competence in young children.* Champaign, IL: Human Kinetics.

National Center for Health Statistics, Vital Statistics of the United States, Mortality, Underlying and Multiple Causes of Death, Public Use Files (2000). Hyattsville, Maryland: Author.

Suggested Readings

American Red Cross. (1993). *Swimming & diving.* St. Louis, MO: StayWell.

Branche, C., & Stewart, S. (Eds.). (2001). *Lifeguard effectiveness: A report of the working group.* Atlanta: Centers for Disease Control and Prevention, National Center for Injury Prevention and Control.

Elder, T., & Campbell, K. (1997). *Aquatic fitness for everyone,* 2nd ed. Winston-Salem, NC: Hunter Textbooks.

Katz, J. (1996). *The aquatic handbook for lifetime fitness.* Boston: Allyn & Bacon.

Laughlin, T. (1997). *Total immersion: The revolutionary way to swim better, faster, and easier.* New York: Simon & Schuster.

Maglischo, E.W., & Ferguson-Brennan, C. (1985). *Swim for the health of it.* Palo Alto, CA: Mayfield.

Thomas, D.G. (1996). *Swimming: Steps to success.* Champaign, IL: Human Kinetics.

YMCA of the USA. (2001). *On the guard II: The YMCA lifeguard manual.* Champaign, IL: Human Kinetics.

6

Self-Defense

Ray Wood and Bridget Wilson

The study and practice of a martial art may be approached as (1) a physical discipline or form of exercise, (2) a spiritual discipline or way of life, (3) a competitive sport, and (4) a means of self-defense. The self-defense applications of martial arts have been used to promote the study of martial arts for many years. However, the introduction of self-defense classes into physical education curriculum at the postsecondary level is a relatively recent phenomenon. Most often, self-defense programs have been geared primarily toward women and toward meeting the perceived increase in sexual assault in an increasingly violent society. Teaching women and men to protect themselves has also been used as a means of increasing self-confidence and personal empowerment.

Self-defense courses at the postsecondary level generally teach strategies and tactics to avoid threat situations and the skills needed to disable an attacker if avoidance fails. One of the most neglected aspects of self-defense training is attitude adjustment. Basic self-defense skills are relatively easy to teach and learn, but they are ineffective and potentially counterproductive if the defender is not willing and able to injure the attacker. Teaching basic self-defense skills without fostering the development of an aggressive mind-set and aggressive behaviors promotes a false sense of competency and confidence. Coaches or physical educators would not teach aggressive behaviors or attitudes as used in self-defense in a competitive sport or a recreationally oriented physical education class, but these attitudes and behaviors are needed for the effective application of self-defense skills. Teaching aggression as part of a physical education class may be difficult for some educators. In addition, it is incumbent upon the instructor to be familiar with the legal aspects of the use of physical force to defend oneself.

Self-defense techniques that may be employed when escape and avoidance strategies and tactics fail can be broadly grouped into five classes: (1) strikes and kicks to incapacitate or render unconscious; (2) joint locks that incapacitate or control; (3) chokes to induce unconsciousness or achieve control; (4) throws to control, disadvantage, or injure; and (5) instinctive actions such as biting, clawing, and scratching.

Self-defense training or instruction generally teaches skills that are characteristic of the style and philosophy of the parent martial art in training. Few if any martial art styles equally stress learning all of the five skill groups, and thus no one style meets all self-defense situations optimally. Karate and striking arts tend to emphasize the use of striking and kicking skills in their approach to self-defense. Aikido or Japanese Ju-Jitsu styles of martial arts favor the use of joint locks as an integral aspect. Grappling arts such as judo and Brazilian Ju-Jitsu incorporate competitive throws, chokes, and joint locks in combination with basic strikes and kicks in their approach to self-defense training. A complete and comprehensive approach to self-defense should incorporate skills from a variety of martial arts that enable a student to deal with a wide range of self-defense situations.

Purpose of the Course

The purpose of self-defense and combatives training at the U.S. Military Academy is to enable men and women to understand and cope with physical or sexual assault in daily life or in their role as a professional soldier. Self-defense training produces benefits in all three of the educational domains. In the psychomotor domain, self-defense skills depend on a wide variety of motor abilities such as gross and fine hand, foot, and body coordination; dynamic and static balance; agility; and kinesthetic awareness. In the cognitive domain, acquiring the cognitive strategies and tactics to escape and neutralize a physical assault and the ability to recognize and read threat behavior are crucial to a successful defense. Perhaps the most important personal benefit of self-defense training is in the affective domain. Confidence, fear management, and the ability to function effectively while engaged in fear-producing activities are products of a rational and comprehensive training program. Self-defense skills may be used as a vehicle to develop confidence in a woman's ability to defend herself through an understanding of the nature of violence and through learning how to cope with physical assault.

Instructional Area

The size and makeup of the instructional area depend on the specific skills, type and intensity of drills, and the number of students. Falling, throwing, and ground grappling skills require a larger instructional area. A 42- by 42-foot (13- by 13-meter) matted area allows 16 to 18 students to practice grappling, throwing, and falling skills safely, provided that the instruction and drills are structured and that the activities are monitored closely by the instructor. If students are allowed to practice on their own or engage in live-action activities, a 42- by 42-foot mat will accommodate 10 to 12 students safely with instructor supervision.

If the curriculum consists primarily of skills such as striking, punching, kicking, and blocking, then the same-size mat can handle 22 to 24 students in a structured drill format. A hardwood floor like that of a basketball court is acceptable for striking skills provided that no throws or takedowns are practiced.

If there isn't room to spread students out far enough to avoid contact, then padding the walls of the instructional area is advisable. Wrestling rooms are good facilities for self-defense instruction, and basketball courts may be readily adapted to self-defense instruction by the use of portable mats.

Equipment

Expensive and high-tech equipment is nice to have but not necessary for teaching basic self-defense. Four types of equipment are recommended: striking dummies, protective gear, mats, and mirrors. Striking dummies are simple and effective aids for teaching students to strike and block effectively. Teaching proper striking or kicking form is relatively easy, but to develop effective and powerful strikes and kicks requires that students hit an object that has mass, provides resistance, and will not cause injury if used properly. Resistance and mass are also needed to condition the limbs and body to execute these techniques safely and without injury. A wide variety of commercial striking aids are useful for developing powerful striking and kicking techniques. Boxing focus mitts, punching bags, and dummies shaped like humans are all readily available commercially (see figure 6.1). Cylindrical foam-filled football tackling dummies (18 by 50 inches [.45 by 1.3 meters]) are an all-purpose striking and kicking teaching aid.

Cylindrical tackling dummies are light enough (24 pounds [11 kilograms]) to be held and tough enough for safe practice of full-force strikes and kicks if used properly. Tackling dummies are effective teaching aids provided that students receive instruction on how to use the bags safely and to coach their partner.

There is a saying in karate that a block is a strike and a strike is a block. This means that if a block is executed properly, it will inflict pain or discomfort. Protective gear is needed for the safety and comfort of the partner who is striking, not the partner who is blocking (see figure 6.2).

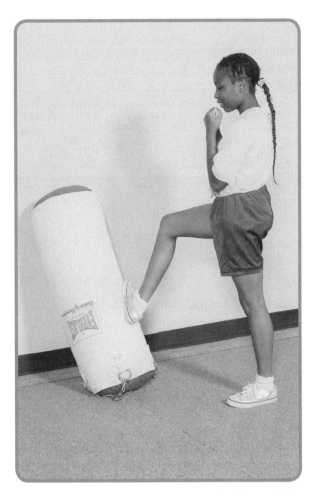

FIGURE 6.1 A punching bag or cylindrical foam-filled tackling dummy are useful for developing striking or kicking skills.

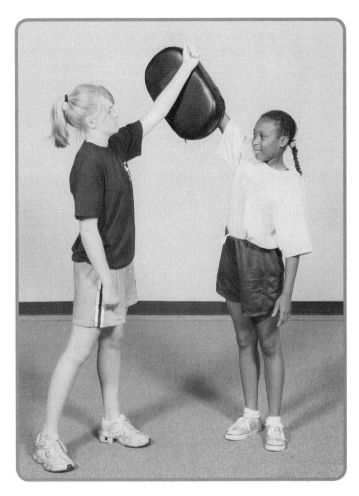

FIGURE 6.2 Use protective pads to protect the hand, wrist, and forearm.

Foam pads that protect the forearm, elbow, and upper arm are inexpensive and allow students to practice full-force blocks safely and with minimal discomfort to either partner.

Mats are a valuable teaching aid. A comprehensive and advanced course in self-defense should include defenses for attacks that are initiated on the ground or end up on the ground. A well-matted surface is necessary for teaching falling or throwing skills and any ground-based skills. The degree of impact protection that the mats need to provide is dictated by the skills and intensity of the training. One-inch folding mats are generally adequate for ground-based skills that start on the ground, and wrestling mats are well suited for ground grappling skills. Throwing techniques or defenses for throws and takedowns require mats with a higher degree of impact protection and are specifically designed for that use. Mats and proper falling skills can reduce, but not totally eliminate, the risk of injury when one is teaching skills that involve throws and takedowns.

Risk Management

Students and parents should be informed about the risks inherent in self-defense training. An informed consent and safety and warning statement (see p. 94), as well as information about risk identification and reduction (see table 6.1 on page 95), should be available or should be part of a course overview or orientation. The use of an informed consent form ensures a knowledgeable and willing student. A risk assessment is a guide for the instructor to use to anticipate possible training issues and sources of risk, as well as to develop preventive measures and emergency action plans.

INFORMED CONSENT FORM

PURPOSE OF THE WARNING

The purpose of the following is to inform students of the risk and nature of potential injuries in combatives and self-defense so that students may participate with an understanding and knowledge of risks involved. The risk of injury in activities involving the acquisition and simulated application of techniques designed to incapacitate an attacker can be minimized, but not eliminated entirely. Information regarding proper conditioning and safety tips is provided to create a realistic, safe, and productive learning experience. The injuries and risks listed in table 6.1 are meant to be representative of the risks involved in these activities, and the listing is not exhaustive or all-inclusive.

NATURE OF THE ACTIVITY

Self-defense instruction is designed to provide students with an opportunity to acquire offensive and defensive combatives and self-defense skills. These skills include striking, blocking, kicking, throwing, choking, joint locking, movement techniques, and their application in a wide variety of self-defense and combat scenarios. Realistic self-defense skill training involves intense and extended physical effort and has an inherent risk of injury, especially when one is practicing potentially injurious skills with a partner. The risk of injury in realistic training can be minimized but cannot be eliminated.

RISK REDUCTION STRATEGIES

Instruction and practice will be conducted at a pace, skill level, and intensity commensurate with the student's skill level, experience, and level of conditioning. Training sessions will include a warm-up period prior to participation and a cool-down period after each class, commensurate with the training intensity level, for safety and comfort. An active skill-specific stretching regimen may be added if appropriate. The following strategies will help safeguard participants: (1) progressive instruction (instructor responsibility), (2) professionally accepted training methods (instructor responsibility), (3) an appropriate level of physical conditioning (student responsibility), (4) exercise of physical control while working with a partner (student responsibility), (5) attention to safety concerns (instructor and student responsibility), and (6) periodic inspection and maintenance of equipment and facilities (instructor responsibility).

I have read and understand the preceding information and certify that I am physically fit to participate in self-defense instruction and training. If I incur any physical injuries, illnesses, or impairments now or during the course of this training, I agree to immediately notify the instructor. I understand that no amount of instruction, precaution, and supervision will totally eliminate all risk of serious, catastrophic, or even fatal injury. I fully understand and accept the risks inherent in self-defense and martial arts training, and any questions have been addressed satisfactorily.

_____   _____   _____
      (Printed name)   (Signature)   (Date)

From M. LeBoeuf and L. Butler, eds., 2008, *Fit & active* (Champaign, IL: Human Kinetics).

Table 6.1　Possible Risks in Self-Defense

Risk identification	Reduction strategies
Muscle, tendon, and ligament sprains	• Adequate warm-up and cool-down periods • Exercise intensity commensurate with student's level of conditioning and experience • Drill and skill progressions commensurate with student's level of expertise and experience • Instructor supervision of practice
Impact injuries to eyes from striking or grappling	• Proper use of eye safety glasses and goggles • No contact lenses • Proper instruction in practice of strikes to the head and face • Instructor supervision of practice • Peer coaching emphasizing safe and correct execution of skill
Impact injuries to mouth, face, teeth, and jaw from striking, kicking, or falling	• Use of headgear, hand protection, and mouthpieces and instruction on proper use • Proper instruction in practice of strikes to the head and face • Drill complexity and skill progressions commensurate with student's experience, level of expertise, and conditioning • Peer coaching, emphasizing safe and correct execution of skill • Instructor supervision of skill practice
Impact injuries to internal organs from striking, kicking, or falling	• Use of body protector gear and instruction on proper use • Peer coaching techniques emphasizing safe and correct execution of skill • Use of safety mats • Instruction and practice of appropriate falling skills • Drill complexity and skill progressions commensurate with student's experience and level of expertise and conditioning • Instructor supervision of skill practice
Impact injuries to head, neck, arms, shoulders, back, hips, legs, and feet from striking, kicking, or falling	• Use of safety mats • Instruction and practice of appropriate falling skills • Use of body protector gear and instruction on proper use • Drill complexity and skill progressions commensurate with student's experience and level of expertise and conditioning • Peer coaching techniques emphasizing safe and correct execution of skill • Instructor supervision of skill practice
Dislocations of the neck, spine, shoulders, elbows, wrist, fingers, hips, knees, ankles, feet, and toes from striking, kicking, or falling	• Use of safety mats • Instruction and practice of appropriate falling skills • Use of body protector gear and instruction on proper use • Drill complexity and skill progressions commensurate with student's experience and level of expertise and conditioning • Peer coaching techniques emphasizing safe and correct execution of skill • Instructor supervision of skill practice
Fractures of the bones of the skull, face, jaw, neck, shoulder, arm, wrist, fingers, spine, hips, legs, knee, ankle, feet, or toes from striking, kicking, or falling	• Use of safety mats • Instruction and practice of appropriate falling skills • Use of protective gear and instruction on proper use • Drill complexity and skill progressions commensurate with student's experience and level of expertise and conditioning • Peer coaching techniques emphasizing safe and correct execution of skill • Instructor supervision of skill practice

(continued)

Table 6.1 (continued)

Risk identification	Reduction strategies
Cuts and abrasions	• Attention to personal hygiene • Prohibiting wearing of jewelry, hair accessories, or articles that may cause injury during instruction and practice • Use of safety mats with nonabrasive covering • Proper use of equipment
Equipment-related injury	• Instruction in the proper use of equipment • Periodic inspection and maintenance of equipment • Maintaining a plan for rotation and replacement of equipment • Archiving results of inspection, maintenance, repair, and replacement of equipment
Facilities-related injury	• Periodic inspection and maintenance of facilities • Maintaining a plan for the repair and upgrading of facilities based on time and use • Archiving results of inspection, maintenance, repair, and upgrading of facilities
Illness or injury due to environmental conditions	• Daily inspection of the classroom environment • Daily evaluation of health of students • Not allowing ill students to actively participate
Risk of communicable disease from bodily fluids or medical waste	• Daily inspection of the classroom environment • Daily evaluation of health of students • Educating all students and staff on approved procedures for dealing with potentially infectious body fluids or medical waste • Maintaining materials for cleanup of bodily fluids or medical waste on site • Action plan for disposal of bodily fluids or medical waste on site
Aggravation of an existing condition or illness that contraindicates participation	• Pre- and postclass medical screening by instructor • Requiring students to report all injuries, illnesses, and conditions that may affect participation to the instructor before class • Educating students not to exceed their limits when injured • Not allowing ill students to actively participate
Inadequate emergency action plan	• Having first aid equipment • Maintaining and having available for inspection a plan for the care and transport of people in medical emergencies
Inadequate instructor and staff medical training	• Periodic first aid training for instructors and staff • Maintaining and having available for inspection certifications of training

Course Overview

The purpose of the course overview is to familiarize students with the course content and provide them with a brief description of the activities in each lesson (see table 6.2).

Skills and Techniques

The following lesson plan outlines show examples of the skills that may be taught and of ways to structure a class. The information presented here is meant to serve as a conceptual framework for developing a self-defense course. Self-defense knowledge, training, and skills should be gained from face-to-face instruction from an experienced and qualified instructor.

Table 6.2 Overview of Self-Defense Lessons

Lesson	Skills
1	Course overview, awareness and avoidance training for assault
2	Back break fall progression, ground defense, two-hand stand up in base, and double-leg takedown
3	Dive roll-out progression and high set break fall
4	Circular punch defense 1: forward movement, outside block, forward strikes, and knee strike
5	Circular punch defense 2: rear movement, outside block, forward strikes, and knee strike
6	Circular punch defense 3: forward movement, inside blocks, rear strikes, and front kicks
7	Straight punch defense 1: rear movement, inside block, and front kicks
8	Straight punch defense 2: rear movement, outside block, and front kicks
9	Review: drill of straight and circular punch defense
10	Midterm skills test and falling assessment
11	Ground defense 1: two-hand choke in front mount and guard
12	Ground defense 2: slap, punch, and wrist pin in front mount and guard
13	Ground defense 3: high and low rear tackle and referee's position
14	Front and rear garrote strangle and front two-hand strangle
15	Rear forearm strangle defense and choking headlock defense
16	Push-down strangle and wall choke
17	Lifting and static rear bear hug defense
18	Wrist escapes and review
19	End-of-course situational test

The Self-Defense I curriculum (Combatives II) focuses on five skill areas and their applications in situational attacks that women frequently encounter. The criteria for selecting techniques are (1) effectiveness, (2) wide range of application, (3) level of teaching difficulty, (4) how easy the technique is to learn, and (5) how safe the technique is to execute and practice.

Striking

Four basic strikes are taught to cadets. The groin slap is an openhanded rising slap to the groin followed by a grab and squeezing motion. The heel palm strike is delivered with an open hand, and the striking surface is the heel of the palm. The throat strike is an openhanded strike, and the striking surface is the area between the base of the thumb and the tip of the forefinger. The elbow strike is the most powerful upper body strike. It is executed with an open hand, and the striking surface is the front of the elbow on the lower forearm.

Blocking

Two basic blocks are taught. The basic blocks are easily adapted for strikes to the head and torso. The inside block is named for a blocking action that takes place as the blocking surface moves toward the midline of the body. The blocking surface extends from the base of the little finger to the elbow. The outside block is named because of the opposite blocking action; that is, the blocking action takes place as the blocking surface moves toward the outside limits of the body. For high, middle, or low strikes, the blocking surface is raised to the level of the strike.

Leg Strikes

Two basic kicks and a knee strike are taught. The front snap kick is a speed kick that is executed with a snapping motion of the lower leg from the knee. The striking surface is the toe of a shoe or the ball of the foot. The kicking action is similar to that of snapping a towel, except that it is executed as though the towel were between the toes (see figure 6.3). The front kick is a simple stomping motion executed in a horizontal plane. The striking surface is the ball or heel of the foot. The vertical knee strike is the most powerful leg strike and the most effective at close quarters. The striking surface is the top of the knee (see figure 6.4).

Falling

Basic falling skills include the rear break fall and the dive rollout. Falling skills are taught to counter situational attacks in which a woman is thrown, pushed, or knocked to the ground. The dive rollout is very similar to the shoulder roll taught in gymnastics (see figure 6.5). The back break fall is a judo skill that is used to prevent injury from a pushing attack or a fall to the rear.

Movement Skills

The movement skills we discuss next include forward, rear, lateral, and oblique movements. The ability to move forward, laterally, backward, and at oblique angles (i.e., at a 45-degree angle to the line of attack) with speed, balance, and power is the foundation of effective offense and defense skills. Forward movements are used more often in offensive or attacking sequences. Lateral and rear movements are generally defensive and are used in conjunction with blocking skills.

Standing Front Choke

Defensive responses are taught for three variations of the front choke: (1) two-hand choke—the defender is choked as two hands are placed around his or her neck; (2) garrote choke—the choke is applied with a rope or cord from the front; (3) wall choke—the defender may be choked with both hands after being pinned against a wall.

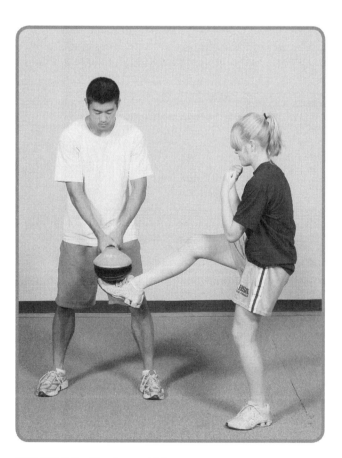

FIGURE 6.3 Front snap kick.

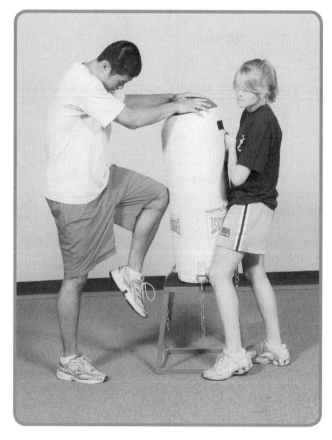

FIGURE 6.4 Vertical knee.

Standing Rear Choke

Defensive responses are taught for three variations of a rear choke: (1) rear forearm choke—the defense is against a choke executed with the arm wrapped around the throat; (2) garrote choke—the choke may be applied with a rope or cord from the rear; (3) two-hand choke—the defender is choked as two hands are placed around his or her neck from the rear.

Ground Chokes

Defensive responses are taught for a two-handed choke with the attacker sitting astride the defender (see figure 6.6).

Strikes, Punches, and Grabs

Defensive responses are taught for open-hand slaps, roundhouse punches, or straight punches to the face and head.

Front and Rear Tackles

Defensive responses are taught for football tackle attacks from the front or rear.

Rear Bear Hugs With Arms Free and Pinned

Defensive responses are taught for situations in which a woman is grabbed in a bear hug from the front or rear and with the arms pinned or free.

Wrist Grabs

Defensive responses are taught for single, double, and cross-wrist grabs.

Sample Lesson Plans

The following lesson plans provide a format for the sequence of a class session. The normal class session includes (1) student accountability; (2) lesson overview; (3) warm-up; (4) skills, drills, practice, assessment, and feedback; (5) cool-down; (6) lesson summary; and (7) class dismissal. Each lesson has a major skill theme, such as falling and pushing; hand striking with speed and power; or defending against the choke. The amount of time allocated for each activity may be adjusted to the needs of your unique setting.

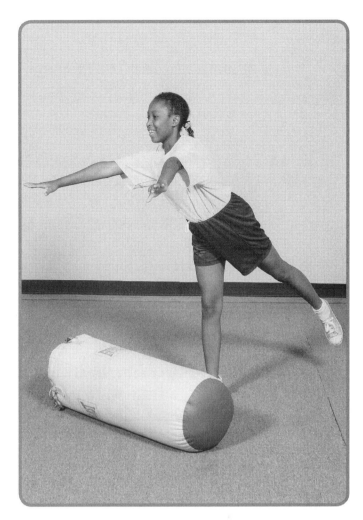

FIGURE 6.5   Dive rollout.

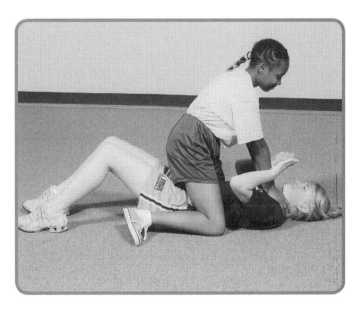

FIGURE 6.6   Two-handed choke.

Back Fall

SEQUENCE (40-MINUTE CLASS)

1. Lesson overview (3 minutes)
2. Warm-up (5 minutes)
3. Back fall progression (26 minutes)
   a. Back position of landing (5 minutes)
   b. Sitting back fall (3 minutes)
   c. Squatting back fall (3 minutes)
   d. Standing back fall (5 minutes)
   e. Push back fall (10 minutes)
4. Cool-down (2-4 minutes)
5. Lesson summary (2 minutes)

MAJOR SKILL THEME

Learning a back fall as a response to a pushing attack

SUGGESTED LEARNING ACTIVITIES

1. Demonstration: The teacher models the proper execution of the back fall and explains the application and value of the skill.
2. Explanation: The instructor explains the learning strategy for skill progression and demonstrates each phase of the progression. The proper execution of each step of the progression is described, and teaching cues are presented for each step.
3. Drill: The skill sequence is drilled by the numbers, with the instructor providing both group and individual feedback as needed. As students' skill develops, the progression is condensed until the students are performing the skill or sequence as one complete movement and not as a series of discrete movements.
4. Free practice: Once the students can perform the skill sequence without resorting to a by-the-numbers approach, they are allowed to practice the skill with partners at their own pace. Free practice includes one partner acting as an attacker and simulating a pushing attack. The instructor provides behavioral performance standards that facilitate self-assessment and peer coaching. The instructor monitors practice and provides group and individual feedback as needed.

Heel Palm Strike

SEQUENCE (40-MINUTE CLASS)

1. Lesson overview (3 minutes)
2. Warm-up (5 minutes)
3. Heel palm strike (26 minutes)
4. Cool-down (2-4 minutes)
5. Lesson summary (2 minutes)

MAJOR SKILL THEME

Learning to strike with speed and power using a hand technique

SUGGESTED LEARNING ACTIVITIES

1. Demonstration: The teacher models the proper execution of the heel palm strike in combination with forward movement and an outside block. The applications of the skill are discussed.

2. Explanation: The instructor explains the learning strategy for skill progression, models each phase of the progression, and explains proper execution of each phase including teaching cues for each movement.

3. Drill: The skill is drilled by the numbers, with the instructor providing both group and individual feedback as needed. As the students' skill develops, the progression is condensed until the students are performing the skill as one complete movement and not as a series of discrete movements.

4. Free practice: Once the students can perform the skill without resorting to a by-the-numbers approach, they practice the skill with partners at their own pace. The instructor models the methods for practice, emphasizes safe practice procedures for the drill, and provides behavioral performance standards that facilitate self-assessment and peer coaching. The instructor monitors practice and provides group and individual feedback as needed.

Knee Strike

SEQUENCE (40-MINUTE CLASS)

1. Lesson overview (3 minutes)
2. Warm-up (5 minutes)
3. Knee strike (26 minutes)
4. Cool-down (2-4 minutes)
5. Lesson summary (2 minutes)

MAJOR SKILL THEME

Learning to knee strike with speed and power

SUGGESTED LEARNING ACTIVITIES

1. Demonstration: The teacher models the proper execution of the knee strike in combination with forward movement and the outside block and discusses the application of the skill.

2. Explanation: The instructor explains the learning strategy, which is to add the knee strike to the previously acquired move, block, and strike sequence. The instructor explains and models the proper execution of the knee strike and provides teaching cues for correct performance.

3. Drill: The knee strike is drilled separately by the numbers, with the instructor providing both group and individual feedback as needed. The knee strike is added to the move, block, and strike sequence, and the entire sequence is drilled by the numbers. The move, block, and strike sequence is now a single

count; and the knee strike is added as a second count in the numbers drill. As the students' skill develops, the progression is condensed until the students are performing the entire sequence as one complete movement.

4. Free practice: Once the students can perform the skill without resorting to a by-the-numbers approach, they practice the skill with partners at their own pace. The instructor models the methods for practice, emphasizes safe practice procedures, and provides behavioral performance standards that facilitate self-assessment and peer coaching. The instructor monitors practice and provides group and individual feedback as needed.

Standing Two-Hand Choke Defense

SEQUENCE (40-MINUTE CLASS)

1. Lesson overview and application (3 minutes)
2. Warm-up (5 minutes)
3. Standing two-hand choke (26 minutes)
4. Cool-down (2-4 minutes)
5. Lesson summary (2 minutes)

MAJOR SKILL THEME

Learning to defend against a standing choke

SUGGESTED LEARNING ACTIVITIES

1. Demonstration: The teacher models the proper execution of the two-hand choke, the defense for the two-hand choke, and situational variables.
2. Explanation: The instructor explains the proper execution of defense, possible variations of the attack, and the corresponding response to each variation.
3. Drill: The attack and defense sequence is broken down into a series of discrete movements and drilled by the numbers, with the instructor providing both group and individual feedback as needed. As the students' skill develops, the drill sequence is condensed until the students are performing the offensive and defensive response in one smooth, complete movement.
4. Free practice: Once the students can perform the skill without resorting to a by-the-numbers approach, they practice the skill with partners at their own pace. The instructor models selected free practice drills, emphasizes safe practice procedures, and provides behavioral performance standards that facilitate self-assessment and peer coaching. The instructor monitors practice and provides group and individual feedback as needed.

Program Applications

The information in this section is geared to a self-defense program for a senior high school or college level activities course. Although both men and women can benefit from self-defense instruction, many self-defense courses are designed for women. The information in this chapter is designed as a conceptual framework and a guide for developing a self-defense course for either men or women.

Cognitive Components

A well-designed self-defense program should address and integrate the cognitive, psychomotor, and affective components of instruction in order to be effective. There are four approaches to the cognitive instructional component: (1) awareness, (2) avoidance, (3) escape, (4) and physical resistance. The first three cognitive components pertain to nonphysical coping strategies to physical assault, and the training is qualitatively different from the cognitive training crucial to resistance training. The awareness approach involves exposing and defining the problem. Most men and women are aware that physical assault is a possibility; however, it may not be perceived as a problem by people who have not been exposed to an environment where the possibility of physical assault is a day-to-day realistic concern.

1. The element of awareness in a self-defense program has to do with educating students on the nature, extent, and adverse consequences of physical assault for themselves, their family, friends, and society. Awareness strategies are introduced in Lesson 1 and integrated throughout the course. The strategies include defining and understanding the nature of the criminal act; differentiating between the types of physical and sexual assault and their consequences for the victim, family, and friends; and exposure to the profiles of perpetrators of the different types of sexual assault. Additional subjects for discussion are statistics on the frequency of common forms of assault for the target student population, the perpetrator's response to the victim's reactions to the assault, environmental vulnerability, the perpetrator's predatory habits, and tips on what to do and what not to do if one is confronted with a potential threat situation.

2. Avoidance centers on learning and practicing strategies and behaviors that enable a student to avoid being placed in a potential threat situation. If the strategies and tactics of avoidance are successful, the student should not encounter or have to deal with a physical threat. Avoidance teaching strategies require students to know and implement the safety behavior tips described in the awareness training. To be effective, the student must know the psychological, environmental, and behavioral signs of assault and adapt new behaviors or change existing behavior patterns to limit exposure to threat situations.

3. Awareness and avoidance education and training do not have to involve actual contact with a perpetrator. Escape education and training are needed when awareness and avoidance strategies are not effective or when unique circumstances are encountered. Teaching effective escape strategies and tactics involves teaching students to deal with and control fear. The fear and high level of physical arousal engendered by face-to-face contact with a perpetrator may cause some individuals to freeze up physically and psychologically. Students must know in a general sense what perpetrators will say, how they will behave, what their affective or emotional response will be, and how to manage the fear and arousal that will occur. Affect or fear management is absolutely necessary in order for a coping strategy to be effective. Fear is a tool of the perpetrator, who depends on it to diminish the will and ability of the victim to resist. If the student is paralyzed psychologically or physically, knowledge of self-defense strategies and techniques is useless.

Interactive role playing training is an effective means of acquiring and perfecting escape skills. If you have ever seen a movie and have been frightened or emotionally moved by the actors, then you know the purpose of interactive role playing. This approach to training is sometimes called vaccination therapy. A vaccination for polio or smallpox introduces dead or weakened germs into the body at a level that allows the immune system to develop antibodies to ward off or prevent the disease. A vaccination approach to self-defense training involves scaling down affect during role playing to a level that students can handle. Students assume the roles of victim and perpetrator and act out generic threat situations. The "perpetrator" acts out the language and behaviors of physical assault at a level that allows the victim to develop, refine, and reinforce coping strategies and behaviors. To be effective, the language and behavior of the perpetrator must closely mimic the behavior and verbalizations that are likely to occur during an actual assault. Effective role playing can elicit more realistic affective responses and higher levels of arousal than would normally occur in just skills training. Students experience realistic but manageable emotions and levels of arousal similar to what they will encounter in a real situation. Training must be realistic and must be reinforced to allow students to develop confidence in their ability to deal with the arousal and affect of a real attack.

4. Resistance or fighting is the response of last resort. Not all perpetrators allow the victim the opportunity to avoid or escape using nonphysical resistance measures. In some assaults, direct violence may be used initially to preempt victim resistance and gain compliance. Most perpetrators are looking for a victim. They expect the victim to resist, but do not expect effective and organized resistance. If the victim fights with purpose and skill, the perpetrator may change his or her psychological orientation to the intended victim. He or she may view the intended victim as a direct physical threat instead of just a victim and end up inflicting greater physical damage than originally intended. Once physical resistance is employed, it is rarely possible to fall back on nonphysical resistance strategies.

Surprise is a woman's first weapon. Success for a woman in a self-defense situation is not the amount of physical damage that she can inflict, but the extent to which she can extract herself from the situation unharmed. Avoidance is an even greater measure of success, but it may not be realistic or even possible in some instances.

Self-defense skills may be easily gleaned from books or videos, but the coping skills for fear and arousal management are best acquired through guided practice by a knowledgeable and qualified instructor familiar with self-defense and combative applications of martial arts. All martial arts have self-defense applications, but they are generally taught in an open-ended training regimen over an extended period. The average woman may not want to study the art and may be interested only in the self-defense applications. A focused self-defense course is the answer for most women.

Self-defense training encompasses a variety of skills. People do not attain real-life proficiency by taking a semester course and then ignoring the skills until a situation develops. Skills must be periodically reinforced so that they are effective when needed. Remember, no one knows when she will be attacked. Physical assault is a violent act, and a student must be prepared to meet such violence with an appropriate and legally allowable violent response.

Psychomotor Skill Component

Teachers can incorporate self-defense into the curriculum in several ways, such as implementing a survey course with a small amount of time spent on a lot of skills, or teaching mastery with a lot of time spent on a few skills. Other options include teaching skills and situations using the tool skill model or the embedded skills model.

Survey Versus Mastery Several fundamental questions face an instructor who is designing a skill module or course. Will it be a survey course in which the students are exposed to a variety of self-defense techniques but are not expected to gain functional competence, or will it be oriented toward mastery of selected skills? Time and instructor expertise are probably the most important determinants in answering these questions. Traditional martial arts training is open-ended, meaning that students are expected to train 2 hours a day, two or three times a week, for months or years. Self-defense training is only part of a traditional training regimen, but the time on task is significantly greater in a traditional as opposed to a classroom setting. Regardless of the orientation, the instructor must make the students aware of what they can reasonably expect to accomplish and the limits of their capabilities and training. Overconfidence or unrealistic assessments of what they can do can get students in trouble.

Tool Skill Model Versus Embedded Skills Model The Tool Skill Model and the Embedded Skills Model are two common approaches to teaching self-defense techniques. The skills and situations may be taught with either model. The difference between the two approaches is in how the individual skills are introduced and practiced. In the Tool Skill Model, the skills are practiced initially independently of the context in which they may be applied. For example, students may practice their punching form without a partner, or they may seek to develop punching power by hitting a heavy bag. In either case, the focus for the student is the mastery of the technical aspects of the technique. How the technique may be applied in a given situation is not an immediate concern. There are numerous situations in which a punch can be used, but at this stage mastery of the skill is the goal. When a set of component skills has been acquired, applications or situations that can be handled with the skill set are introduced.

The major advantage of the Tool Skill Model is that it produces high levels of proficiency in basic skills and applications, and enterprising students may draw from their toolbox and apply skills to situations not covered during class. The strength of this approach is also its major limitation as far as physical education instruction is concerned. A significant investment of time on task is needed to produce high levels of proficiency. The time on task and the repetition needed to produce effective skill levels can be boring, and students may lose interest before learning what they need or want to know. The discipline inherent in the Tool Skill Model may be daunting or counterproductive in a class taught in a physical education curriculum. From a methodological perspective, the instructor needs to make the connection between individual skills and their proper applications to ensure that students do not misapply the skills.

The Embedded Skills Model approaches learning from a whole-part-whole perspective. A self-defense situation is envisioned, and the response or responses are generated. A subset of skills is determined for each response, and the skills are taught sequentially in the context of the response to the situation. The advantage of this approach is that the connections between the situational applications and use of the individual skill(s) are apparent and tend to hold the students' interest. This training model tends to be more motivating for students. Extended practice of the skills within the context of the situation produces high levels of proficiency. However, the major caveat to this approach is that individual skills may come to be associated with a specific application and may not generalize to new or novel applications easily. The instructor must take care to teach a wide range of situations and applications to ensure that students have a comprehensive repertoire of situations and skills applications to meet their needs.

Affective Component

Fear management and the need for aggression training are crucial and often-misunderstood aspects of self-defense training. Fear and aggressive behavior are occupational hazards for soldiers, police officers, and firefighters. For most of us, fear and aggression management isn't a part of our daily life. However, fear and aggression management is the foundation of success in self-defense training. If an instructor teaches only the self-defense skills but does not teach students to control their fear and aggression, the students are being set up for failure. As socially unacceptable as it may seem, students must be taught to manage their fears of assault and injury and to understand that aggressive behavior is a viable option for dealing with violence. In addition to being taught aggressive behavior, students must be taught to control their aggressive action and be taught responsibility for the social consequences of its use.

Students who legitimately respond aggressively must know and accept the responsibilities for their actions. Not all attempts to defend against assault are successful. If a student is taught to act aggressively, it is incumbent upon the instructor to inform the student of the consequences of failed aggression. In a case of failed aggression, what can the student expect to happen and how can he or she cope?

When developing a self-defense curriculum or course, the instructor should at the very least include information and advice on how to deal with fear and aggression. Teaching fear and aggression management is beyond the scope of this book, but is the foundation for the success of any aggressive response to a threat. One will not work without the other.

Adapting This Course for Your School

The ability of the students, time allocated for class, equipment and facilities, and teacher qualifications are all areas that one must address when considering teaching self-defense. However, with careful consideration and some creativity, a high quality self-defense course can be taught both safely and effectively.

Students' Abilities

The age, physical abilities, and maturity level of the students are the primary variables that affect the design of the curriculum. Emotional maturity and physical maturity are functions of age and experience. A program designed for a senior high school class or a college-level activity course can be more physically oriented than a program for older or out-of-shape students. The level of maturity also affects the delivery of the information. Information about physical or sexual assault can produce anxiety. Instructors need to be aware of the sensitive nature and possible disconcerting effects of this type of information. If someone in the class has been exposed to physical or sexual assault, talking about it can elicit an unexpected and unpleasant emotional response in that student. It would be advisable to announce the nature of the awareness and physical techniques before starting the class and to discreetly screen students for possible adverse reactions to the course content.

Student interest in a self-defense course is generally favorable, but as a rule most women are not knowledgeable about the physical and emotional demands of realistic and comprehensive defense instruction. Interest does not equal commitment to a program of instruction. Student interest should be surveyed, and then the course requirements should be explained in detail so that there are no surprises or misunderstanding as to the course goals, curriculum, and performance requirements.

Time

The length of the class period and the number of lessons proposed are limitations that must be factored into the design of the course. A typical lesson plan would include a warm-up and cool-down phase and a review period to reinforce previously learned skills. Noninstructional activities such as time to change clothes and shower may reduce the instructional portion of the class by 15 or 20 minutes. A short instructional period affects the level of physical activity, types of techniques taught, and the time on task.

Equipment and Facilities

Equipment and facilities also have significant impact on the curriculum in terms of the types of skills taught and the levels of activity. The availability of a matted surface will support a curriculum that includes ground grappling skills and standing attacks and defenses. Padded walls are a plus for grappling sessions. If throws or takedowns are taught, the mats should be rated to accommodate high-amplitude throws safely. Wrestling mats are suitable for ground work but are not a good choice for practicing judo or high-amplitude throws. Judo mats are expensive. A 14- by 14-meter judo competition mat may cost between $9,000 and $10,000. A gymnastics spring floor overlaid with a wrestling mat and vinyl cover, or 2 inches (5 centimeters) of closed-cell foam and a vinyl cover, may be used as an alternative surface for throwing.

A hardwood floor, like that of a basketball court, is suitable for teaching standing attacks and defenses in self-defense, provided that throws or takedowns are not used in combination with punches, kicks, or escapes. Fold-out mats may be laid out if students are to be taught ground grappling skills, but these mats are usually not suitable for throws or takedowns.

The use of teaching aids such as punching bags and protective gear for head, chest, arms, and groin allows limited contact in training and adds a degree of realism to self-defense training. Punching bags or various forms of striking dummies allow students to strike something that provides resistance and thus help them develop striking and kicking technique and power. Students must be taught the proper drill and the striking techniques, and attackers wearing gear must have a clear idea of their role in the drill. The purpose of protective gear is to prevent injury to the attacker, but complete protection is impractical. If the attacker is completely protected and not very mobile, the student might as well hit or kick a punching bag or dummy.

The most obvious drawback to using protective gear and other teaching aids or equipment is cost. A complete set of full-body protective body armor may cost $700 to $800. Although interaction with an attacker in protective gear adds a degree of realism and intensity, there are trade-offs with regard to time. Putting on, taking off, and changing gear may take a significant amount of class time. The protection afforded by the gear and use of the gear must be balanced against the time needed to put it on and take it off. Student safety is a consideration when students role play in contact drills. This type of training is usually done one-on-one and may not be time efficient for large numbers of students and short instructional periods. As a final caveat regarding the use of protective gear, instructors must realize that the attacker is an active part of the learning process. Attackers are surrogate teachers whose role is to facilitate the learning process as part of a structured drill. The attacker must be trained to perform his or her role correctly and safely to optimize learning in the drill.

Teacher Qualifications

The instructor's expertise and experience are the most important factors in the successful conduct of a self-defense course. How does a physical education teacher gain these skills? One may study a martial art with four goals in mind: (1) as a mental discipline or "way of life," (2) as a physical discipline or form of exercise, (3) as a competitive sport, or (4) as a means of self-defense or combat. A traditional approach to study incorporates all of these goals, but the emphasis placed on each goal will vary from art to art, from instructor to instructor, and even across time. Martial arts have taught self-discipline, confidence, and physical development as benefits of study.

No one martial arts system meets all self-defense situations optimally. Self-defense instruction especially for women should use an eclectic approach to the subject and include techniques from a variety of systems that enable a woman to meet common threat situations.

Self-defense applications do not automatically transfer from combative sports as readily as most people believe. There is no doubt that boxing, wrestling, or judo teachers or coaches can teach skills that are useful in self-defense. However, there are unique aspects of the self-defense training that must be studied independent of the sport or other applications of a martial art. This is where the difficulty in gaining experience and competence lies for physical educators. Many traditional arts advertise self-defense applications but train for the competitive aspect of the sport during most of the training period. Training for self-defense applications is not the same as training for sport competition.

We draw from five basic categories of self-defense techniques to develop self-defense applications: (1) strikes, any part of the body; (2) chokes or strangles; (3) joint locks, any joint in the body; (4) throws or takedowns; and (5) instinctive techniques—biting, scratching, or clawing. The following are criteria for selecting a skill: (1) Is it effective? (2) Is it easy to learn? (3) Can it be used in a wide variety of situations and applications? (4) Is it easy to teach? (5) Is there a low potential for injury to the student in practice and actual use? The five categories of techniques are drawn from different martial arts, and they tend to emphasize learning through different sensory modalities. The skills and abilities needed for mastery in striking and grappling differ significantly. Grappling skills are learned primarily through kinesthetic awareness, although vision is an asset. Striking skills are based primarily on hand–eye and foot–eye coordination. Success in learning skills from one category does not guarantee easy mastery or learning of skills drawn from another category. It is easier to teach visually-based skills to individuals involved in the grappling arts than it is to teach grappling or kinesthetic-based skills to individuals involved in the striking arts.

Clothing Requirements

Uniform requirements depend upon the type of skills being taught and the level of intensity of training. Shorts, athletic shoes, and a T-shirt are adequate for teaching striking and kicking skills at low levels of exertion. Ground grappling is more strenuous, and the pulling and tugging involved require more rugged apparel. A sweatshirt and sweat pants could be added to shorts and T-shirt for ground grappling.

Classroom Safety

Equipment and facilities used in self-defense training must be checked for wear and tear to ensure viability. Instructors should have a plan, available for outside review, to periodically inspect and maintain training facilities and the equipment used in class. The equipment should be cleaned and sanitized daily to prevent transmission of any diseases. Students should be screened daily before class for any illness or condition that may be transmitted to another student. Uniforms should be cleaned and checked for wear and tear after each class. Realism and safety are training concepts on opposite ends of a continuum. The risk of injury increases as the training becomes more realistic.

Regardless of the type of training, instructors should have an Emergency Action Plan to cover all reasonable foreseeable medical conditions that might arise. It would be advisable to have students fill out a brief medical history form before participating to screen for conditions and injuries not immediately apparent that might be aggravated by the training.

Legal Guidelines

The right to defend ourselves is an accepted part of our culture, and it has been upheld through codification into state and federal laws. What is legally acceptable defensive behavior varies from state to state and from state to federal law, but generally reflects the prevailing moral-ethical climate of the legal entity that enforces the law. Traditional martial arts have codes of conduct that provide guidelines for self-defense, but these guidelines may not reflect the legal and moral-ethical expectations for self-defense in our society. Instructors should know the basic precepts of self-defense in the state or location of instruction; they do not have to have the detailed knowledge of a criminal lawyer, but they should be able to give basic legal guidelines for self-defense.

The law provides guidelines for self-defense. However, there may be differences between what is legal and what is thought to be morally and ethically justifiable. For instance, in many self-defense classes, students are told that if you are attacked, your first course of action is to run away. Good advice! However, if running away is not feasible, then you must try to reason with your assailant. If that doesn't work, then physically resist, but hurt before you maim, and maim before using lethal force.

Aside from the legal ramifications of self-defense, instructors, students, and parents should be aware of the moral-ethical and personal consequences of the use of aggressive behavior and skills.

Key Terms

affective domain—The type of emotions and level of arousal generally associated with specific neuromuscular skills acquisition.

cognitive domain—The knowledge of consequences, strategies, and tactics that direct and influence the application of learned neuromuscular skills.

embedded skills teaching model—A teaching model in which the component skills of a motor sequence are taught sequentially within the context of the movement outcome.

fear vaccination—A type of training intended to prepare the student to maintain physical performance and to minimize the disruptive effect of high levels of emotion and physical arousal. Training begins at low levels of arousal. As the students' proficiency increases, systematic and progressive increases in the emotional and physical arousal are introduced into training and practice.

group feedback—Knowledge of results gleaned from observation and analysis of the collective performance of the class during drills and practice and given to the class as a whole rather than to an individual.

individual feedback—Knowledge of results gleaned from observation and analysis of the individual's performance during drills and practice and given to the individual, not the group.

interactive role playing—A teaching model for threat scenarios in which students assume and act out the roles of both attacker and potential victim.

mastery course—An activity course in which the course goal is a specific level of skill proficiency. The level of proficiency is a function of instructional time and students' entry-level proficiency and experience, and is measured against an observable performance criterion.

psychomotor domain—Neuromuscular skills associated with a specific movement activity.

survey course—An activity course in which the course goal is to inspire further student involvement. The range of course skills and training techniques is sampled to give the student an understanding of the commitment needed to attain a given level of mastery. Inspiring the student to further participation and knowledge takes precedence over the actual skill development.

tool skill teaching model—A teaching model in which motor skills are initially taught and mastered independent of an applied context.

7

Fitness Boxing

Ray Barone

Great Britain brought boxing to America during colonization because the British viewed boxing as a means to stay fit, build character, develop courage, and learn poise under pressure (Sammons, 1982; Wakefield, 1997). The British believed that this activity would help them cope with the hard knocks, bruises, and challenges of the New World. As America developed, so did boxing, from the bare-knuckle street brawls used to settle disputes to its present status as an amateur and Olympic sport (Gorn, 1986; Sugden, 1996; Wakefield, 1997).

Exercise leaders, personal trainers, and teachers have adopted many of the drills of a typical boxing training regimen, using them as a fun way to achieve fitness. As a result, courses such as boxing for fitness have developed and grown rapidly. Boxing for Fitness was developed at West Point as an "offshoot" of the contact boxing program so that cadets could get the benefits of boxing without the contact in a coeducational setting. Boxing for fitness is different from Tae Bo and other aerobic boxing routines because it closely replicates an actual boxer's workout. Not only do students learn how to stand, move, defend, and punch like a boxer; but skills such as "no-rope" jump roping, quick feet, mitt work, and noncontact sparring are also integrated into the workout.

Boxing for fitness is a noncontact activity that students can enjoy regardless of their height, weight, age, income, gender, or level of fitness or coordination. Since boxing for fitness incorporates a great deal of movement, the routine can include music to add to student enjoyment and help the instructor monitor the tempo of the workout. This fitness activity appeals to a wide range of people because it works, is easy to learn, and is fun to do and because no one participant has an advantage over another. Everyone can readily participate. The limiting factor is the student's motivation to reach a desired level of fitness.

Purpose of the Course

At West Point, we teach Boxing for Fitness because of its many health benefits and its widespread appeal among the students. In addition to contributing to the development of hand-and-eye coordination and reflexes, this activity improves muscular endurance and cardiovascular fitness, increases lean body mass, and reduces stress—a great bargain for the busy student and the health-conscious individual!

Both students and teachers subscribe to boxing for fitness for numerous reasons. Students find it appealing because of the wide variety of movement patterns. Because of the number of options available for practice, students can exercise individually, with a partner, or as a group, and the student controls the tempo. Teachers can utilize this low-cost activity because the action is nonstop and maximizes time on task. Everyone is a "player" for the entire workout. Moreover, the flexibility of fitness boxing allows it to be used as a stand-alone activity or in conjunction with other workout modalities such as resistance training. Additionally, the minimal equipment requirements permit conducting this workout virtually anywhere indoors or out. Finally, boxing for fitness is structured so that one teacher can teach the entire class or divide the space into stations or circuits. Students can easily lead a station or a part of a circuit. In addition to these numerous benefits, the ease with which students can perform the exercises can result in a positive impact on their self-esteem.

Because of West Point's mission to develop leaders of character, the Academy tries to gear all classes toward this common goal. Boxing for Fitness meets this criterion for individual leadership and development. Successful trials and the focus task specificity enhance student self-assurance. Even without contact, the "boxing" drills improve the students' self-defense skills and increase self-confidence. The perception of danger inherent in some of the one-on-one drills improves the students' ability to manage fear.

Upon completion of this course, students will

1. demonstrate basic offensive and defensive boxing skills;
2. lead a Boxing for Fitness class;
3. understand the safety precautions involved in a fitness boxing class;
4. improve their muscular endurance, cardio-respiratory endurance, and hand-and-eye coordination;
5. demonstrate teamwork; and
6. enhance their self-confidence through involvement in a combatives course.

Instructional Area

The limited requirements of boxing for fitness permit teachers to conduct class in any clear, flat-surface area. The class size should be no more than 36 students, with each student occupying a space of about 3 square feet (.3 square meters). This space allows for total group instruction or six stations of six people each. Because of the versatility of boxing for fitness, the size of the workout area, the objectives of the class, and the teacher's imagination often determine where the activity is performed and the configuration of the class (either as a whole or in stations).

Indoors

A full-size gymnasium is ideal for teaching boxing for fitness. A gymnasium allows the class to spread out, turn up the music, and start exercising! However, aerobics rooms with mirrored walls are especially effective. Additionally, students can use weight rooms because resistance training exercises integrate well with boxing for fitness drills. With little need for special equipment, even classrooms have proven to be sufficient. Move the desks and chairs to the side and go!

Outdoors

If the weather cooperates, teachers may want to take students outside for class. Open fields, blacktop or court areas, or open parking lots are suitable. Teachers should take extra precautions if conducting class on wet pavement or uneven grassy areas.

Equipment

Boxing for fitness does not require the use of any expensive or safety equipment. In some cases, no equipment is required. The following lists various skills and whether they require equipment:

1. On-guard stance and movement: no equipment required
2. No-rope jump rope: no equipment required
3. Quick feet: no equipment needed
4. Shadow boxing: 12- to 15-inch (30- to 38-centimeter) piece of tape to help students establish the target position
5. Mitt workout
   - Hand gloves: any type of hand glove that one can readily make a fist in
   - Striking mitts: worn one on each hand as targets for students to strike

6. Noncontact sparring: two 12- to 15-inch pieces of tape to help students establish the target position (place lines of tape parallel and 36 inches [.9 meters] apart to keep students from making contact during their workout)

6. make certain that students who perform drills involving striking are far enough apart to preclude contact (use floor tape to guide the placement of the students' feet to provide for their safety).

Risk Management

Sound risk management is essential for the safe operation of any sport. Although boxing for fitness is a noncontact activity, anytime a participant throws punches there is a potential for injury. Table 7.1 lists possible risks and strategies for decreasing risks. To preclude injuries one must

1. be aware of the age and size of the participants and match them accordingly;

2. ensure that students are adequately warmed up;

3. meet the minimum equipment standards—that is, tape, mitts, first aid kit, and so on;

4. ensure that students understand the safety precautions for each lesson;

5. follow the lessons in order of progression; and

Course Overview

The teacher can adjust the course overview presented in table 7.2 to meet the needs of the students. The skills in these lesson plans should be taught according to the progression presented, as skills taught in any lesson build on previous lessons. Formative evaluations are provided to assess student learning. All lessons should begin with a proper warm-up and end with a cool-down to prevent injuries.

Skills and Techniques

Because Boxing for Fitness lessons are designed to provide students with maximum time on task, skills are taught sequentially. Once students learn the individual skills, the instructor may lead classes for the group or may utilize circuit stations.

Table 7.1 Possible Risks in Fitness Boxing

Risk identification	Reduction strategies
Injured hand	Making tight fist when striking mitts
Sprained wrist	Striking mitts without bending wrist
Broken or cracked teeth or any type of head injury	Noncontact sparring, teacher supervision, use of tape to separate boxers
Hyperextended shoulder	Thorough instruction on proper punching techniques, proper warm-up
Pulled muscle in back, shoulders, or legs	Proper warm-up
Excessive weight loss, dehydration	Drinking water before, during, and after workout

Table 7.2 Overview of Fitness Boxing Lessons

Lesson	Course overview
1	• Warm-up • Target position • Make a fist • On-guard stance (OGS)
2	• Warm-up • Review: target position, make a fist, and OGS • Movement (forward, left, right, backward, circle left, circle right) • Quick feet
3	• Warm-up • Review: movement (forward, left, right backward, circle left, circle right) and quick feet • Left jab to head • Left jab with movement
4	• Warm-up • Review: quick feet, left jab to head, left jab with movement • Shadow box • Introduce mitt drills
5	• Warm-up • Review: quick feet, left jab with movement, shadow box • Mitt drills • Introduce noncontact sparring
6	• Warm-up • Review: quick feet, shadow box, mitt drills • Noncontact sparring • Discuss next lesson's formative evaluation
7	• Warm-up • Evaluate: target position, OGS, jab with movement, shadow box, mitt drills, noncontact sparring
8	• Warm-up • Discuss previous lesson's evaluation • Straight right to head • Combinations with left and right
9	• Warm-up • Review: straight right, left and right combinations • Shadow box with left and right • Mitt drills with left and right • Introduce noncontact sparring with left and right
10	• Warm-up • Review: shadow box and mitt drills with left and right • Noncontact sparring with left and right

Lesson	Course overview
11	• Warm-up • Review: shadow box and mitt drills with left and right • Noncontact sparring with left and right • Discuss next lesson's evaluation
12	• Warm-up • Evaluate: shadow box, mitt drills and noncontact sparring using the left and right
13	• Warm-up • Discuss previous evaluation • Left hook to the head • Combinations left–right–left hook • Shadow box • Introduce mitt work with left hook
14	• Warm-up • Review: left hook to the head, shadow box using jab–right–left hook • Mitt work with left hook • Introduce noncontact sparring with left hook
15	• Warm-up • Review: left hook to the head, shadow box and mitt work using left–right–left hook • Noncontact sparring with left hook
16	• Warm-up • Review: left hook to the head, shadow box, mitt drills, and noncontact sparring • Right hook to head • Shadow box • Mitt work • Introduce noncontact sparring with right hook
17	• Warm-up • Review: right hook to the head, shadow box, mitt drills • Noncontact sparring • Introduce right uppercut
18	• Warm-up • Review: right hook to head • Right uppercut • Shadow box • Mitts • Noncontact sparring • Discuss final evaluation
19	• Warm-up • Evaluate: shadow box, mitt drills, and noncontact sparring using the left jab, the straight right, left hook, right hook, and right uppercut

Warm-Up

Each class begins with a 5- to 7-minute warm-up session. Warm-up exercises are designed to physically and mentally prepare students for the day's lesson by raising the body's core temperature and loosening key joints and muscles. Recommended warm-up exercises with the number of repetitions are provided next. Teachers can adjust these exercises to meet individual class or student needs.

TEACHING CUES

- Marching in place while doing 10 arm circles forward and backward
- 20 jumping jacks
- 10 push-ups
- 10 knee bends
- 1/2 minute of no-rope jump rope
- Light stretches for upper and lower body

SUGGESTED LEARNING ACTIVITIES

- While standing still, demonstrate forward and backward arm circles starting with a small range of motion and finishing with a full range of motion. Next, alternate lifting the knees to belt level while doing arm circles.
- Stand erect with feet together and arms at sides. While keeping arms at sides, jump into the air so that the legs land slightly wider than shoulder-width; jump again, and bring legs back together. Progress to jumping and clapping hands overhead.
- Do 10 regular push-ups. Students go to their knees or to their waist to complete 10 repetitions.
- Start and finish in a standing position. Sit with the back against a wall, feet 12 inches (30 centimeters) away from the wall and knees bent at 90 degrees. Knees may extend slightly beyond toes. Advance to squatting and standing without a wall.
- No-rope jump rope, explained next, is a separate skill that can be used in the warm-up or anytime during the workout.

No-Rope Jump Rope

No-rope jump rope (NRJR) is a cardiorespiratory exercise that requires little skill and can be done to the tempo of the group's favorite music. Students must be able to jump up and down, either on one foot or on both feet, and move their arms in a circular motion. Group leaders can introduce innovative variations of NRJR based on their skills and experience. In order to enhance leadership skills, instructors can rotate leadership of the group among students.

TEACHING CUES

- Assume target position (see next section) with hands gripping an imaginary rope.
- Move the arms in a circular motion, either forward or backward.
- Jump in the air on one or both feet when the hands make a complete circle.

SUGGESTED LEARNING ACTIVITIES

- Students practice jumping up and down on two feet without bending their knees.
- Students jump up and down, first on one leg and then on the other, without bending their knees.
- Students make forward full-range arm circles.
- Students combine the jumping in place with arm circles.

Target Position

The target position is the start position for many of the drills that students perform in the Boxing for Fitness workout. Walking in place and assuming the on-guard stance begin from the target position. A 12- to 15-inch (30- to 38-centimeter) piece of tape placed on the floor enables students to establish the target position. Keeping feet parallel to each other, students set the left toe on the left edge of the piece of tape and the right toe on the right edge. The knees should have a slight bend; the hips and shoulders are square to the front; and the arms are relaxed at the sides with the hands loosely clenched. The head is in a neutral position. Body weight is evenly distributed on the balls of the feet. Once students can assume this position quickly, they no longer need the floor tape.

TEACHING CUES

- 12- to 15-inch piece of tape on the floor
- Feet parallel, left toe on the left edge of tape, right toe on right edge
- Knees slightly bent
- Hips and shoulders square to the front
- Arms relaxed at the sides
- Hands loosely clenched
- Head in neutral position
- Body weight evenly distributed on balls of the feet

SUGGESTED LEARNING ACTIVITIES

- Students stand with feet shoulder-width apart and bounce up and down on the balls of their feet.
- Students stand on the balls of their feet and rise up as high as possible on their toes.
- Working in pairs, students provide individual feedback on the target position.

On-Guard Stance

The on-guard stance (OGS) is the basic boxing stance (see figure 7.1). All movement starts and finishes in the OGS. All punches start and finish in the OGS. The OGS allows skilled boxers to maintain balance while throwing the basic punches (left jab, right cross, left hook, right hook, and right uppercut). To assume the OGS, students start in the target position with their feet on the left and right edges of the piece of tape,

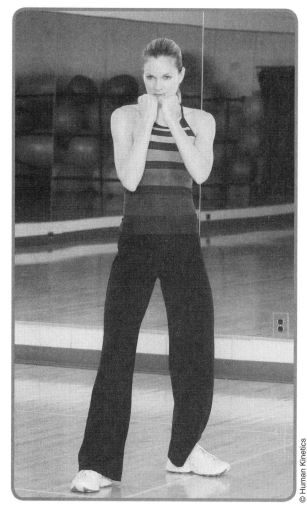

FIGURE 7.1   On-guard stance.

© Human Kinetics

facing forward, looking at the teacher. Working from the feet up, students take an 8- to 12-inch (20- to 30-centimeter) step forward with the left foot and turn it to the left 25 degrees. (To keep the lessons consistent, all students will have their left foot forward while in the OGS.) The right toe remains on the right side of the floor tape and is angled to the right 40 degrees. The right heel is 1/4 inch (.6 centimeters) off the ground. The knees are slightly bent. The left hip and shoulder are forward, and the right hip and shoulder are back. The left hand is "high," level with the eye, and the right hand is "in," even with the chin. Palms face toward each other. The forearms are parallel to each other and perpendicular to the ground. The chin is level in a neutral position. Body weight is evenly distributed over the balls of the feet. The overall body is relaxed, and the boxer's line of sight is between his or her hands.

TEACHING CUES

- Start in the target position.
- Turn left foot right 25 degrees and step forward 8 to 12 inches.
- Right toe remains on tape and is angled to the right 40 degrees.
- Right heel is 1/4 inch off the ground.
- The knees are slightly bent.
- Left hip and shoulder are forward, right hip and shoulder are back.
- Left hand is "high," level with the eye; right hand is "in," even with the chin.
- Palms face toward each other.
- Forearms are parallel to each other and perpendicular to the ground.
- Elbows are touching the sides of the body.
- Chin is level in a neutral position.
- Body weight is evenly distributed over the balls of the feet.
- Body is relaxed.

SUGGESTED LEARNING ACTIVITIES

- Take an 8- to 12-inch step with the left foot and throw an imaginary ball with the right hand so that the right heel comes 1/4 inch off the ground.
- Rotate the shoulders and hips to a 45-degree angle (left shoulder and hip forward).
- Hold the arms at shoulder height, parallel to the ground, elbows locked; bend elbows until they are touching the sides of the body.
- Working in pairs, students provide individual feedback.

Movement

All movement starts and finishes in the OGS. When students are moving, the feet should neither cross nor come together and should slide-shuffle on the floor rather than being picked up. The foot closest to the direction of movement moves first. For example, if the boxer moves forward, the left foot (front foot) moves first and then the right foot. If the boxer moves to the right, the right foot moves first and then the left foot. Body weight is evenly distributed on the balls of the feet for balance.

TEACHING CUES

- Start in a good OGS (relax).
- Slide the feet rather than pick them up.
- The foot closest to the direction of travel moves first.
- Never cross feet.
- Never bring feet together.
- Body weight is evenly distributed on the balls of the feet.
- Move left by moving the left foot first, then the right foot.
- Move right by moving the right foot first, then the left.

SUGGESTED LEARNING ACTIVITIES

- Take a 12- to 18-inch (30- to 46-centimeter) step with the left foot and throw an imaginary ball with the right hand so that the right heel comes 1/4 inch (.6 centimeters) off the ground; drop hands and arms so they rest on the sides.
- From this position, move in all four cardinal directions without crossing the feet or allowing the feet to come together.
- Assume the OGS and continue.
- Move the length of the classroom.
- Work with a partner to provide feedback.

Left Jab

Since the left jab, or just "left," is the most important punch in boxing, boxers either move and throw the left or stay still and throw the left. The punch starts and finishes at the left side of the boxer's face. When throwing a left, students should punch straight, above the shoulder, at the target and return their fist straight back to the left side of the face. Because our OGS has the left foot forward, students will perform all jabs with the left hand.

TEACHING CUES

- Assume OGS.
- Start punch from the left cheek.
- Punch straight out at target.
- Left arm is slightly above the shoulder when extended.
- Twist the fist palm facing down and knuckles up at the point of full extension.
- The left hip and shoulder should twist slightly.

- Return jab to the left side of the face.
- During moving, one step requires one jab.
- Return to OGS.

SUGGESTED LEARNING ACTIVITIES

- Have the class practice the punch in slow motion.
- Check them at the extended position (jab fully away from body).
- Check to make sure they bring the jab back high and resume OGS.
- From OGS, students move 2 to 4 inches (5-10 centimeters) forward, backward, left, and right and throw jab.
- Students move the length of the classroom while jabbing.

Straight Right

The straight right is the first of the power punches and is thrown after a left jab. The right arm and fist are the vehicles of force. The power for this punch comes from shifting the body weight from the right foot to the left foot by rotating the hips and shoulders.

TEACHING CUES

- Assume OGS.
- Pivot on the ball of the right foot (think of screwing a screw counterclockwise into the ground with the ball of the foot).
- Rotate the right hip so that it is forward and in front of the left hip.
- Rotate the right shoulder forward and past the left shoulder.
- Right hand comes out from the chin.
- At full extension, the palm is down and the knuckles are up.
- Boxer pivots back to the OGS and returns the hand to right side of the face.

SUGGESTED LEARNING ACTIVITIES

- Have the class practice the punch in slow motion.
- Check them at the extended position (right fully away from body).
- Check to make sure they bring the right back high and resume OGS.
- Students assume OGS with the right heel 2 inches (5 centimeters) from the wall and practice throwing straight right—right heel should hit the wall when right arm is fully extended.
- From OGS, they move 2 to 4 inches forward, backward, left, and right and throw left followed by right.

Left Hook

The left hook is the first of the bent-arm punches and is thrown after a straight right. Students should transfer the body's weight forward to the left foot when throwing a straight right and then transfer weight from the left foot to the right foot when throwing the left hook. To throw the left hook, the boxer pivots on the ball of the left foot, rotates the torso to the right, and drives the right heel into the ground by putting the chin over that foot; simultaneously, the boxer bends the lead arm at 90 degrees and brings it across the body, parallel to the ground at shoulder height with the thumb up and palm facing toward the boxer.

TEACHING CUES

- Assume OGS.
- Transfer body weight to the left foot (left foot is flat) by rotating hips, torso, and shoulders left; right heel is off the ground, chin over left knee.
- Rotate the hips, torso, and shoulders to the right to shift the body weight from the left foot to the right foot; left heel is off the ground, right foot flat, chin over right knee.
- The left arm is bent at 90 degrees at the elbow and parallel to the ground.
- The wrist is rigid (not bent).
- Thumb knuckle points up and the palm faces toward the boxer.
- Return to OGS.

SUGGESTED LEARNING ACTIVITIES

- Students assume OGS and practice shifting their weight from their right leg to their left leg by rotating their hips and shoulders and placing their chin over the knee of the weight-bearing leg (like dancing!).
- Have students practice the punch in slow motion by the numbers:
  - On count 1, students shift their weight to their left foot. On count 2, they move their left hand (made in a fist 4 inches [10 centimeters] from their face), bend their arms 90 degrees, and hold them parallel to the ground.
  - On count 3, they shift their body weight from their left foot to their right foot by rotating their hips and shoulders and moving their chin over their right knee; left heel is off the ground, and right heel is on the ground.
  - On count 4, students shift back to the OGS.
- Next, they put counts 1 and 2 together and 3 and 4 together:
  - Execute left hook in slow motion.
  - Execute left hook at normal speed.

Right Hook

The right hook is the second of the bent-arm punches. It is thrown after a left jab or left hook. When the boxer throws a right hook, the body's weight is transferred forward to the left foot. Students should then pivot on the right foot, as if they were throwing a straight right, and land the hook with thumbs up and palms facing toward them.

TEACHING CUES

- Assume OGS.
- Pivot on the ball of the rear foot (think of screwing a screw counterclockwise into the ground with the ball of the foot).
- Twist the rear (right) hip so that it is square to the front with the left hip.
- Twist the rear shoulder so that it is even with the lead shoulder.
- Bend right arm 90 degrees at the elbow and hold parallel to the ground.
- The wrist is rigid (not bent).

- At completion, the palm faces toward the student and the thumb knuckle points up.
- Pivot back to the OGS and return the hand to right side of the face.

SUGGESTED LEARNING ACTIVITIES

- Students assume OGS and practice shifting their weight from their right leg to their left leg by rotating their hips, torso, and shoulders and placing their chin over the knee of the weight-bearing leg.
- Have students practice the punch in slow motion by the numbers:
  - On count 1, students move their right hand (made into a fist) 4 inches (10 centimeters) from their face, bend their arm 90 degrees, and hold it parallel to the ground.
  - On count 2, students shift their weight to their left foot by rotating their hips and shoulders and moving their chin over their left knee; left heel is flat on ground, and right heel is off the ground.
  - On count 3, students shift back to the OGS.
- Next, they put counts 1 and 2 together:
  - Execute right hook in slow motion.
  - Execute right hook at normal speed.

Right Uppercut

The right uppercut is the third of the bent-arm punches and is generally thrown upward after a left jab or left hook. When the boxer is throwing this punch, the body weight transfers to the left foot and the shoulders are squared to the front (see figure 7.2). The boxer pivots on the right foot (this is similar to throwing a straight right or right hook), driving the right hand upward above eye level with the palm and forearm facing toward the boxer and knuckles pointed upward.

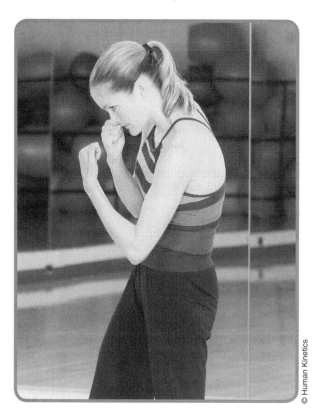

TEACHING CUES

- Assume the OGS.
- Pivot on the ball of the right foot.
- Twist the right hip so that it is square to the front with the left hip.
- Square the shoulders by rotating the left shoulder back and the right shoulder forward.
- Right arm is bent less than 90 degrees.
- Palm and forearm face toward the exerciser.
- Knuckles face up.
- Punch to above eye level.
- Return to the OGS by unsquaring the shoulders and returning the right hand to the side of the chin.

© Human Kinetics

FIGURE 7.2 Uppercut punch.

SUGGESTED LEARNING ACTIVITIES

- Have the class practice the punch in slow motion.
- Students assume OGS with right heel 2 inches (5 centimeters) from wall and practice throwing the right uppercut; right heel should hit the wall when right arm is fully vertical above eye level.
- Check boxers at the vertical position; arm should be bent, palm facing exerciser, knuckles pointing up.
- Check to make sure students bring the right hand to the chin and resume OGS.

Quick Feet

Quick feet is another cardiorespiratory exercise that requires little skill and that students can practice to the group's favorite music. Boxers work in pairs. Standing in the OGS, they attempt to step on their partner's lead left foot with their lead left foot. They see how many points can be acquired in 1 minute and then rest for 30 seconds and resume.

TEACHING CUES

- Boxers assume the OGS.
- On "Go," boxers move about in the OGS and attempt to acquire points by lightly stepping on their partner's lead left foot with their own lead left foot.
- Boxers cannot walk, hop, or jump—they must shuffle.
- Boxers must lift the left foot slightly off the ground when attempting to step on the partner's lead left foot.

SUGGESTED LEARNING ACTIVITIES

- Place a mark on the ground (floor).
- Have the students assume the OGS one shuffle step away.
- On "Go," students see how quickly they can shuffle forward and place their left foot on the spot and then shuffle back to their original position.
- Have partners try to shuffle step onto the same spot.

Shadow Boxing

Shadow boxing drills improve all boxing for fitness punching and moving skills while improving eye-and-hand coordination and muscular endurance. Punching in combinations (putting several punches together in sequence) seems to work best for these drills. In most cases, students start and finish each combination with the lead left hand. Fitness boxers must perfect shadow boxing skills prior to noncontact sparring.

TEACHING CUES

- Start in the OGS.
- All punches and movements start and finish in the OGS.
- Suggested combinations to practice:
  - Left
  - Left–left

- Left–left–left
- Left–right–left
- Left–right–left hook
- Left–right–left hook–right uppercut
- Left–right–left hook–right hook–left
- Left–right–left hook–right hook–left hook
- Left–right uppercut–left hook
- Left–right uppercut–left hook–right hook–left

SUGGESTED LEARNING ACTIVITIES

Students perform punch combinations by the numbers in slow motion:

- On count 1, they throw a left.
- On count 2, they throw a right.
- On count 3, they throw a left hook.

Mitt Work

The mitts work all facets of boxing for fitness, and mitt work is a logical progression from shadow boxing. Mitt holders place boxing mitts on their hands and assume the target position. Keeping their elbows pointed over their knees, they raise their hands until the hands are 4 to 6 inches (10-15 centimeters) in front of the shoulders. The puncher puts on striking gloves and assumes the OGS at a range from which he or she can touch the mitt holder's right mitt with the lead left fist (see figure 7.3).

The drill is controlled by the group leader or the mitt holder. The puncher throws the left jab and all right punches into the mitt holder's right hand and throws the left hook into the mitt holder's left hand. Note that when the puncher throws the left hook, the right hook, or the right uppercut, the mitt holder needs to move his or her hands into a position facing the punch. For example, when receiving a left hook, the mitt holder holds the left hand out 18 to 24 inches (45-60 centimeters) from the left shoulder with the palm of the hand facing toward the center of the body. When receiving a right hook, the mitt holder holds the right hand out 18 to 24 inches from the right shoulder with the palm of the hand facing toward the center of the body. When receiving a right uppercut, the mitt holder holds the right hand out 4 inches (10 centimeters) from the body with the palm of the hand facing the ground. Punch combination drills are similar to those used for shadow boxing.

TEACHING CUES

- Mitt holder assumes target position.
- Mitt holder places hands 4 to 6 inches in front of shoulders, with elbows over knees.
- Puncher assumes OGS with striking gloves on hands.
- Puncher touches mitt holder's right mitt with closed left fist.
- Group leader or mitt holder controls drill.
- Left jab and all right punches are thrown to the mitt holder's right hand.
- Left hook is thrown into mitt holder's left hand.

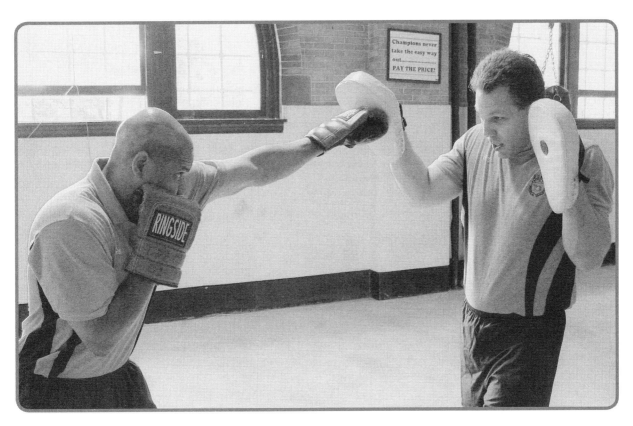

FIGURE 7.3 On-guard stance for mitt work.

- To receive the left hook, the mitt holder holds the left hand 18 to 24 inches from the left shoulder, palm facing toward the center of the body.
- Right hook is thrown into mitt holder's right hand.
- To receive the right hook, the mitt holder holds the right hand 18 to 24 inches from the right shoulder, palm facing toward the center of the body.
- To receive the right uppercut, the mitt holder holds the right hand 4 inches from the body, palm facing toward the ground.

SUGGESTED LEARNING ACTIVITIES

- Practice mitt work in slow motion.
- Punch in combinations.
- Practice groups of small combinations, then put groups together:
  - Left–right
  - Left hook–right hook
  - Left–right–left hook–right hook

Noncontact Sparring

Noncontact sparring builds finesse, eye–hand coordination, and self-confidence. Boxers work together to improve each other's offensive and defensive skills. To keep boxers separated, place two pieces of tape on the ground, parallel to each other, at least 36 inches (.9 meters) apart. Boxers are not permitted to cross either their piece of tape or their partner's piece of tape. One boxer punches while the other boxer defends. The defending boxers coordinate their movements with the offensive boxers' punches. Either the group leader or the defending boxer calls out punch sequences.

1. When the group leader calls for a "left" (lead hand jab), the offensive boxer throws a left; and the defending boxer, while staying in the OGS, shifts the body to the left foot by moving the chin over the left knee.

2. When the group leader calls for a "right" (straight right), the punching boxer throws a straight right; and the defending boxer, while maintaining a good OGS, shifts his or her body weight to the right foot by moving the chin over the right knee.

3. When the group leader calls for a left hook, the defending boxer shifts his or her weight to the left foot by placing the chin over the left knee, then bends both knees so that the thighs are at a 45-degree angle, moves the chin over the right knee, then straightens both knees. The defender has made a letter "U" by moving the chin over the left knee, squatting, moving the chin over the right knee, and then standing straight up again.

4. When the group leader calls for a right hook, the defending boxer shifts his or her weight to the right foot by placing the chin over the right knee, then bends both knees so that the thighs are at a 45-degree angle, moves the chin over the left knee, then straightens both knees. The defender has made a letter "U" by moving the chin over the right knee, squatting, moving the chin over the left knee, and then standing straight up again.

5. When the group leader calls for an "uppercut" (right-hand uppercut), the punching boxer throws a right-hand uppercut; and the defending boxer, while maintaining a good OGS, shifts his or her body weight to the right foot by moving the chin over the right knee.

TEACHING CUES

* Assume OGS.
* Place two pieces of tape at least 36 inches apart on the ground, parallel to each other.
* Do not permit boxers to cross either piece of tape.
* Defending boxers coordinate movements with offensive boxers' punches (for example, if the offensive boxer throws a left, the defending boxer moves left).
* Group leader or defensive boxer calls punches.
* Offensive boxer throws a left; the defending boxer, while staying in the OGS, shifts body weight to the left foot by moving the chin over the left knee.
* Offensive boxer throws a right; the defending boxer, while maintaining a good OGS, shifts body weight to the right foot by moving the chin over the right knee.
* When the offensive boxer throws a left hook, the defending boxer shifts his or her weight to the left foot by placing the chin over the left knee, then bends both knees so that the thighs are at 45 degrees, moves the chin over the right knee, and then straightens both knees.
* When the offensive boxer throws a right hook, the defending boxer shifts his or her weight to the right foot by placing the chin over the right knee, then bends both knees so that the thighs are at 45 degrees, moves the chin over the left knee, and then straightens both knees.

- When the offensive boxer throws a right-hand uppercut, the defending boxer, while maintaining a good OGS, shifts body weight to the right foot by moving the chin over the right knee.

SUGGESTED LEARNING ACTIVITIES

- Group leader calls out punch, and class performs punch.
- Group leader calls out punch, and class moves away from punch.

Adapting This Course for Your School

Boxing for fitness is an appropriate activity for any age group. These are some factors to consider when offering this course:

- Class size and time
- Equipment and facilities
- Safety and risk management
- Teacher experience or education
- The target audience (school year)

Class Size and Time

One of the fundamental problems in teaching physical education is lack of equipment, which may result in decreased time on task as students wait to share equipment. However, due to the number and variety of movement drills, boxing for fitness has a minimal wait time as students rotate through the various drills. Effective class planning and smooth transitions to routines are essential to maximizing time on task. In order to improve safety, the teacher-to-student ratio should be no greater than 1:36.

Equipment and Facilities

A distinct advantage of boxing for fitness is the minimal equipment and facility requirements. The instructor with a couple of student helpers can easily carry any equipment required for the day's lesson (i.e., mitts, tape, first aid kit, boom box) to the workout area. In most cases, a gymnasium or outdoor area that can adequately hold the class is all that is necessary.

Safety and Risk Management

To avoid injuries, teachers should ensure that students are closely supervised and sufficiently warmed up prior to exercising. Instructors must teach a logical sequence of skills progression. Table 7.1 on page 111 provides sound recommendations for safety issues that may arise.

Teacher Qualifications

The utility of boxing for fitness is that instructors need little combatives experience to conduct a fitness- and character-developing class. The Boxing for Fitness course described in this chapter provides all of the basic skills required to successfully teach each lesson. Suggested lesson plans can be modified to meet the needs of the students based on their level of fitness or combatives experience.

Teaching Students of All Ages and Abilities

Coaches can safely tailor the Boxing for Fitness program to meet the needs of any age group. Teachers can develop fitness themes according to the physical abilities and maturity level of the students participating in the class. This program is an effective way to include all students in the physical education program. The following sections address adjusting this program according to age group.

Elementary and Middle School Students The development of gross motor skills, muscular endurance, hand-and-eye coordination, and teamwork constitutes suggested goals for school-age children. As with many motor skill activities, correct performance and high repetitions often bring success. Boxing for fitness allots time for student practice and time on task. Students enjoy the short, intense workouts and are encouraged by the success, both physically and psychologically, that comes from performing high repetitions of the skills. In order to maintain student interest and to introduce students to leadership challenges, it is advisable to continually change the routines and also the exercise leaders. For example, a session that progresses from three 1-minute rounds of quick feet to three 1-minute rounds of no-rope jump rope to three 1-minute rounds of shadow boxing, with different students leading the group in exercises, keeps students on task and fresh while simultaneously encouraging them to develop flexibility. To make this work, teachers must plan routines that require minimal or seamless transitions between skills.

Since the left hook, right hook, and right uppercut are higher-level skills, they may not be appropriate for students of elementary and middle school age. Teachers can readily alter routines such as shadow boxing, mitt work, and noncontact sparring to eliminate these skills. The following is a suggested routine.

Suggested Routine for a 45-Minute Class

- Warm-up: 5 to 7 minutes
- Quick feet: three 1-minute rounds; 1-minute rest between rounds
- No-rope jump rope: three 1-minute rounds; 1-minute rest between rounds
- Shadow boxing: three 1-minute rounds; 1-minute rest between rounds
- Mitt work (first student): three 1-minute rounds; 1-minute rest between rounds
- Mitt work (second student): three 1-minute rounds; 1-minute rest between rounds
- Noncontact sparring: three 1-minute rounds; 1-minute rest between rounds
- Cool-down

High School and College Students Since boxing for fitness involves high-intensity workouts, music of choice, and a varied routine, high school and college students enjoy the high-paced variety that the class has to offer. Learning basic self-defense skills while getting in shape is a big factor in the success of this program. Both men and women at West Point are quick to enroll in this course because it provides a great workout and does not promote contact or competition among students for a grade. In order to meet the fitness needs of the students, the intensity of the workout and the routines can be adjusted. High school and college students enjoy the additional challenges that the left- and right-hand hooks and the right uppercut bring to a workout. The following is a suggested circuit routine.

Suggested Routine for a 45-Minute Class

- Warm-up: 5 to 7 minutes
- Station 1: quick feet
- Station 2: jumping jacks
- Station 3: no-rope jump rope
- Station 4: push-ups
- Station 5: shadow box
- Station 6: mitt work
- Station 7: rocky sit-ups
- Station 8: noncontact sparring
- Cool-down

Boxing for fitness is a fun way to get fit by using a boxer's training regimen without the contact. Students enjoy it because of the variety of activities involved, and teachers appreciate the high level of time on task and the minimal needs for facilities and equipment.

Key Terms

mitt workout—Drill in which one student holds a pair of boxing mitts while the other student strikes them.

noncontact sparring—Sparring in which opposing boxers do not strike each other.

no-rope jump rope—The performance of a jump roping routine without the rope.

on-guard stance (OGS)—The basic boxing stance.

quick feet—A drill in which opponents accumulate points by stepping on a target with their left foot while in the OGS.

shadow boxing—A timed activity in which students practice boxing skills against an imaginary opponent.

target position—The start position for many of the drills that students perform in a Boxing for Fitness workout.

References

Gorn, E.J. (1986). *The manly art: Bare-knuckle prize fighting in America.* Ithaca, NY: Cornell University Press.

Sammons, J.H. (1982). *America in the ring: The relationship between boxing and society.* Chapel Hill, NC: University of North Carolina.

Sugden, J. (1996). *Boxing and society.* New York: Manchester University Press.

Wakefield, W. (1997). *Playing to win: Sports and the American military, 1898-1945.* New York: State University of New York Press.

Suggested Readings

Burns, T. (1934). *Scientific boxing and self-defense.* London: Athletic Publications, Ltd.

Fleischer, N. (1979). *Training for boxers.* New York: Ring Athletic Library.

Haslett, E.L. (1940). *Boxing.* New York: Barnes.

LaFond, E., & Menendez, J. (1959). *Better boxing.* New York: Ronald Press.

Sugar, B.R. (1982). *100 years of boxing.* New York: Galley Press.

Thomas, C. (1976). *How to create a super boxer.* New York: Exposition Press.

United States Amateur Boxing. (1995). *Coaching Olympic style boxing.* Carmel, IN: Cooper Publishing Group.

United States Amateur Boxing. (2002). *Official rules.* Colorado Springs, CO: Colorado Publishing Group.

United States Military Academy. (2003). *Boxing manual.* West Point, NY: U.S. Military Academy.

Walsh, J.J. (1951). *Boxing simplified.* New York: Prentice-Hall.

Obstacle Courses

Thomas Horne

No two obstacle courses are exactly alike. Obstacle courses vary significantly in difficulty, length, obstacle type, risk level, course layout, and administrative procedures. Teachers may design courses to accomplish a variety of objectives depending on the program objectives and the target audience. Obstacle courses that focus on meeting a specific goal or objective are called "theme obstacle courses." Physical development theme obstacle courses are popular and often include obstacles to develop physical components, such as strength, muscular endurance, agility, balance, and coordination. Other courses focus more on affective themes like self-confidence, teamwork, trust, or just having fun. Most obstacle courses are used in physical education classes, recreational settings, outdoor adventure programs, and recreational camps or as commercial entertainment and in military development.

Risk Management

Obstacle courses are fun and can add variety to any movement course. However, because students will be moving quickly under and over obstacles as well as climbing, jumping, and vaulting, there is opportunity for injury. As with any physical activity, injuries can be prevented or mitigated with some preplanning and attention to potential hazards (see table 8.1).

Obstacle Courses at West Point

The obstacle courses used at West Point are similar to those used by the U.S. Army and other branches of the military. Military obstacle courses are not usually designed to develop specific components of fitness. They are used to add variety to soldiers' physical training programs and tend to focus on the skill-related components of fitness including speed, agility, coordination, balance, reaction time, and power. Military courses may also provide opportunities for soldiers to plan strategies, make split-second decisions, learn teamwork,

Table 8.1 Possible Risks in Obstacle Courses

Risk identification	Reduction strategies
General falling injuries	Train and utilize spotters. Construct landing pits or use protective matting under obstacles. Install protective netting under high obstacles. Inspect and keep all obstacles in good repair.
Obstacle failure	Inspect and keep all obstacles in good repair.
Splinters	Inspect and keep all obstacles in good repair.
Cuts, scrapes, bruises, or abrasions	Inspect and keep all obstacles in good repair. Eliminate sharp points or corners. Participants wear appropriate clothing.
Rope burns	Participants receive rope climbing instructions before negotiating an obstacle with a rope. Participants wear appropriate clothing.
Knee and ankle injuries	Construct landing pits or use protective matting under obstacles.
Muscle strains	Do warm-ups and stretching prior to activity.

and demonstrate leadership. Success in combat may depend on a soldier's ability to perform skills learned in the military obstacle courses.

The two obstacle course themes most often found in military courses are physical conditioning and confidence building. Conditioning courses have relatively low obstacles that are negotiated quickly and require good basic motor skills and physical conditioning. Confidence courses focus on the affective domain and have higher, more difficult obstacles designed to build self-confidence and cultivate a spirit of daring.

Students at West Point are exposed to many training opportunities within these obstacle courses. Some courses are part of military training during the summers, and others are embedded in formal classes. West Point's obstacle courses are excellent examples of established obstacle courses designed to meet specific training goals and objectives. Most schools, colleges, recreation programs, and camps do not have permanently constructed obstacle courses like those at West Point, but they do have established physical education or recreation goals and objectives that may be accomplished using less permanent obstacle courses. The obstacle courses used by West Point provide examples of how courses can be structured to accomplish specific objectives for a defined user group. This section presents a brief overview of some of the courses at West Point.

Indoor Obstacle Course

The Indoor Obstacle Course at West Point is a series of 14 obstacles designed to develop applied military skills and a variety of health- and skill-related components of physical fitness. Freshmen learn how to negotiate the Indoor Obstacle Course as part of their Military Movement class, a gymnastics-based applied movement class. The obstacle course is also used during the sophomore, junior, and senior years as an individual test, called the Indoor Obstacle Course Test (IOCT).

Some features of this course include the following:

- Tests are timed and graded.
- Students attempt all obstacles.
- Specified standards are set for most obstacles.
- Time penalties are assessed if an obstacle is incorrectly negotiated.

See table 8.2 for a description of the course's components and figure 8.1 for course setup.

Balance Sequence

The Balance Sequence is an example of a general motor fitness obstacle course taught during the freshman year in the Military Movement class. The

Table 8.2 Indoor Obstacle Course Components

Obstacle	Description	Objectives
Low crawl	Do alligator-type crawl under a barrier about 18 in. high.	Coordination and military skill
Tire run	Touch the center of each tire in a series of 8 linked tires.	Agility
Two-hand vault	Vault over a side horse touching only with the hands.	Power and military skill
Shelf	Mount a wooden shelf that is 7 ft off the ground without using the shelf supports.	Strength and military skill
Climb to track	Move from the shelf to an elevated track by climbing over the railing.	Strength, agility, and military skill
Horizontal bar traverse	Traverse across the top of five horizontal bars while holding on to the support structures.	Balance, agility, and fear management
Hanging tires	Pass, feetfirst, through suspended tires.	Coordination and body control
Balance beam walk (3)	Traverse three balance beams, each higher than the previous one.	Balance
Vertical wall	Climb over a 7 ft high wall.	Strength and military skill
Horizontal ladder	Traverse a horizontal ladder supporting the weight on each rung of the ladder.	Strength and military skill
Vertical rope	Climb a 2 in. rope and mount a 20 ft high shelf and climb over the railing onto a track.	Strength and military skill
Medicine ball carry	Carry a 10 lb medicine ball around an indoor track.	Strength and anaerobic conditioning
Baton carry	Carry a baton around an indoor track.	Anaerobic conditioning
Run	Run 3/4 lap to the finish line.	Anaerobic conditioning

Balance Sequence is taught at one end of the gymnasium while a Movement Sequence is taught at the other end. Students execute both of these obstacle courses while wearing battle dress uniform (BDU, a camouflage uniform), combat boots, and helmet.

Balance is developed through negotiation of a sequence of events that focus on the student's ability to remain kinesthetically aware while attempting unfamiliar and challenging obstacles. Two lanes of the Balance Sequence are set up at one end of the gymnasium. Each student runs through the obstacles independently, except where a spotter is required. The Balance Sequence obstacles may be modified by the instructor in charge of the class since this is a nongraded activity. The instructors are continually looking for new and more effective obstacles and procedures. The obstacles and procedures of most obstacle courses may be modified to meet program goals, group size and ability, equipment available, and site size.

Some features of this course include the following:

- Students are not graded or timed.
- Discovery is encouraged.
- Spotting stations are set up on the course.
- Students may bypass an event.

See table 8.3 for a description of the course's components and figure 8.2 for course setup.

Confidence Obstacle Course

The Confidence Obstacle Course consists of 23 outdoor obstacles constructed with logs, ropes, and iron support beams in a natural setting. All students complete the course during summer training after their freshman year. The intent of the course is to build student confidence by challenging the students on obstacles that put them in awkward

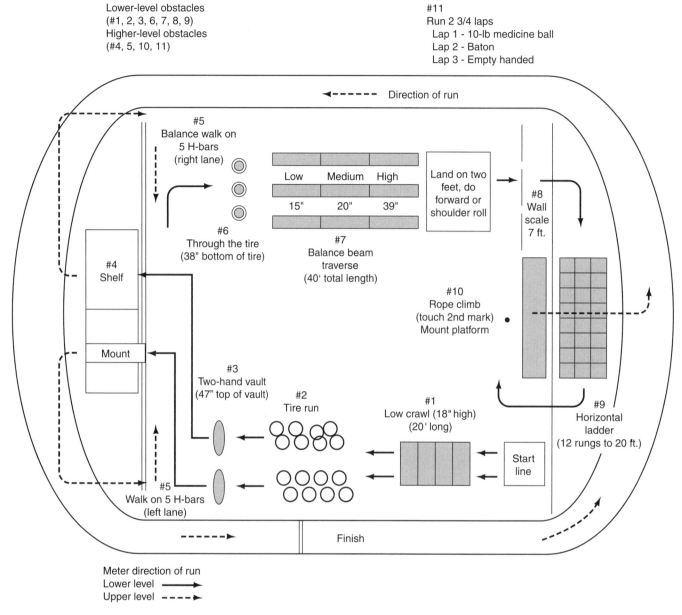

FIGURE 8.1 Indoor obstacle course.

Table 8.3 Balance Sequence Components

Obstacle	Description	Objectives
Stair climb	Run up the stairs.	Leg strength and endurance
Horizontal bars	Walk along the top of five horizontal bars.	Balance and fear management
Rope ladder	Transition to rope ladder and descend to the floor.	Coordination and balance
Rope swing	Swing from a spotting block, then swing on a rope onto another spotting block.	Arm strength and balance
Rope-to-rope swing	Swing from suspended rope with a foot loop to next rope and repeat four times.	Coordination, balance, and arm strength

Obstacle	Description	Objectives
Elevated horizontal rope	Climb rope ladder to shelf and commando crawl along the top of the rope (cable covered with rubber hose); spot required.	Balance and fear management
Island hopper	Hop from one floor disc to another using various hopping methods.	Agility and balance
Balance beams	Traverse three balance beams at different heights using various methods.	Balance and agility

body positions at varying heights. Students are challenged to attempt all the obstacles, thereby overcoming fear and developing self-confidence. The body movements needed are similar to those movements the students will need to master as future Army officers.

The following are some features of this course:

- Students are not graded or timed.
- Obstacles are optional.
- Skill and safety training is required.
- Specialized obstacles require safety netting.
- Spotting and spotting instruction are required.

See table 8.4 for a description of the course's components and figure 8.3 for illustrations.

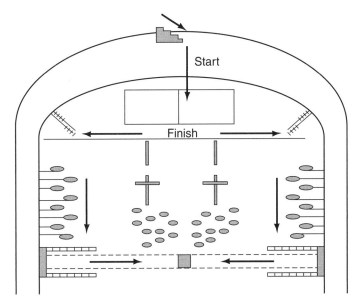

FIGURE 8.2 Balance sequence setup.

Table 8.4 **Confidence Obstacle Course Components**

Obstacle	Description	Objective
Swing, stop, and jump	Swing on elevated rope to a stand on a log and jump to the ground.	Confidence and balance
Belly buster	Get over a mobile log 4 ft high. The log is set so that it rolls when pushed.	Power and upper body strength
Reverse climb	Climb up the underside, over the top, and down the other side of a log ladder at a 60-degree slant.	Confidence and climbing skills
Weaver	Move over and then under a series of logs.	Confidence, coordination, and strength
High step-over	Step over logs with the hands on the head.	Flexibility and balance
Balancing logs	Walk along three logs that may roll.	Confidence and balance
Low belly over	Jump from a low log over an elevated log and drop to the ground.	Power and agility

(continued)

Table 8.4 *(continued)*

Obstacle	Description	Objective
Island hopper	Traverse a series of logs set on end at varying heights.	Balance
Confidence climb	Climb the inclined ladder to the vertical ladder, climb up and over the top and down the other side.	Fear management and agility
Low wire	Crawl 10 ft under barb wire set at about 18 in. high.	Crawling skills
The tough nut	Step over a series of crossed logs in an "X" pattern.	
Dirty name	Higher version of Low Belly Over, with larger distance between logs.	Confidence, power, and strength
Hip-hip	Step over elevated logs keeping hands on head.	Flexibility and balance
Tarzan	Traverse the top of three progressively higher logs (4, 6, and 8 ft) and traverse a 40 ft horizontal ladder, hand over hand.	Fear management, balance, and grip strength
Log walk	Climb to a log that is secured 25 feet above the ground. Walk the length of the log and climb down. A safety net is required!	Confidence and fear management
Swinger	Climb over a swinging log and onto the ground.	Power and agility
Incline wall	Climb from the underside of a 6.5 ft high wall that is leaning at a 30-degree angle.	Strength and climbing skills
Six vaults	Vault over six barriers that are 4 ft high and 6 ft apart, touching with the hands only.	Power
Easy balance	Walk up a nonfixed log, elevated on one end to 3.5 ft, then down another log.	Balance
Jump and land	Climb, with the hands on the head, up a log ladder to a 9 ft high platform; jump to the ground.	Confidence and landing skills
Belly robber	Climb onto five large rolling logs 4.5 ft high and crawl over the logs in the prone position.	Coordination and agility
Skyscraper	Team members help each other climb a multistory structure.	Teamwork and confidence
The tough one	Climb a 15 ft rope, walk across a log platform, climb a log ladder, and descend down a rope.	Confidence and climbing skills

Obstacle Courses for Schools

Unlike most other sports and activities covered in this book, obstacle courses are rarely taught as a separate class or unit designed to make participants more proficient in a specific sport or activity. Successfully negotiating obstacles is more often a means to accomplish broader program goals and objectives. Providing a typical instructional program with lesson plans, skill progressions, course outlines, and specific administrative procedures is not practical for this chapter on obstacle courses. This section focuses on selecting obstacles, adapting West Point obstacle courses to a high school teaching situation, and presenting obstacle course scenarios.

Selecting Obstacles

The most important consideration for designing and developing an obstacle course is selecting obstacles that will contribute to the goals and objectives of the lesson, unit, or program. Each individual obstacle should contribute to at least one identified

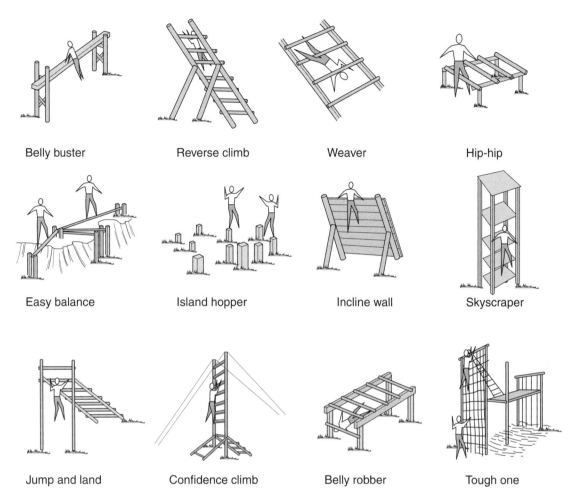

Belly buster   Reverse climb   Weaver   Hip-hip

Easy balance   Island hopper   Incline wall   Skyscraper

Jump and land   Confidence climb   Belly robber   Tough one

FIGURE 8.3   Confidence obstacle course components.

objective. Obstacles that do not contribute to the objectives may be included, however, if they aid in transition from one obstacle to another, make a positive contribution to a nonspecified worthy objective, add desired variety, or simply make the course more interesting and enjoyable.

Sequencing of the selected obstacles is also important in the development of an obstacle course. This is especially true if the obstacles in the course must be negotiated in a specific order. If this is the case, the first and last few obstacles are often less challenging than those in the middle of the course. This allows students a short warm-up prior to negotiating the most demanding obstacles and allows them to complete the final obstacles even when they are fatigued. Obstacles that tax the same muscle group should be dispersed throughout the course to allow for some muscle recovery time. Proper sequencing of the obstacles facilitates movement from one obstacle to another. The paramount consideration when sequencing obstacles

is safety. If an obstacle requires a spotter, a large landing area, or a safety net, sufficient space must be designated for the obstacle.

When developing obstacles, consider the age and skill level of the participants, the nature of the obstacle, its intended purpose, and the level of risk deemed appropriate and acceptable. Carefully selecting and sequencing the obstacles are essential in managing risks and meeting intended outcomes.

Planning obstacles that can be successfully completed at a variety of difficulty levels provides options for students negotiating the course. Obstacles that can be successfully completed at varying difficulty levels have the following advantages:

- Participants can complete the obstacle course but not complete every obstacle at the most difficult level. Those not completing an obstacle at the highest difficulty level will nevertheless be able to complete the course.

- A single course can be used by participants of different ages, sizes, and skill levels.

- Students with disabilities can participate.
- Risk factors can be reduced.

Providing an alternate, less challenging method of completing an obstacle allows participants to complete all of the obstacles on the course and gives them a better sense of accomplishment.

An endless number of obstacles are possible, so providing a detailed discussion of each is not practical. When developing obstacles, an instructor must be sure that the obstacle accomplishes the desired results, is appropriate for the students' ages and skill levels, and does not pose an unacceptable safety risk.

Applying West Point Obstacle Course Concepts

West Point employs more obstacle courses than most schools and universities. Similar to programs of other military organizations, the courses at West Point focus on conditioning, confidence, and leadership development. These are themes that apply to many school, college, and recreational settings. Using obstacle courses provides schools, colleges, and recreation programs with a versatile tool to meet program goals.

Conditioning Obstacle Courses

West Point's Indoor Obstacle Course is an example of a conditioning-type obstacle course. the Indoor Obstacle Course is used to develop and assess a wide variety of health- and skill-related components of fitness. Similar courses are appropriate if the objective is to develop or assess multiple components of fitness, like speed, strength, power, agility, and coordination. The Indoor Obstacle Course is normally completed in fewer than 4 minutes, so a similar course will have limited use in developing cardiorespiratory fitness.

Confidence and Leadership Obstacle Courses

If program objectives are oriented toward self-confidence, problem solving, or leadership development, an obstacle course similar to the Balance Sequence or Confidence Obstacle Course may be a useful template. Negotiating these courses requires some degree of physical prowess, but the focus of these courses is on developing self-confidence, courage, teamwork, and initiative. Adventure courses with high ropes courses, low ropes courses, and initiative challenges provide applications similar to the confidence course at West Point.

Obstacle Course Scenarios

Obstacle courses can be designed to accomplish a wide variety of goals and objectives. This section describes two sample obstacle course applications for a high school class or unit.

Adventure Obstacle Course

Adventure programs are becoming more popular in secondary schools. This high school level obstacle course scenario includes adventure program components. Adventure programs often include initiative games and activities, low ropes courses, high rope courses, climbing walls, and rappel towers. Some adventure programs are specifically designed in an obstacle course format, and almost all have components that can easily be utilized as part of an obstacle course.

SCENARIO

Middle America High School has a physical education requirement for all students. One of its most popular classes is a "Fun and Fitness" class. The Fun and Fitness instructors want to add a conditioning-type obstacle course that also requires some teamwork. The high school has a modest adventure program that includes some outdoor trails, a low ropes course, a low wall (12 feet or 3.7 meters high), and some lumber and rope. The teachers have designed an obstacle course using these materials and a variety of natural obstacles. The Fitness and Fun class has a maximum class size of 24 students who meet for a 50-minute class period.

APPLICATION

The concept for integrating the obstacle course into the Fun and Fitness class is to take two class periods for teaching, practicing, and then running the course. On the first day, the entire class is given an explanation, demonstration, and safety orientation for each obstacle. After the students receive a detailed explanation of how to complete each obstacle safely, they are divided into teams of four. The teams of four are dispersed along the course and given an opportunity to negotiate each obstacle at a moderate pace. During the second day, the students run the entire obstacle course at least once in their groups of four. If time permits, the instructor may have the students run through the course again with new team members or different teams, or the students may continuously run the obstacles for the entire class time.

The course designed by the instructors uses an existing trail, a small natural stream, some logs, an initiative element called the Four-by-Four Walk (two boards with four sets of ropes on each board), a few low ropes course obstacles, a tension wire (a tightly strung wire between two low posts), a wall climb, a rope swing, and a suspended tire. See table 8.5 for a description of the course's components and figure 8.4 for a course diagram.

Table 8.5   Adventure Obstacle Course Components

Obstacle	Description	Objective
Run	From the start line, run to the stream jump area.	Warm-up and elevating heart rate
Jump creek	Either individually or with partner assistance, jump over the small stream.	Teamwork and leg power
Log stand	Mount the low end of the log and walk up the log. Stay on the log until all teammates are on the log, and then jump off.	Teamwork and balance
Boulder climb	Climb to the top of the large boulder and remain until all teammates are on the top. Climb down carefully.	Teamwork, courage, and strength
Tension wire	Traverse a tightly strung cable while holding a suspended rope. Have a teammate spot. All team members must traverse the cable.	Balance, upper body strength, and teamwork
Wall climb	All team members must climb over a 12 ft wall onto a platform. Those already on the platform may help others up.	Teamwork and upper body strength
Hanging tire	Climb through a large suspended tire, preferably headfirst to avoid clothing being pulled up.	Upper body strength and agility

(continued)

Table 8.5 *(continued)*

Obstacle	Description	Objective
Rope swing	From a small platform, swing across the small stream on a suspended rope.	Upper body strength
Under log	The team members must join hands and go under the log without breaking grip.	Teamwork
Over log	All team members must climb over a log mounted 6 ft high.	
4 by 4 walk	Using two 4 in. by 4 in. by 12 ft wooden beams with rope handholds, all team members stand on the beams, hold the rope handles, and walk around a tree.	Balance, grip strength, and teamwork
Sprint to finish	Run to the finish line as a group.	Speed and cardiovascular endurance

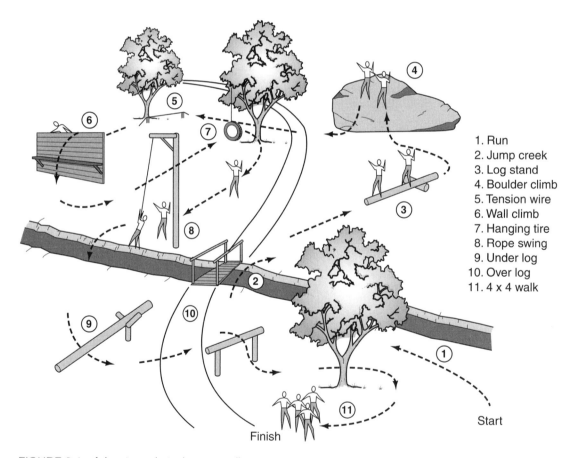

1. Run
2. Jump creek
3. Log stand
4. Boulder climb
5. Tension wire
6. Wall climb
7. Hanging tire
8. Rope swing
9. Under log
10. Over log
11. 4 x 4 walk

FIGURE 8.4 Adventure obstacle course diagram.

The instructors can easily make the course more physically demanding by adding calisthenics, having teams carry a heavy object, or increasing the space between obstacles. This obstacle course uses the available resources, achieves the desired goals and objectives, and can be modified to meet changing conditions or different objectives. Adventure course obstacles must meet industry standards for construction and design safety.

Push Ball Obstacle Course

SCENARIO

Middle Town High School wants to have a Play Day for its students. The event will be at the school's track and will include a variety of individual and team relay races. The teachers would like to have an activity that requires teamwork, is physically demanding, includes competition, and is fun. The teachers inventory the equipment at the track to determine what resources are available to conduct an activity that would meet their objectives. The track has some adjacent field space, numerous hurdles, some large wooden steeplechase barriers, a dozen marking cones, and some large landing mats (15 by 10 by 3 feet [4.6 by 3 by .9 meters]) used for pole-vaulting. The physical education teachers have some round rubber marking dots and a push ball, a very large canvas ball.

APPLICATION

The teachers decide to set up an obstacle course using the space and equipment available to meet the desired objectives (see table 8.6). The concept is to use the hurdles, steeplechase barriers, and a large landing mat as obstacles and have teams of four push the push ball over or around the obstacles while following a prescribed path marked with the large rubberized dots.

The course is shown in figure 8.5. All four team members start at the start/finish line. When signaled to begin, teams push the cage ball through a chute created with hurdles. They roll the ball to the right and go between a hurdle and a marking cone.

Table 8.6 Play Day Obstacle Course

Obstacle	Description	Objective
Hurdle chute	Team moves the cage ball out the hurdle chute.	Teamwork, strength, and fun
Around cones	Control the cage ball between a hurdle and a marker cone.	Teamwork, control, and fun
Over landing mat	Move the ball and all four team members over the landing mat.	Teamwork, strength, and fun
Around cones	Control the cage ball between a hurdle and a marker cone.	Teamwork, control, and fun
Over steeplechase	Members move the ball over the steeplechase barrier and the members go under the barrier.	Teamwork, strength, and fun
Around cones (turn around)	Control the cage ball between a hurdle and a marker cone.	Teamwork, control, and fun
Over steeplechase	Members move the ball over the steeplechase barrier and the members go under the barrier.	Teamwork, strength, and fun
Around cones	Control the cage ball between a hurdle and a marker cone.	Teamwork, control, and fun
Over landing mat	Move the ball and all four team members over the landing mat.	Teamwork, strength, and fun
Around cones	Control the cage ball between a hurdle and a marker cone.	Teamwork, control, and fun
Chute to finish line	Guide the cage ball back through the chute to the finish line.	Teamwork, control, and fun

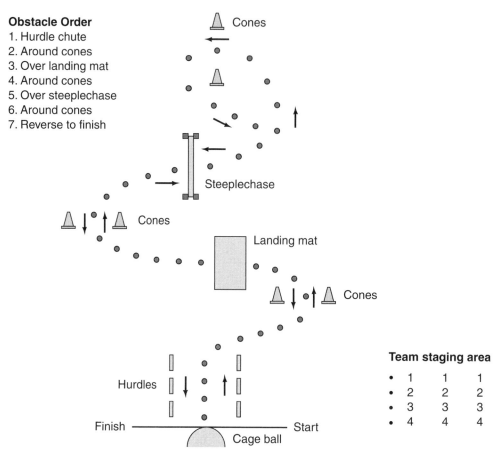

Obstacle Order
1. Hurdle chute
2. Around cones
3. Over landing mat
4. Around cones
5. Over steeplechase
6. Around cones
7. Reverse to finish

FIGURE 8.5   Play Day obstacle course diagram.

The ball then must be rolled back to the middle of the course, and the ball and all team members must go over the large landing mat. The team and the ball must then pass between another hurdle and a marking cone. The team must now take the cage ball over the steeplechase barrier; team members may go over, under, or around the barrier. The ball is then taken around the turnaround point. The team then simply follows the course in reverse as diagrammed.

The Push Ball Obstacle Course requires teamwork, is physically demanding, can be timed for competition, and is a lot of fun. Depending on time constraints, the course can be run multiple times or as a single event in a series of other races.

Obstacle courses are a versatile tool that can be used in a wide range of applications. The obstacles can be developed to meet specific program goals and objectives, adjusted for different ages and skill levels, and designed to promote a specific theme. A careful review of the program goals and objectives provides the basis for selecting, design-ing, and building obstacles. Specific equipment and materials may need to be procured for some obstacles, but most obstacles can be constructed with existing equipment and materials. The only limiting factors when course developers are design-ing and developing an obstacle course are their imagination and creativity.

PART III

Wellness and Personal Fitness Courses

9

Focus on Fitness

William Brechue, Mike Buckley, Ray Barone,
Todd Crowder, Sandor Helfgott, and Jon Liba

The West Point Physical Development Program incorporates Army fitness doctrine, contemporary exercise science, and sound risk management procedures to provide training that develops physically fit Army officers. Additionally, the cadets develop a lifetime commitment to physical fitness and wellness. The Physical Program provides cadets with an academic foundation concerning the principles of fitness, as they will bear the primary responsibility for the physical readiness of their unit.

This chapter presents the philosophical basis for developing fitness, explains how this philosophy is applied by the U.S. Military Academy (USMA) and the Department of Physical Education (DPE) to produce the Physical Program for cadets, and outlines how this philosophy can be adapted to an elementary or secondary physical education curriculum. The chapter's three sections deal with the fundamentals of fitness development, the West Point Physical Program, and assessing fitness. The section on the fundamentals of fitness covers the philosophy and basic scientific principles for developing fitness. The two subsequent sections outline the background and the programming employed by DPE to administer the Physical Program and assess the physical readiness of cadets. Each of these sections includes a discussion of how the principles and program presented may be adapted for an elementary or secondary physical education curriculum.

Developing a Teaching and Training Plan

Physical training is the process by which we teach the physical, whether in relation to development of skill or biological adaptation. The level of physical training is dictated by goals and objectives as expressed in the physical continuum from physical health to athletic performance. Education of the physical is based on a sound teaching and training plan. The plan must be logical and controlled—a systematic approach to moving the body with or without external loading to produce a specific desired level of skill and metabolic function. Exercise and physical training are stresses; and, according to the General Adaptation Syndrome (Selye, 1951), learning is specific to the stress and can be positive or negative depending on the nature and duration of the stress. The physical teaching and training plan defines the nature and duration of the stress to be applied, and for efficient and optimized learning it should be structured, programmed, and supervised.

Structured Teaching

A physical development plan must include goals, objectives, desired outcomes, and the process for achieving each. The overall teaching and training plan provides the blueprint for how physical teaching and training will be applied and advanced to ensure learning and development. The physical development plan should provide a general overview of a teaching and training strategy and goals for a year-to-year sequence, then be divided into a by-year plan. The yearly plan should again provide an overview of the teaching and training sequence, strategies, and goals. Both plans should include timing of evaluations and competition—a general overview in the year-to-year plan and a specific schedule in the yearly plan. The yearly plan should then be divided into a series of intervals or phases arranged in units or cycles. It is at this level that the plan details specific skill development; exercise selection; and training volume, intensity, and duration. Each phase and cycle has a specific goal and outcome to which teaching and training are directed. These phases and cycles are then arranged to facilitate, enhance, and optimize the learning process and physical development to achieve the desired outcome. This arrangement of phases and cycles is known as periodization, a concept that was introduced by the Russians in the 1960s and developed in the United States in the 1970s.

Programmed Teaching

The Physical Program is designed through application of a series of definitional principles that specifically address the nature and duration of the stress that will be applied to stimulate adaptation and learning—what will actually be done and how.

The overlying variable in program development is teaching and training *volume,* which refers to the overall exposure to a skill or the amount of work that will be performed in a particular unit. This variable takes into account the intensity and duration of teaching and training. Intensity and duration of activity vary inversely, such that increasing intensity is generally accompanied by decrements in repetitions or duration. The last variable is frequency—how many times per month, week, or day the teaching and training will take place. The specific application of volume is accomplished through the training principles of overload, progression, novelty, specificity, and recovery.

Overload   To apply stress, one must expose the biological system to an overload, a physical or energetic demand that is beyond what the system normally encounters. Examples of overload include exposure to a new skill; changing the length of stride during running; altering head position during throwing; lifting an external load to stress muscles, bones, tendons, and ligaments; and swimming to overload the cardiorespiratory system. Another way to accomplish overload is to alter the training volume (intensity, duration, or both). Appropriate and repeated exposure to physical or energetic loads will result in specific adaptations. Once a system has adapted to a particular demand, an overload must be reinstated to stimulate additional adaptation. This can be accomplished using the principles of progression or novelty.

Progression   Progression refers to the advancement of skill level or the training load. Progression must be controlled; appropriate progression of skill sequencing or training load is paramount to optimizing teaching and the response to training. With controlled progression, every aspect of teaching and training is planned and serves as preparation for the next skill or load phase. Controlled progression of skill level and exercise complexity should focus on the technical aspects of the given movement. Thus, progression should be based on skill mastery, although this is not always easy in the face of time constraints in an academic or athletic setting. Progression of training load, whether expressed as number of repetitions, speed of movement, distance or duration, or load lifted, is the main mechanism for reestablishing overload once biological adaptations have occurred. Although appropriate progression of training load is essential to optimizing the response to training, the real key to controlled progression is to ensure that no student attempts any skill or training load that he or she is not physically or mentally prepared to perform. This is paramount to efficient skill acquisition, training adaptation, and safety. Ultimately, controlled progression of skill level and training volume is a key to individualizing instruction and training.

Novelty   Novelty refers to the use of a variety of techniques in teaching a skill or exposing a system to an overload. For skill development, this can involve implementation of various drills that teach and reinforce the same skill. Novelty can also involve performing different exercises that stress the same system. For example, squats, jumps, and sprinting all improve leg power; running, swimming, and cycling are quite different actions that stress the cardiovascular system. Another way to provide novelty is to change the volume or intensity of training. In essence, the principles of progression and novelty are conceptual extensions of overload.

Specificity The principle of specificity reflects the idea that learning is related to the lesson taught—to a matching between the teaching and training and the intended outcome. The exercises and skills practiced have a direct impact on the variable being taught and trained. Specificity simply means that students must engage in the exact activity that they are going to compete in or be tested on. For people to jump higher, the training must include jumping; for them to run faster, the training must include sprint work; for them to improve at golf, they must play golf. Teaching and training must specifically match the desired outcome; that is, particular activities are selected to execute the teaching and training plan. But additionally, skills and exercises must be chosen to supplement the teaching and training process. Skills are broken down into parts and taught through the use of drills. Biological systems can be trained in a variety of ways. Thus, the modes or types of skills and exercises are chosen to have both a direct (specificity) and an indirect (novelty) effect on attaining the desired outcome. All this is combined to enhance the teaching and training process and achieve the outcome.

Recovery The principle of recovery is the most often overlooked and least understood aspect of any teaching and training program. According to the General Adaptation Syndrome, the stress of physical training can be positive or negative. The negative aspect is expressed as overtraining, in which skill execution or training adaptation is impaired by excessive fatigue or prevention of the system's accommodation due to continual overloading. In most cases, biological adaptation to stress follows the application and removal of the stress. For example, during running, blood volume is significantly decreased. However, following a bout of running, blood volume is restored to a level higher than preexercise. If training bouts are imposed at a frequency that limits the recovery of blood volume, then adaptation and future training bouts will be impaired. Thus, the teaching and training plan must include appropriate amounts of recovery.

To facilitate recovery, it is important to understand the impact of the exercise on the system being stressed and the recovery potential of the person being trained. Despite much research on recovery, there are still very few, if any, simple markers of recovery that practitioners can use. Thus, it is left to the teacher or coach to "guess" when sufficient recovery has occurred and new teaching and training can be administered. Recovery can be either active or passive. With proper planning, instructors can use active recovery and actually continue the teaching and training process. With use of periodization and novelty, they can accomplish recovery by rotating periods of high-volume training with low-volume training, or by having exercisers swim instead of run or do body weight calisthenics instead of lifting weights. Despite the many methods of providing active recovery, there is still a clear-cut necessity for passive recovery, or complete cessation of all activity, to ensure the realization of complete recovery and adaptive changes.

Supervised Teaching

Supervision of teaching and training is of cardinal importance for two reasons. First, supervision implies watching. As a teacher you must watch training to evaluate technique and progress and to provide immediate and appropriate feedback. This will ensure efficient skill acquisition and proper performance of the training. Secondly, supervision is a primary factor in risk mitigation as discussed later (see "Safety and Risk Management").

Stage Sequence for Teaching and Physical Training

The training principles just discussed are the same across the physical spectrum, but are applied differently depending on the desired goals, outcomes, or level of physical competency. Thus, it is the goals and desired outcomes that dictate the exercise prescription. Matching the application of these training principles to teaching and training physical competency outcomes can be accomplished using a four-stage developmental model, which

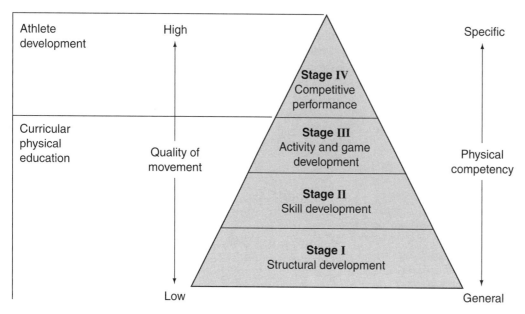

FIGURE 9.1   The four-stage developmental model.

includes Stage I, Structural Development; Stage II, Skill Development; Stage III, Activity and Game Development; and Stage IV, Athlete Development and Competitive Performance (see figure 9.1).

Stage I: Structural Development

The primary focus of Stage I is to develop the body's structure and function. This stage is the foundation of all teaching and training and is defined by its emphasis on the basic attributes of physical expression: physical structure and work capacity. Developing the physical structure emphasizes musculoskeletal development, here called structural strength and postural strength. Structural strength refers to the integrity of the musculoskeletal system with a general emphasis on developing muscle mass, bone mineral density, tendons, and ligaments. Postural strength refers to a general ability to manipulate the body to attain and hold various postures. These postures serve as a physical and technical prelude to skill development (Stage II) toward incorporating more complex movement and physical activity. The teaching and training of postural strength provides important introductory lessons toward an understanding of body position and movements in space, weight bearing, balance, transfer of body weight, and kinesthetic awareness.

Work capacity refers to the amount of work that people can perform without undue physical and psychological fatigue. Development focuses on improvement of energy supply systems to meet the needs of increasing levels of work. Energy supply systems, for our purposes, can be conveniently divided into short-term (oxygen independent) and long-term (oxygen dependent) energy supply. The element of time with reference to energy supply systems reveals the inverse relationship between time and intensity of exercise and provides clues to how to stimulate adaptation of each aspect of work capacity. Short-term energy supply depends on the utilization of creatine phosphate and the production of lactic acid to provide energy and is associated with high-intensity effort. The capacity of this system has been termed anaerobic capacity. Thus, expression and training of this system require high-intensity, short-duration bouts of work (<2 minutes).

In contrast, the long-term energy system depends on aerobic metabolism to provide the major percentage of energy during work. Aerobic metabolism includes both creatine phosphate and lactic acid metabolism for energy supply, but at a low percentage of the total energy supplied. Aerobic metabolic function includes significant support from the cardiovascular, respiratory, and endocrine systems for energy supply and transport. The capacity of the aerobic system is indicated by maximal oxygen uptake ($\dot{V}O_2$max). Expression and training of the aerobic system typically require lower-intensity work performed for a longer duration (>20 minutes). However, it is important to note that when applied in a training setting, repeated bouts of high-intensity, short-term work provide significant stimulation toward the development of aerobic metabolic function. To effectively develop work capacity, both energy systems must be advanced, but the ultimate level of development must be based on goals and desires.

Stage II: Skill Development

In Stage II the emphasis is on the acquisition of skill. The focus shifts toward expression of higher levels of force and power as skills, but importantly, to the application of power to produce more complex motor patterns and sequenced movements leading to improved technique and skill proficiency. Additionally, emphasis on the level and specialization of metabolic development increases. Basic skills include jumping, hopping, skipping, sliding, tumbling, throwing, catching, and kicking. These basic skills are then applied to sequenced movements such as tumbling, gymnastics, swimming, skating, running, and sprinting. This advances the Stage I lessons of body awareness, balance, body weight transfer, and coordination. Incorporated in this stage is a teaching and training emphasis on smooth, efficient movement along with an understanding of the movement quality with respect to force, speed, power, and effort.

Stage III: Activity and Game Development

Stage III emphasizes the application of skills to physical activity and games. Stage III includes a higher level of skill proficiency and physical competency than Stages I and II, but the focus is not extreme specialization toward competition. The level of skill proficiency and physical competency is based on enjoyment of the activity and on expanding the development of physical health and fitness. Stage III game development can be extended to include lifetime sports and intramural sports, or can be a part of athlete development programs.

Lifetime Sports   Lifetime sports are played purely for social benefits and physical health and fitness pursuits, with a focus on involvement throughout life. However, a discussion of lifetime sports raises the question of skill proficiency versus enjoyment of the game. Typically, the enjoyment of many sport activities requires a minimal level of skill proficiency. Practicing for skill proficiency is inherent in playing the game. But how much additional practice is required? What level of skill proficiency is required? In the case of lifetime sports, the answer always has to do with enhancing the level of enjoyment. For example, tennis would not be enjoyable or fitness promoting if each player could hit the ball only once per volley. While this may be desirable for competition, it would be dissatisfying from the perspective of a lifetime activity and physical health and fitness. The level of skill proficiency in Stage III is directly linked to the desired outcome, enjoyment of sport with a physical health or fitness goal.

Intramural Sports   At most academic institutions in the United States there is an appreciation for competition and the values that competition instills. Intramural competition plays an important role in physical education in that it provides a controlled exposure to competition without a necessarily high level of skill and training specialization. The value of intramural sports is discussed in more detail later (See "Adapting This Course for Your School" and also chapter 2, "Sport Education").

Athlete Development Programs   With young athletes it is important to incorporate a wide variety of skills into their development prior to sport specialization. This will ensure their broadest physical development. One way to do this is to involve athletes in a variety of games and sports. Games and sports can also be used for *novel* training and as part of the athlete's active recovery program.

Stage IV: Athlete Development and Competitive Performance

In Stage IV, teaching and physical training become very specific and focused on the highest level of physical competency: specialization of skill development and metabolic adaptations for optimization of performance for competition. Individuals at this stage are competing at the interscholastic, intercollegiate, international, or professional level.

Obviously, each stage involves a particular set of attributes and physical competencies that can be taught and trained in a particular way. However, the stages are not necessarily discrete; rather there is a blending as one stage transitions to the next. These stages represent the same general-to-specific physical continuum as for physical development (from physical health to athletic performance) and reflect increasing levels of physical competency, but are expressed in terms of attributes and skills. Also reflected in these stages is the implicit progression of physical education regardless of desired outcome; thus the stages provide a model for designing any teaching and training physical program that can be matched to the desired outcome.

Developing an Exercise Prescription and Training Plan

With use of the four-stage model, the exercise prescription (training plan) can be developed by matching the desired outcome to the particular stage and then programming to meet the given physical competency. Recall that the principles for training are the same across the physical spectrum; the application of those principles changes to attain the level of physical competency defined by the desired outcome—physical health, fitness, or performance. Thus, physical education for physical health is not oriented toward skill but rather toward anatomy and biochemistry, whereas physical education for sport performance requires a high level of specialization or physical competency. A physical education curriculum takes an intermediate view, focusing on generalized physical and skill development toward a moderate level of physical competency to enhance lifetime activity.

Designing a training program for physical health or fitness should be based on the concept of well-roundedness (Brechue, 1995; Pollock, Feigenbaum, & Brechue, 1995). The well-rounded program includes exercise and activity that address both structural and metabolic development. This is reflected in the guidelines for exercise prescription published by the American College of Sports Medicine (2000), the Centers for Disease Control and American College of Sports Medicine (Pate et al., 1995), and the American Heart Association (2002).

Training for Physical Health

Training for physical health requires a focus on Stage I development. Because physical health is based on anatomical and biochemical markers, the exercise prescription should promote changes in these markers. The training program for physical health includes resistance exercise and 30 minutes per day of accumulated physical activity on most, if not all, days of the week (Pate et al., 1995). From a resistance exercise standpoint, Stage I training should focus on structural strength. The planned training overload should emphasize maintenance of muscle mass accumulation and the development of strength. The suggested prescription is to perform resistance exercise two or three days per week and to work every major muscle group of the body—typically about 13 exercises. Each exercise is performed for one set to exhaustion with between 8 and 12 repetitions. Changes in muscular strength will be noted given the mode of training, but increased muscular strength is not the goal. Resistance exercise and increased muscle mass lead to increased bone mineral density and abatement of metabolic syndrome, with positive influences

on resting metabolic rate (which increases with increased muscle mass) and glucose metabolism and insulin sensitivity.

Training for Physical Fitness

Physical fitness has been defined in a variety of ways over the years, but in general reflects an ability to meet daily demands and to participate in vigorous activity without an inordinate amount of fatigue. Physical fitness typically implies a higher level of physical competency, Stage II level development, than does physical health. Work on body composition emphasizes accumulating muscle mass while minimizing body fat. This would be an advancement of Stage I structural development. The focus on flexibility is toward increasing and optimizing range of motion necessary for higher levels of activity. The increased level of physical competency for physical fitness reflects an active, vigorous lifestyle, which may include participation in sport as a lifetime activity.

The exercise prescription for physical fitness also reflects an increased level of vigor and activity. The prescription for resistance exercise for fitness is essentially the same as for physical health (American College of Sports Medicine, 2000). One major difference is the progression of load. For fitness, the load lifted during exercise should be incremented when the person can perform 12 repetitions. This will ensure increases in muscular strength. This prescription reflects the minimal level of training to facilitate physical fitness; many fitness programs involve higher volumes of resistance exercise training through increases in the number of exercises, the number of sets of each exercise, and the total number of repetitions performed. People should participate in these higher-volume programs according to their personal interests and goals.

Metabolic development for physical fitness involves more intense levels of physical training. Training is typically prescribed based on a percentage of $\dot{V}O_2$max, heart rate reserve, or maximal heart rate. The frequency of training recommended by the American College of Sports Medicine (ACSM) is a minimum of three days per week and as much as five days per week at an intensity of 50-60 to 90 percent of maximal heart rate or 40-50 to 80 percent of heart rate reserve or $\dot{V}O_2$max. Exercise duration ranges from 20 to 60 minutes per bout. This prescription can be applied in general across modes of exercise (e.g., running, swimming, cycling). Recall the inverse relationship between intensity of training and duration and frequency. Thus higher-intensity exercise is associated with lower duration and frequency. See the ACSM guidelines (2000) for further details.

The issue of developing fitness for performance is unique to the Army. Military performance is neither optimized skill development nor highly specialized physical development; rather it requires a general but high level of physical condition (fitness) and competency to meet the unique demands of military performance. Hence, the West Point physical education program is more demanding physically than a typical secondary or university-level physical education program. This presents unique challenges for developing and administering the Physical Program for cadets at West Point and for the Army in general.

The West Point Physical Program

Students arrive at West Point with a broad range of levels of physical fitness and prior athletic experience. Although many are highly accomplished athletes, few have been exposed to the wide array of physical and mental challenges they will face in developing skills specific to military function at West Point and in the Army. To accomplish this development, the West Point Physical Program incorporates each of the four stages of the stage sequence model for teaching and physical training.

• Stage I: Stage I development (physical structure and work capacity) is accomplished in a manner that is unique to West Point. First cadets participate in Cadet Basic Training (CBT). Cadets report to West Point the first week of July (eight weeks before beginning academic coursework) to begin their military preparation and careers. This is a very intense introduction to the Army and to physical development and fitness training. Cadet Basic Training focuses on developing base levels of muscular strength and work capacity through participation in military drill exercises and planned periods of exercise. Strength training comes in the form of traditional calisthenic exercises such as push-ups, pull-ups, sit-ups, and rope climbing. Development of work capacity is accomplished through marching, company runs, and incorporation of grass and guerilla drills (see pp. 150-153).

Following CBT, Stage I development is an implicit personal responsibility of each cadet and is supported by academic courses offered through DPE. The philosophical basis for this self-directed physical training is that, as future military leaders, the cadets should understand and embrace the importance of their own physical preparation as part of their personal and professional responsibility. Also, this training produces cadets with an academic basis for teaching others about physical development. As future officers, cadets will be responsible for the physical development and military readiness of the units they lead. At the core of this philosophy are two axioms of all educational pursuits at West Point—"lead from the front," which means teach by example, and "Be, Know, Do."

Cadets plan personal and company-level (group) physical training programs and are responsible for evaluation of their own and others' level of physical fitness. These two courses are described in detail in chapters 11 and 18.

Through the Personal Fitness courses and electives, cadets also receive basic instruction in weight training and cardiovascular fitness leading to the development of Stage I physical competency.

• Stage II: Stage II development focuses on acquisition of skill, and at West Point this includes skills specific to military function. During the plebe year, cadets enroll in Basic Movement (chapter 4), Swimming (chapter 5), and Combatives (Self-Defense for female cadets, chapter 6; Boxing for male cadets). These courses are basic physical education courses, but skills are applied to a military setting.

• Stage III: To promote the objectives of lifetime fitness and wellness, DPE offers a variety of lifetime fitness courses as part of the cadet elective program. All cadets must take one lifetime fitness course during their academic career. The elective course selection includes Tennis (chapter 12), Golf (chapter 13), Soccer (chapter 16), Volleyball (chapter 17), Group Fitness (chapter 18), Cross-Country Skiing (chapter 19), and Downhill Skiing and Snowboarding. Many of these courses, while focusing on lifetime activity, support Stage I development throughout the Physical Program.

• Stage IV: Athletic participation plays a central role in the physical education of cadets. Every cadet is required to participate in the athletic program. There are three levels of involvement for cadets at the Military Academy:

1. Corps Squad Athletics—National Collegiate Athletic Association (NCAA) intercollegiate athletics competition

2. Club Sports—extramural competition with other clubs throughout the United States

3. Company Athletics—a sport intramural program administered within the Corps of Cadets

Next we provide details on Stage I, including the drills and exercises done in CBT, the Strength Development course, the Cardiovascular Fitness course, and the Fitness Foundations course.

Basic Training Exercise Circuits

At West Point we use several forms of circuit training to motivate our students with program variety. Circuits can be designed in a limitless variety of ways to address specific components of fitness. This section presents examples of circuits that we incorporate at West Point and suggestions as to how you might use circuits in your setting. These drills are taken from the U.S. Army Field Manual 21-20 (1992).

Grass Drills

Grass drills are a great way to improve fitness levels in a challenging, motivational environment. Few resources are needed other than a grassy or matted area large enough to accommodate your entire class. These drills are used extensively during Cadet Summer Training at West Point and throughout the U.S. Army. They are an excellent method of building cohesion and provide variety in physical training. By incorporating these drills into a fitness curriculum, you can teach students the value of maintaining physically active lives as well as the importance of incorporating variety into a fitness plan. The list of exercises provided is by no means exhaustive. Use your creativity in developing additional skills.

Because these skills can be extremely strenuous, they should last for short periods of time, approximately 30 to 45 seconds per exercise. It is important that you emphasize correct form and tailor the intensity level to allow for this. The two drills described here each contain four or five exercises. You can develop additional drills as you see fit.

As soon as students are familiar with the drill, they do all the exercises as vigorously and rapidly as possible, and they do each exercise until the next command is announced. Students should do a thorough warm-up before performing grass drills and should perform a cool-down and stretch afterward to prevent injuries. Most movements are done in place. An extended-rectangular formation is best for a class size greater than 30 students. The circular formation is more suitable for smaller groups.

After the warm-up, bring the students to a standing position with a command such as "Attention." The drills begin with the command "Go" or on a whistle signal. Other basic commands are "Front," "Back," and "Stop." The following are the positions associated with each command:

- "Go": Students run in place at top speed on the balls of the feet. They raise their knees high, pump the arms, and bend forward slightly at the waist.
- "Back": Students lie flat on their back with their arms extended along the sides and the palms facing downward. The legs are straight and together and the feet face the teacher.
- "Front": Same as the "Back" position, but students lie flat on their chest, stomach, and front of the thighs.
- To assume the "Front" or "Back" position from the standing "Go" or "Stop" position, students change positions vigorously and rapidly.

The following grass drills are adapted from U.S. Army, 1992.

GRASS DRILL 1

- **Bouncing Ball.** Lying facedown, push up and support the body on the hands (shoulder-width apart) and feet. Keep the back and legs generally in line and the knees straight. Bounce up and down in a series of short, simultaneous upward springs from the hands, hips, and feet.
- **Supine Bicycle.** From the back position, flex the hips and knees. Place the palms directly on top of the head, and interlace the fingers. Bring the knee of one leg upward toward the chest. At the same time, curl the trunk and head upward while touching the opposite elbow to the elevated knee. Repeat with the other leg and elbow. Continue these movements, alternating opposite legs and arms.
- **Knee Bender.** From the attention position, do half-knee bends with the feet in line and the hands at the sides. Make sure the knees do not bend to an angle less than 90 degrees.
- **Roll Left and Right.** From the front position, roll in one direction and continue to do so until told to change direction. Then return to the front position.

GRASS DRILL 2

- **The Swimmer.** From the front position, extend the arms forward. Move the right arm and left leg up and down; then move the left arm and right leg up and down. Continue in an alternating manner.
- **Bounce and Clap Hands.** This is similar to the bouncing ball in grass drill 1. However, while in the air, clap the hands. This action requires a more vigorous bounce or spring.
- **Leg Spreader.** From the back position, raise the legs until the heels are no higher than 6 inches off the ground. Spread the legs apart as far as possible, then put them back together. Keep the head off the ground. Throughout, place the hands under the upper part of the buttocks, and slightly bend the knees to ease pressure on the lower back. Open and close the legs as fast as possible.
- **Forward Roll.** From the stop position, place both hands on the ground, tuck the head, and roll forward. Keep the head tucked while rolling.
- **Stationary Run.** From the attention position, start running in place at the "go" command by lifting the left foot first. Follow the instructor as he or she counts two repetitions of cadence. For example, "One, two, three, four; one two, three, four." The instructor then gives commands such as the following: "Follow me," "Run on your toes," "Speed it up," "Raise your knees high," and "Slow it down."

To end the circuit session, the teacher gives the command "Go" and then counts two repetitions of cadence as the left foot strikes the ground: "One, two, three, four, one, two, three, halt." Remember to conduct an adequate cool-down session at the conclusion of the drills.

Guerrilla Drills

Guerrilla drills combine individual and partner exercises to improve work capacity, agility, cardiorespiratory fitness, and, to some degree, muscular strength. These exercises require students to change their positions quickly and to perform various basic skills while moving forward. The group moves in a circular formation while performing the drills. If the group exceeds 30 students, you can use concentric circles. After forming the circle, move to its center to issue subsequent voice or whistle commands. Students progress by shortening the marching periods between exercises and by doing all exercises for a second or a even third time. This produces an overload that improves fitness.

The following guerrilla drills are adapted from U.S. Army, 1992.

- **All-Fours Run.** Face downward, supporting the body on the hands and feet. Advance forward as fast as possible by moving the arms and legs forward in a coordinated manner.
- **Bottoms-Up Walk.** Assume the front-leaning-rest position, and move the feet toward the hands in short steps while keeping the knees locked. When the feet are as close to the hands as possible, walk forward on the hands to the front-leaning-rest position.
- **Crab Walk.** Sit with the hips off the ground and hands and feet supporting the body's weight. Walk forward, feet first.
- **The Engine.** Stand with the arms straight and in front of the body. The arms should be parallel to the ground with the palms facing downward. While walking forward, bring the left knee up to the left elbow. Return to the start position. Continuing to walk forward, touch the right knee to the right elbow. Return to the start position. Be sure to keep the arms parallel to the ground throughout the entire exercise.
- **Double Time.** Do a double-time run while maintaining the circle formation.
- **Broad Jump.** Jump forward on both feet in a series of broad jumps. Swing the arms vigorously to help with the jumps.
- **Straddle Run.** Run forward, leaping to the right with the left foot and to the left with the right foot.
- **Hobble Hopping.** Hold one foot back with the opposite hand and hop forward. On the command "Change," grasp the opposite foot with the opposite hand and hop forward.
- **Two-Man Carry.** For two-man carries, students are designated as number one (odd-numbered) and number two (even-numbered). A number one and a number two work as partners.
- **Fireman's Carry.** Two students do the carry. On command, the number-two student bends at the waist with feet apart in a balanced stance. The number-one student moves toward his partner. He places himself by his partner's left shoulder and bends himself over his partner's shoulders and back. When in position, the number-two student, with her left hand, reaches between her partner's legs and grasps her left wrist. On command, they move forward until they hear the command for changeover. They then change positions.
- **Single-Shoulder Carry.** Two students do the carry. On command, the number-two student bends at the waist with feet apart in a balanced stance. At the same time, the number-one student moves toward her partner. She places her abdominal area onto her partner's right or left shoulder and leans over. The number-two student puts his arms around the back of his partner's knees and stands up. On command, they move forward until they hear the command for changeover. They then change positions.
- **Cross Carry.** On command, the number-two student bends over at the waist. He twists slightly to the left with feet spread apart in a balanced position. At the same

time, the number-one student moves toward her partner's left side and leans over her partner's back. The number-two student, with his left arm, reaches around his partner's legs. At the same time, he reaches around his partner's back with his right arm, being careful not to grab his partner's neck or head. He then stands up straight, holding his partner on his back. On command, they move forward until they hear the command for changeover. They then change positions.

- **Saddle-Back (Piggyback) Carry.** On command, the number-two student bends at the waist and knees with his hands on his knees and his head up. To assume the piggyback position, the number-one student moves behind her partner, places her hands on her partner's shoulders, and climbs carefully onto her partner's hips. As the number-one student climbs on, the number-two student grasps his partner's legs to help support her. The number-one student places her arms over her partner's shoulders and crosses her hands over her partner's upper chest. They move forward until they hear the command for changeover. They then change positions.

Strength Development Course

Using weight training for the development of Stage I and II physical competency is the foundation for the Strength Development course. In this course students are exposed to elements of three competitive forms of weightlifting (weightlifting, powerlifting, bodybuilding) and learn how to apply the basic skills and techniques from these competitive forms, as well as the basic fitness principles, to develop work capacity, muscle mass, muscular strength, and explosive power.

The strength training course is taught at a beginner to intermediate level. The variables of training—frequency, intensity, time, and type—are used to prescribe strength training programs at West Point. Typically with beginners, two or three workouts per week is sufficient. However, as experience and training increase, the frequency can be increased if desired. At West Point the strength training program is designed to train students five times every two weeks. Intensity of training is based on the goal of the training and in resistance exercise can be determined in either of two ways: by percentage of the 1-repetition maximum (1-RM) or by number of repetitions. Training for muscular strength is best accomplished using loads between 85 and 100 percent of the 1-RM, while training for power is best accomplished with loads of 70 to 80 percent of the 1-RM. Training focused on muscular enlargement is best accomplished with 60 to 70 percent of the 1-RM training load. Repetition counts are most frequently used to set training intensity for beginners, as determining their 1-RM

is difficult and unreliable. Thus, the training plan could be based on selecting weights that allow the participant to accomplish a given number of repetitions with good technique. Whether using percent 1-RM or repetitions, the relationship between percent 1-RM and repetitions performed is expressed as follows:

1 rep = 100 percent

2 reps ~95 percent

3 reps ~90 percent

4 reps ~85 percent

5 reps ~80 percent

6 reps ~75 percent

7 reps ~65 percent

8 to 12 reps to failure ~50 to 55 percent

The duration of resistance training is typically determined by the number of sets and repetitions and the rest interval rather than by setting a specific time to accomplish a workout. The time to complete a workout will increase as the number of sets, repetitions, and exercises increases. By and large, these variables are selected by desired outcome rather than training duration. One aspect of training duration that is planned is the rest interval, the time between sets and exercises. The rule of thumb for rest intervals is that it should be more than 5 minutes in training for strength, 3 to 5 minutes in training for power, and 1 to 3 minutes when the training goal is muscle enlargement.

Type refers to the mode of resistance training used to complete a workout. While the major emphasis of this course is free weights, partner-resisted exercises, body weight manipulation exercises (calisthenics), dumbbells, kettle bells, machines (MedX, Nautilus, Hammer Strength, etc.), medicine balls, or plyometrics are incorporated as novel means for providing overload. These techniques can be included in a resistance exercise program to facilitate training goals.

A sample 10-week resistance exercise program designed to provide base levels of muscular strength and power follows. Using the principles described here, this program is divided into four phases, each with a specific goal. Phase I provides a general foundation for work capacity and strength training. Phase II is designed to improve muscular strength with additional work capacity training (increased number of repetitions). Phase III provides an introduction to power exercises. Phase IV focuses specifically on the development of explosive muscular power.

RESISTANCE EXERCISE TRAINING— GENERAL PROGRAM

BEGINNER OR INTERMEDIATE 10-WEEK RESISTANCE TRAINING PLAN

The following is a suggested general resistance training program that focuses on Stage I and Stage II development: improvement of work capacity, postural strength, muscular strength, and explosive two-dimensional power.

Phase I (Weeks 1-3): Establish a Foundation for Strength Training

Week 1

MONDAY, WEDNESDAY, FRIDAY	
Exercise	**Duration**
Warm-up (includes stretching)	5 minutes
Push-ups	60% of 1-minute max, 2 sets
Sit-ups	60% of 1-minute max, 2 sets
Body weight squats	60% of 30-second max, 2 sets
Medicine ball throws	20 repetitions each arm
Medicine ball dead lifts	10 repetitions, 2 sets
Partner-resisted exercise (PRE) bench press	10 repetitions, 2 sets
Partner-resisted exercise (PRE) lat pull-down	10 repetitions, 2 sets
Partner-resisted exercise (PRE) biceps curl	10 repetitions, 2 sets
Partner-resisted exercise (PRE) triceps extension	10 repetitions, 2 sets
Cool-down (includes stretching)	5 minutes

Week 2

TUESDAY, THURSDAY	
Exercise	**Duration**
Warm-up (includes stretching)	5 minutes
Push-ups or pull-ups	70% of 1-minute max, 2 sets
Sit-ups	70% of 1-minute max, 2 sets
Body weight squats	70% of 30-second max, 2 sets
Medicine ball throws	25 repetitions each arm
Medicine ball dead lifts	10 repetitions, 2 sets
PRE bench press	12 repetitions, 2 sets
PRE lat pull-down	12 repetitions, 2 sets
PRE biceps curl	12 repetitions, 2 sets
PRE triceps extension	12 repetitions, 2 sets
Cool-down (includes stretching)	5 minutes

Week 3

MONDAY, WEDNESDAY, FRIDAY	
Exercise	**Duration**
Warm-up (includes stretching)	5 minutes
Push-ups or pull-ups	80% of 1-minute max, 2 sets
Sit-ups	80% of 1-minute max, 2 sets
Body weight squats	80% of 30-second max, 2 sets
Medicine ball throws	30 repetitions each arm
Medicine ball dead lifts	10 repetitions, 2 sets (heavier ball)
PRE bench press	8-10 repetitions, 2 sets
PRE lat pull-down	8-10 repetitions, 2 sets
PRE biceps curl	10 repetitions, 2 sets
PRE triceps extension	10 repetitions, 2 sets
Cool-down (includes stretching)	5 minutes

Phase II (Weeks 4-6): Develop Work Capacity and Muscular Strength

Week 4

TUESDAY, THURSDAY	
Exercise	**Duration**
Warm-up (includes stretching)	5 minutes
Medicine ball throws	25 repetitions each arm (heavier ball)
Sit-ups	80% of 1-minute max, 2 sets
Back squats	60% of 1-RM till muscle failure, 2 sets
Dead lifts	60% of 1-RM till muscle failure, 2 sets
Bench press (machine/weights)	60% of 1-RM till muscle failure, 2 sets
Seated lat pull-down (machine)	60% of 1-RM till muscle failure, 2 sets
Biceps curl (machine/weights)	60% of 1-RM till muscle failure, 2 sets
Triceps extension (machine/weights)	60% of 1-RM till muscle failure, 2 sets
Cool-down (includes stretching)	5 minutes

Week 5

MONDAY, WEDNESDAY, FRIDAY	
Exercise	**Duration**
Warm-up (includes stretching)	5 minutes
Medicine ball throws	Monday: 25 repetitions each arm (heavier ball) Wednesday, Friday: 30 repetitions each arm (heavier ball)
Sit-ups	80% of 1-minute max, 2 sets
Back squats	60% of 1-RM till muscle failure, 3 sets
Dead lifts	60% of 1-RM till muscle failure, 3 sets
Bench press (machine/weights)	60% of 1-RM till muscle failure, 3 sets
Seated lat pull-down (machine)	60% of 1-RM till muscle failure, 3 sets
Biceps curl (machine/weights)	60% of 1-RM till muscle failure, 3 sets
Triceps extension (machine/weights)	60% of 1-RM till muscle failure, 3 sets
Cool-down (includes stretching)	5 minutes

Week 6

TUESDAY, THURSDAY	
Exercise	**Duration**
Warm-up (includes stretching)	5 minutes
Medicine ball throws	30 repetitions each arm (heavier ball)
Sit-ups	90% of 1-minute max, 2 sets
Back squats	70% of 1-RM till muscle failure, 2 sets
Dead lifts	70% of 1-RM till muscle failure, 2 sets
Bench press (machine/weights)	70% of 1-RM till muscle failure, 2 sets
Seated lat pull-down (machine/weights)	70% of 1-RM till muscle failure, 2 sets
Biceps curl (machine/weights)	70% of 1-RM till muscle failure, 2 sets
Triceps extension (machine/weights)	70% of 1-RM till muscle failure, 2 sets
Cool-down (includes stretching)	5 minutes

Phase III (Week 7): Transition to Power Phase

Week 7

MONDAY, WEDNESDAY, FRIDAY	
Exercise	**Duration**
Warm-up (includes stretching)	5 minutes
Front squats	Monday, Wednesday: 50% 1-RM, 8-10 reps, 2 sets Friday: 60% 1-RM, 8-10 reps, 2 sets
Calf raises	Monday, Wednesday: 70% 1-RM, 12 reps, 2 sets Friday: 70% 1-RM, 12 reps, 1 set
Monday, Wednesday: Hang clean pulls on the thigh	2-3 reps, 3 sets*
Monday, Wednesday: Hang clean on the thigh	2-3 reps, 3 sets*
Monday, Wednesday: Hang clean pulls above the knee	2-3 reps, 3 sets*
Hang clean above the knee	Monday, Wednesday: 2-3 reps, 3 sets* Friday: 2-3 reps, 2 sets*
Wednesday, Friday: Hang clean below the knee	Wednesday: 2-3 reps, 3 sets* Friday: 2-3 reps, 2 sets*
Friday: Clean from the floor	2-3 reps, 2 sets*
Standing press behind the head (snatch and clean grip)	Same weight as front squat, 8 reps, 2 sets

(continued)

Week 7 *(continued)*

Exercise	Duration
Monday, Wednesday: Back squats	80% of 1-RM till muscle failure, 1 set
Monday, Wednesday: Dead lifts	80% of 1-RM till muscle failure, 1 set
Monday, Wednesday: Bench press (machine/weights)	80% of 1-RM till muscle failure, 1 set
Friday: Hang snatch pulls from the thigh	2-3 reps, 3 sets*
Friday: Hang snatch from the thigh	2-3 reps, 3 sets*
Friday: Hang snatch pulls from above the knee	2-3 reps, 3 sets*
Friday: Hang snatch from above the knee	2-3 reps, 3 sets*
Cool-down (includes stretching)	5 minutes

* Student uses a bar and focuses on technique.

Phase IV (Weeks 8-10): Develop Muscular Power

Week 8 (focus on clean and snatch technique)

TUESDAY, THURSDAY	
Exercise	**Duration**
Warm-up (includes stretching)	5 minutes
Front squats	65% of 1-RM, 8-10 reps, 2 sets
Calf raises	70% of 1-RM, 12 reps, 2 sets
Hang clean above the knee	2-3 reps, 2 sets*
Hang clean below the knee	2-3 reps, 2 sets*
Clean from the floor	2-3 reps, 2 sets*
Standing press behind the head (snatch and clean grip)	Same weight as front squat, 8 reps, 2 sets
Tuesday: Hang snatch pulls from the thigh	2-3 reps, 3 sets*
Hang snatch from the thigh	2-3 reps, 3 sets*
Hang snatch pulls from above the knee	2-3 reps, 3 sets*
Hang snatch from above the knee	2-3 reps, 3 sets*
Hang snatch from below the knee	2-3 reps, 3 sets*
Cool-down (includes stretching)	5 minutes

* Student finds a weight he or she can handle; focus is on technique.

Week 9

MONDAY, WEDNESDAY, FRIDAY	
Exercise	**Duration**
Warm-up (includes stretching)	5 minutes
Front squats	65% 1-RM, 8-10 reps, 2 sets
Calf raises	Monday, Friday: 75 % 1-RM, 12 reps, 2 sets Wednesday: 75% 1-RM, 12 reps, 3 sets
Hang clean above the knee	2-3 reps, 3 sets*
Clean from the floor	2-3 reps, 3 sets*
Standing press behind the head (snatch and clean grip)	Same weight as front squat, 8 reps, 3 sets
Monday: Hang snatch from the thigh	2-3 reps, 3 sets*
Hang snatch from above the knee	2-3 reps, 3 sets*
Snatch from the floor	2-3 reps, 3 sets*
Cool-down (includes stretching)	5 minutes

* Student finds a weight he or she can handle.

Week 10
(power and strength exercises in same workout)

TUESDAY, THURSDAY	
Exercise	**Duration**
Warm-up (includes stretching)	5 minutes
Tuesday: Front squats Thursday: Standing press behind the head (snatch grip)	65% 1-RM, 8-10 reps, 2 sets Same weight as front squat, 8 reps, 3 sets
Calf raises	Tuesday: 75 % 1-RM, 12 reps, 2 sets Thursday: 75 % 1-RM, 12 reps, 3 sets
Tuesday: Hang clean above knee Thursday: Hang snatch above knee	2-3 reps, 3 sets* 2-3 reps, 3 sets*
Tuesday: Cleans from the floor Thursday: Snatch from the floor	2-3 reps, 3 sets* 2-3 reps, 3 sets*
Tuesday: Dead lift Thursday: Back squats	70% 1-RM till muscle failure, 2 sets 70% 1-RM till muscle failure, 2 sets
Tuesday: Seated lat pull-down (machine/weights) Thursday: Bench press (machine/weights)	70% 1-RM till muscle failure, 2 sets 70% 1-RM till muscle failure, 2 sets
Tuesday: Biceps curl (machine/weights) Thursday: Triceps extension (machine/weights)	70% 1-RM till muscle failure, 2 sets 70% 1-RM till muscle failure, 2 sets
Cool-down (includes stretching)	5 minutes

* Student finds a weight he or she can handle.

Cardiovascular Fitness Course

Cadets are exposed to the elements of teaching and training cardiovascular fitness through jogging and running as part of Fitness Leader-I and -II, the Cadet Fitness Challenge, and various aerobic training classes offered in small units (e.g., spinning, rowing).

Running is the form of exercise that has been traditionally utilized and is one of the most effective ways to improve cardiorespiratory fitness. Whether the goal is to improve health or physical appearance, relieve stress, or spend some time with friends, many people choose to run. Adults have learned to add running to their lifestyles in order to achieve desired goals. What many people have forgotten is that to a small child, running is simply a fact of life. Athletes often talk of training methods, periodization, running injuries, equipment, and races, whereas a child simply "wants to chase a ball around." Physical educators can capitalize on this exuberance in their physical education classes. By incorporating the variables of training into games that are fun, you can solve the problem of inspiring children and adolescents to improve their physical being and do it in the most beneficial manner.

Long Slow Distance and Easy Runs It is perhaps easiest to divide general aerobic conditioning into two run types: the easy run and the long run. The key difference is that the easy run allows the runner to recover from a strenuous period of training, while the long run builds an aerobic base. Easy runs should be conducted at a heart rate not exceeding 70 percent of the student's maximal heart rate (Daniels, 1998), which the runner can determine with use of a heart rate monitor. It is important to note that the benefits of an easy run are more a function of time spent exercising than of intensity. Long runs are similar to easy runs except for their length. In both cases, people run at a pace 20 to 25 percent slower than race pace and are able to carry on a conversation with a running partner (Noakes, 1991). Easy runs are generally under an hour in duration, whereas long runs exceed 1 hour. Long slow distance running might be the most important type of activity in the entire plan, allowing people the opportunity to gradually improve and increase their level of fitness.

Interval Runs Interval run training is difficult. It demands that students depart from their "comfort zone" and run much harder than they typically do. However, if this type of training is performed properly, the level of improvement in fitness can be substantial. One of the biggest challenges with intervals is to determine their length and duration. At most, each work interval should not be longer than 5 minutes, as this will result in too great an accumulation of blood lactate, which frequently results in shortening of the workout (Daniels, 1998). Typically, interval running should be performed once per week, with intervals ranging from 30 seconds to no more than 5 minutes. Intervals are performed at a pace at which the runner cannot talk comfortably but that on the other hand will not lead to exhaustion. Intensity of the interval is determined more by the rest time between bouts than by intensity. Take into account the physical condition of the student, the goal of the program, and the duration of the interval when adding interval training to a program.

Fast Continuous-Tempo Runs A tempo run is a steady 20-minute run at a pace approximately 80 to 85 percent of maximal heart rate (Daniels, 1998). Always begin the workout with a good warm-up and end with a cool-down. The greatest benefit of tempo running is that it allows the body to learn to run at greater speeds and the runner to concentrate on biomechanics and form. A tempo run is difficult but controlled. Intensity and prior rest are the most important aspects, not the duration or the speed, which can vary substantially with the environment. Perform tempo runs once a week after students have completed approximately four to six weeks of basic foundation running (three times per week, 30 minutes per session). The best structure for a tempo run workout consists of 20 percent of the total time on warm-up, 70 percent on hard running, and 10 percent on cool-down. Conducting tempo-style running sessions after a solid aerobic base has been developed leads to substantial improvement in overall performance and fitness.

Fartlek Runs The term "fartlek," roughly translated, means "speed play." It is a combination of tempo running, intervals, sprints, and strides, all combined to make a very individualized workout. It is an effective and often satisfying form of training that many students should enjoy. The greatest benefit of fartlek running is the informal structure, which allows students to have some fun during their workout. A typical approach is to choose a landmark or object seen during the run and sprint to it, then recover. Runners might sprint from one telephone pole to another or from one golf course hole to another. The student determines the distance and the pace. Depending on the situation, a fartlek workout might be the hardest or the easiest workout of the week. This workout builds strength and endurance, develops the race pace, and, if students are preparing to run a local race, assists in developing race tactics and strategy.

These concepts are incorporated into the following 10-week jogging and running program.

JOGGING AND RUNNING PROGRAM

The following 10-week program is intended for the novice runner and is structured to include basic running principles. Definitions of running types are as follows:

- Easy: An easy run is at 60 to 65 percent of the student's maximal heart rate. Another way to evaluate this pace is to have students run with partners and ensure that they can talk to one another in a conversational manner.

- Rest or cross-training: Students should take the day off or perform another physical activity such as cycling, swimming, resistance training, walking, or stretching, at an easy pace.

- Long: This run is the key to the entire week's schedule. The long run builds work capacity, increases cardiorespiratory fitness, enhances slow-twitch muscle fiber development, strengthens connective tissue, and improves heart stroke volume.

- Tempo: The tempo run is a key run for enhancing performance. It is performed at 90 percent of maximal heart rate, lasts approximately 20 minutes, and requires a minimum of a 10-minute warm-up and cool-down. The benefits include optimal aerobic benefits and improvement in the student's ability to handle blood-level lactate at a faster pace. Include this type of running in a training plan only after the student has completed approximately 6 to 10 weeks of base endurance training.

See table 9.1 for a sample training schedule.

Table 9.1   Sample 10-Week Running Program

	Sunday	Monday	Tuesday	Wednesday	Thursday	Friday	Saturday
1	Off	Easy (2 miles)	Rest/CT	Easy (2 miles)	Rest/CT	Easy (3 miles)	Rest/CT
2	Off	Easy (2 miles)	Rest/CT	Easy (3 miles)	Rest/CT	Easy (3 miles)	Rest/CT
3	Off	Easy (3 miles)	Rest/CT	Easy (3 miles)	Rest/CT	Easy (4 miles)	Rest/CT
4	Long (5 miles)	Easy (3 miles)	Rest/CT	Easy (4 miles)	Rest/CT	Easy (4 miles)	Rest/CT
5	Long (5 miles)	Easy (3 miles)	Rest/CT	Easy (4 miles)	Rest/CT	Easy (4 miles)	Rest/CT
6	Long (5 miles)	Easy (3 miles)	Rest/CT	Easy (4 miles)	Rest/CT	Easy (4 miles)	Rest/CT

(continued)

Table 9.1 *(continued)*

	Sunday	Monday	Tuesday	Wednesday	Thursday	Friday	Saturday
7	Long (5 miles)	Easy (3 miles)	Rest/CT	Tempo	Rest/CT	Easy (4 miles)	Rest/CT
8	Long (6 miles)	Easy (3 miles)	Rest/CT	Tempo	Easy (3 miles)	Easy (4 miles)	Rest/CT
9	Long (6 miles)	Easy (3 miles)	Rest/CT	Tempo	Easy (3 miles)	Easy (4 miles)	Rest/CT
10	Long (6 miles)	Easy (3 miles)	Rest/CT	Tempo	Easy (3 miles)	Easy (4 miles)	Rest/CT

CT = cross-training

Fitness Foundations Course

If cadets are unable to meet the minimum movement standards of the Physical Program (Stage II skills) because of inadequate requisite conditioning, they are assigned to a remediation program called Fitness Foundations. The Fitness Foundations program was originally designed to help freshman students lacking in muscular strength and has since evolved to include work capacity and cardiovascular fitness (a more complete Stage I development).

The long-term goals of Fitness Foundations are those of any sound physical education program—to teach and facilitate the skills, knowledge, attitudes, and behaviors that lead to regular participation in physical activity. As with the Physical Program in general, the ultimate goal is to generate an appreciation of the importance of physical fitness, craft the mental skills required to increase physical performance, and instill a lifelong passion for physical fitness—and, at West Point, to prepare each student for a successful future as a commissioned officer in the U.S. Army.

Because our faculty expertise is diverse, students are exposed to a wide array of exercises. Students are often presented with activities that are completely novel to them. For example, most cadets have never tried aqua jogging or aerobics. The diversity of the program helps to create a positive environment. Students quickly realize that this program is not merely about doing endless push-ups and sit-ups, but is aimed at exposing them to a variety of exercise modalities that are key to developing well-rounded physical fitness. Instructors

work diligently to present a challenging yet fun and enjoyable program. Variety is a key component of Fitness Foundations and is paramount to the Stage I development of the cadets. The breadth of physical experience stemming from program variety increases the level of appreciation of the program and enhances the effectiveness of preparation for Stage II teaching and training.

It is crucial in any remedial program that students not be viewed negatively or as incompetent. Many think of remedial physical training as punishment rather than an opportunity to receive help and improve their physical condition. Contrary to what cadets might think, the primary goal of Fitness Foundations is for cadets to succeed. Creating a positive environment early in the program is important. All instructors and cadets who assist in running the program are volunteers. They are committed to helping the cadets achieve success. Once this positive atmosphere and trust are established, cadets feel very comfortable in the Fitness Foundations program and frequently ask to remain in it. However, the underlying goal is to get out of the program. There is camaraderie in knowing that the people around you are pulling for you to succeed.

Ideally, Fitness Foundations should meet daily, but because of the cadets' busy academic schedules, classes meet two or three days per week for 2-hour sessions. Daily plans are grouped into three categories. Two of these categories focus on Stage I physical competencies: work capacity and muscular strength. The third category focuses on the cognitive or mental component of fitness. The mental piece is accomplished through the help of the West Point Center for Enhanced Performance (CEP). The CEP teaches cadets utilizing a unique combination of reading, study, and applied performance psychology skills that help them become self-directed learners. Cadets are empowered to actively pursue their full academic, physical and athletic, and military potential. Each of the first five lessons includes work to develop the mental skills required to increase physical performance. Topics include confidence building, stress management, concentration, imagery, and goal setting. Among these topics, goal setting appears to have the greatest benefit early. Often, beginners or weaker performers are discouraged because they don't see immediate results or achieve success quickly enough. Teaching them to set realistic short-term goals helps them understand the level of achievement they attain instead of feeling frustrated by it. Each attained goal serves to further motivate the student and encourages the establishment and accomplishment of future, more difficult goals. The following are training techniques used in Fitness Foundations. See table 9.2 for an overview of the lesson plans.

Table 9.2   Overview of Fitness Foundations Lessons

Lesson	Activities
1	Introduction to Fitness Foundations
2	Pretest evaluation
3	*Cognitive:* CEP 1 (confidence) *Gymnastics:* two dive rolls and a backward roll, handstand against a wall, Indoor Obstacle Course Test (IOCT) shelf obstacle *Muscular strength and endurance:* chin-up and dip workout
4	*Cognitive:* CEP 2 (goal setting) *Gymnastics:* headstand, cartwheel, IOCT horizontal bar *Muscular strength and endurance:* ankles-to-the-bar and push-up pyramid
5	*Cognitive:* CEP 3 (stress management, recovery) *Gymnastics:* vertical rope climb (the lock climb) *Muscular strength and endurance:* 1,000 ropes
6	*Cognitive:* CEP 4 (concentration) *Gymnastics:* techniques on still rings, straight-body inverted hang, IOCT horizontal ladder *Aerobic and anaerobic:* slow-moderate run
7	*Cognitive:* CEP 5 (imagery) *Gymnastics:* vertical rope climb (grapevine climb) *Aerobic and anaerobic:* sprint running
8	*Gymnastics:* horizontal rope climb *Muscular strength and endurance:* push-up and sit-up circuit *Aerobic and anaerobic:* slow-moderate run
9	*Gymnastics:* vaulting *Muscular strength and endurance:* chin-up workout *Aerobic and anaerobic:* hill sprint running
10	*Gymnastics:* horizontal rope climb *Muscular strength and endurance:* Circuit B *Aerobic and anaerobic:* slow-moderate run

(continued)

Table 9.2 *(continued)*

Lesson	Activities
11	*Gymnastics:* trampoline *Muscular strength and endurance:* 1,000 ropes *Aerobic and anaerobic:* aqua jogging
12	*Gymnastics:* gymnastics review *Muscular strength and endurance:* push-up and sit-up smoker *Aerobic and anaerobic:* flat sprints
13	*Muscular strength and endurance:* introduction to fitness corners, pull-up and dip smoker *Aerobic and anaerobic:* diagnostic APFT 2-mile run
14	*Muscular strength and endurance:* 2 minutes of push-ups and 2 minutes of sit-ups *Aerobic and anaerobic:* slow-moderate medium-distance run
15	*Muscular strength and endurance:* grass drills, guerrilla drills *Aerobic and anaerobic:* hill sprint running
16	*Muscular strength and endurance:* 1,000 ropes *Aerobic and anaerobic:* Ultimate Frisbee
17	*Muscular strength and endurance:* push-up and sit-up pyramids *Aerobic and anaerobic:* intervals
18	*Muscular strength and endurance:* pull-up and dip smoker workout *Aerobic and anaerobic:* long slow distance run
19	Posttest evaluation

CEP = Center for Enhanced Performance
APFT = Army Physical Fitness Test

1,000 Ropes

1. Students pair up. Partner 1 sits on a 1-inch mat. Partner 2 stands beside the mat with a jump rope in hand.
2. At the command "Exercise," Partner 1 performs abdominal crunches. Partner 2 performs 100 complete jump rope revolutions. Partner 1 does not stop until Partner 2 has finished the jumps.
3. Members quickly switch positions. There should be no break in exercise. Repeat step 2.

Note: The team continues to repeat steps 2 and 3 until both partners have completed 1,000 revolutions or 12 minutes have elapsed.

Chin-Up and Dip Smoker

1. Students of equal size form pairs. Partner 1 performs the exercise while Partner 2 spots and provides assisted repetitions as necessary.

2. Chin-ups
   - 60 seconds of chin-ups, then partners switch.
   - 30 seconds of chin-ups, then switch.
   - 15 seconds of chin-ups, then switch.
3. Decline dips using a chair or 3-foot (.9-meter) balance beam.
   - 60 seconds of dips, then switch.
   - 30 seconds of dips, then switch.
   - 15 seconds of dips, then switch.

Mixed-Bag Circuit

1. Start at any "a" station and complete all the "a" stations before moving on to any "b" station (see table 9.3).
2. Perform upper body exercises to failure plus three partner-assisted repetitions.
3. Perform lunges back and forth on mat or in open space.

Table 9.3 Mixed Bag Circuit

STATION 1	STATION 2	STATION 3	STATION 4
Push-ups	**Abdominal crunches**	**Upper body**	**Lower body**
a. Max to muscle failure	**a.** 60 s	**a.** Chin-ups	**a.** 60 s jump rope
b. 20-25 reps	**b.** 60 s	**b.** Ankles-to-the-bar	**b.** Lunges
c. 15-20 reps	**c.** 45 s	**c.** Pull-ups	**c.** 45 s jump rope
d. 10-15 reps	**d.** 45 s	**d.** Chin-ups	**d.** Lunges
e. 5 reps	**e.** 30 s	**e.** Ankles-to-the-bar	**e.** 30 s jump rope

Pull-Up and Dip Smoker

1. Students of equal size form pairs. One partner performs the exercise while the other spots and provides assisted repetitions as necessary.
2. 30 seconds of dips, then partners switch.
3. 30 seconds of pull-ups, then switch.
4. 15 seconds of dips, then switch.
5. 15 seconds of pull-ups, then switch.
6. 10 seconds of dips, then switch.
7. 10 seconds of pull-ups, then switch.

Push-Up and Sit-Up Smoker

1. Students of equal size form pairs. One partner performs the exercise while the other spots and provides assisted repetitions as necessary.
2. 60 seconds of push-ups, then partners switch.
3. 45 seconds of push-ups, then switch.
4. 30 seconds of push-ups, then switch.
5. 60 seconds of sit-ups (other partner holds feet), then switch.
6. 45 seconds of sit-ups (other partner holds feet), then switch.
7. 30 seconds of sit-ups (other partner holds feet), then switch.
8. 60 seconds of sit-ups (other partner holds feet), then switch.
9. Both partners perform 45 seconds of abdominal crunches, rest 15 seconds, and then perform 30 seconds of abdominal crunches.

Ankles-to-the-Bar

1. Students of equal size pair up. One partner performs the exercise while the other partner spots and provides assisted repetitions as necessary.
2. Partner 1 performs as many ankles-to-the-bar (ATB) repetitions as possible. Upon reaching muscle failure, Partner 1 performs three more repetitions with the assistance of Partner 2. The partners switch places, then rest for 60 seconds.
3. Repeat step 2.
4. Repeat step 2.

Push-Up and Sit-Up Pyramids

1. Push-up and military press
   - Students perform 20 sets of push-ups, beginning with 10 repetitions and working down to 1, then back up from 1 to 10.
   - Between push-up sets, students kneel and perform a military press movement. Students perform the same number of repetitions as for the push-up.
2. Sit-ups and flutter kicks: Students mirror the push-up and military press pyramid, substituting sit-ups for push-ups and single-count flutter kicks for the military press. Caution students to perform flutter kicks with a slightly bent knee to alleviate strain in the lower back.

Circuit B

This circuit consists of the following exercises, performed in order: push-up with feet (or knees) elevated, abdominal crunches, side hops, pull-ups, dips, ATB, jump rope, and supine bicycle.

1. 45 seconds at each station with 15 seconds rest between stations. Students run to the next station during the rest interval.

2. 30 seconds at each station with 15 seconds rest between stations. Students run to the next station during the rest interval.

Safety and Risk Management

Risk of injury is inevitably associated with any movement, physical activity, or exercise training. However, many steps can be taken to ensure the highest possible safety and mitigate risk. In general, and common to all physical activity or exercise training, two major issues lead to reduced risk and injury: practicing proper technique and supervision.

Proper Technique

Proper technique begins with teaching. It is imperative to teach and reinforce proper technique during practice and throughout all teaching and training. It is equally important that students understand and appreciate the importance of good technique. Poor technique is initiated by fatigue, both physical and mental. Fatigue is a consequence of physical activity and exercise training, but also the product of inadequate recovery due to the premature advancement of training volume or intensity or simply the act of repeating the same action or movement over time. Teachers and coaches constantly struggle with the fine line involved in balancing teaching and training with recovery time. Likewise, inadequate recovery based on repetitive movements presents a teaching and training conundrum since learning should be specific to practice. Here is where planning and novelty in teaching and training become so important. Sufficient time must always be allowed to alleviate the cumulative stress of previous work. If not, the end result is overtraining, injury, or both.

From an injury prevention point of view, the focus of Stage I is the development of structural, postural, and stabilizing strength, allowing proper technique in any movement. Thus, regardless of the purpose, it is essential to reinforce Stage I development throughout the teaching and training cycle to maintain or improve structural and postural strength and work capacity and thus to reinforce foundational development and match growth and development over time.

Supervision

Physical activity and exercise training should be supervised, with the level of supervision greatest with younger participants. Supervision provides the opportunity to teach and reinforce good technique, correct poor technique, and ensure that practice and training follow the training plan, as well as deterring nonessential activity (horseplay). Appropriate development of a teaching and training plan is an important deterrent to inappropriate progression of skill or training load and exposure to risk. Lesson and training objectives should be reviewed with participants so they know what is expected of them.

Another important form of supervision is spotting. However, the use of spotters must be highly judicious. Spotting requires a certain level of skill in and of itself, and if performed improperly endangers both the spotter and the participant. Spotting may involve partners in such activities as gymnastics or weight training or may involve external devices such as belts or harnesses during diving, rock climbing, and so on. However, in some instances, spotting should not be attempted, and safety must be ensured by other means. For instance, attempting to spot a lifting movement as ballistic as the snatch or clean and jerk, or its constituent drills, in actuality jeopardizes both the lifter and spotter. Thus, students using the Olympic lifts must be taught how to drop weights properly and how to get away from weights when they miss an attempt.

The next sections cover additional considerations for mitigating risk during training.

Clothing

Be sure that students wear weather-appropriate clothing and use reflective items when exercising in areas or conditions with poor visibility. When the exercise is in wind or heat, clothing must be porous but must protect against wind and allow removal of heat from the body through sweating. During exercise in cold temperatures, extremities must be protected and the effect of breathing cold air monitored. Clothing should fit properly—that is, neither restrict movement nor fit too loosely. Athletic supporters and jog bras should be worn to provide necessary support. Socks are important for preventing blisters and other foot problems.

Shoes

Ensure that each student has a good pair of quality shoes appropriate to the activity. The shoes need not be expensive, but they must fit properly and should provide appropriate lateral stability and cushioning for the feet. For running, cushioned shoes can minimize ground reaction forces and stress to the feet and legs. Hiking is generally considered a more intense form of exercise, and greater support is needed to protect the body. Movement over rough terrain subjects the feet, knees, and ankles to more stress, especially if people are carrying a knapsack or backpack. Hiking boots provide greater lateral support than walking shoes. A sturdy walking stick or pole assists in maintaining balance and can reduce stress on the feet and knees by transferring some weight to the upper body. With weightlifting, on the other hand, too much cushioning can lead to foot and ankle instability. When lifting weights, participants should use solid-soled shoes, as opposed to running shoes, for stability.

Proper selection of a running shoe is critical for optimal mechanical efficiency in jogging or running and for injury prevention. With runners, leg injury may be associated with the shoes. Check to determine if there has been a recent change in the shoe to a different style or if the shoes are new. If the shoes are not new, do they show signs of excessive wear? These factors can lead to foot, ankle, and leg problems. The major areas of failure in a running shoe are the heel, the midsole, and the outer sole. Running shoes are not indestructible, and after breaking down they can cause injury.

External Supports During Weightlifting

Belts, wraps, and other external lifting supports are not recommended during weightlifting. Such bracing tends to support inadequacies in postural and stabilizing strength. Lifting without external supports from the onset will allow people to develop the necessary musculature and postural and stabilization strength. These external supports tend to offer a false sense of security and allow people to attempt loads for which they are not prepared.

Muscle Soreness and Injury

Muscle soreness is a typical consequence of physical exertion and training. It is generally self-limiting and resolves in two or three days. Gentle stretching may alleviate some of the discomfort; however, excessive stretching may exacerbate the soreness. Pulled muscles are typically associated with inadequate preparation to train.

Hand Care in Weightlifting

Weightlifters should keep their hands clean and always wash and treat their hands after training. They should trim their fingernails on a regular basis. Calluses will develop due to contact with the bar. Weightlifters should treat calluses by filing (e.g., using an emery board) until they are smooth to keep them from building up excessively, and should apply a hand lotion to keep calluses smooth and soft to prevent tearing.

Nonexercising Injury

Always inspect the area to be used for exercise to ensure adequate space. Check floors, fields, running courses, and so on for hazards. Be sure everyone fully understands the objectives and lesson plan for the day and the route of any off-site course or trail. Training surfaces should be nonslip and should be clean. Keep running tracks and weight rooms free of clutter. Keep lifting bars and equipment, and weights on racks, off the floor. Use collars on weightlifting bars.

Skin Infection and Hygiene

Keep all exercise equipment in good repair and clean equipment after use. Participants should always wear the appropriate clothing, for example a shirt and shoes, when participating in a gym or weight room. They should shower after exercise to minimize the spread of germs and bacteria.

Adapting This Course for Your School

In this section we discuss adapting the principles and contents of the West Point Physical Program to an elementary or secondary physical education curriculum. Again, the four-stage sequence for teaching and training provides the framework for implementation into the curricular plan.

One of the biggest challenges at West Point, or of any university program, stems from the fact that students arrive with movement patterns and exercise habits they have already developed. It is within elementary- and secondary-level programs that the structural and biological foundation is formed and the physical future predicted. This is also where teaching and training are the most challenging and have the greatest impact. Incoming cadets with inadequate structural and work capacity development are automatically behind their counterparts. This significantly elevates the stress associated with indoctrination to the Military Academy as a whole, not just the Physical Program.

Table 9.4 is a theoretical model representing the percentage of time in the yearly plan devoted to each stage in the physical education curriculum.

Always incorporate Stage I structural and work capacity development into the curriculum, as this is the basis for all future teaching and learning. Emphasis on this stage (number of lessons) should be greater with younger children, less with high school age students. But as the theoretical model reflects, Stage I development should be neither eliminated nor overlooked. Stage I development in physical education provides the foundation for all future learning. The basis for sound, progressive teaching and the development of physical structure and skill acquisition is in teaching proper technique. This ensures efficient learning and safety. Early in physical development, try to separate Stage II skill development from Stage I work capacity development. Do not use the skills you are attempting to teach when conducting work capacity training. For example, do not develop leg work capacity by having students do high-repetition squats, or train cardiovascular fitness by having them use the basketball defensive gliding posture, or reinforce staying in a low body position by having them do hundreds of yards of duck walk. Early training in each of these will result in postural fatigue, and students will incorporate

Table 9.4 Time Devoted to Each Stage of the Model

	Stage I	Stage II	Stage III
Elementary	55	35	10
Junior high	40	35	25
Senior high	20	25	55

incorrect technique and dynamic compensations to complete the bout. This will interfere with acquisition of proper technique.

Stage I can be incorporated into the physical education curriculum in three ways: preparation for activity and training, the transition phase, and specific teaching units.

Preparation for Activity and Training

Prior to physical activity or exercise training, it is necessary to prepare the body for the structural and metabolic stress of activity and training. "Warm-up" actually includes three warming processes: warming the tissues of the body, increasing blood flow, and "jump-starting" metabolism. However, preparation to train should include more than increasing body temperature; it should also prepare the individual for the ranges of motion and the specific task to be encountered. Thus, warm-up should be dynamic, and the movements should resemble those to be used in the activity.

A way to prepare for the training of the day that will stimulate the relevant capacities is to group four or five relatively low-intensity exercises into one complex exercise. Appropriate selection of complexes, sequencing of complexes into circuits, or use of an obstacle course will progress the preparation for training from general to specific. The intensity is controlled by the selection of activities, the use of external loading, or both. Complexes, circuits, or obstacle courses should always include body weight manipulation (push-ups, pull-ups, crawling, tumbling, crab walk, climbing a cargo net, etc.). External loading can be provided using an empty weightlifting bar, dumbbells, kettle bells, or medicine balls, for example. To get students moving, complexes or circuits can utilize juggling, walking on a balance beam, rope ladders, speed ladders, dot-drill mats, obstacle courses, a treasure hunt in which each article to be found describes a movement or exercise, and so on. The main limitation to incorporating complexes, circuits, or obstacle courses into your program is your own imagination and creativity. You can augment the session with elements such as music, light shows, and video displays. As always, be sure to reinforce correct posture and technique even during preparative activity, as these are part of the training effect. All of these techniques will reinforce body position and postural strength, kinesthetic awareness, and movement quality. This technique of "warming up" will enhance the teaching and training process.

Transitioning Between Activities

Transition phases are essentially breaks in the teaching and training progression that emphasize recovery from previous activity or training and preparation for the next phase—hence the concept of "repair–prepare."

Repair The term "repair" implies recovery, a time to alleviate the cumulative stress of previous work that allows for an improvement in physical condition (adaptation) and permits growth and development. This important aspect of physical training and recovery is commonly ignored, especially with multisport athletes in junior high and high school. The body requires time to recover, grow, and develop; and participating in sport-specific development on a daily basis does not ensure this opportunity. This concept is of cardinal importance especially with younger students and athletes.

The term repair may also imply recovery from injury. This would include rehabilitation programs, which serve two purposes: recovery from injury and preparation for the next teaching and training cycle.

Prepare The second half of the concept is "prepare." Activity performed during transitions should also prepare the student for the specific and unique physical demands of the next unit (e.g., from basketball to swimming—preparative shoulder work; from swimming to load-bearing activity—preparative lower leg work), sport (junior or senior high multisport athlete), or training phase (from strength phase to power phase, power phase to competition phase, etc.). This is also a time to introduce new skills or drills that will be used in the next teaching and training cycle.

Transition phase teaching and training should include Stage I and II development. Many of the same techniques, exercises, complexes, or circuits that were discussed in connection with preparation can be used in the transition phase. However, a key concept in this phase is novelty. To defer physiological and psychological boredom, transition phase activity must involve some movements or exercises that are different from those used in the previous sequence. The number and focus of transition phases should be dictated by age, physical state, stage of growth and development, skill level and training and, in curricular physical education, the number of different activities to be encountered. Transition phases should be repeated throughout the teaching sequence to ensure continual development of the structural, technical,

and "metabolic" foundation. Again, programs for younger students and athletes should include more transitions to allow more time for foundation development and growth.

Academically, transition phases underscore the ongoing necessity to maintain or develop a foundational level of fitness for lifelong health and fitness. Even within everyday life and within active lifetime sport programs, people must incorporate a base program focused on Stage I development. Playing basketball or jogging every day will not provide the necessary stimulus to maintain whole-body muscle and bone mass. Thus, other elements are needed to ensure that all aspects of physical health and fitness are being addressed—this is the concept of a well-rounded program.

Teaching Fitness Units

The third way to incorporate Stage I development into the physical education curriculum is through specific teaching units. In general, each unit or training plan should have three phases:

- Base phase: Stage I development—preparation
- Development phase: Stages I and II—preparation and skill
- Performance phase: optimization of the skill and performance of the skill at a moderate level of proficiency

Cardiovascular Fitness The training program presented on pages 161-162 can be adjusted to form the basis for a teaching unit on cardiovascular fitness (Stage I—work capacity; Stage II—aerobic fitness, or $\dot{V}O_2$max). With adolescent runners, the major concern is how much is too much. One simple plan is to adjust the mileage in the basic plan for each student. Stronger runners should increase their mileage to match their individual fitness level, whereas slower or developing runners should remain at sensible and appropriate levels until they are ready to increase their training load. All adjustments in training volume and intensity should be based on assessment of the specific level of structural and work capacity development within your program. At the high school level, physical educators should provide more individualized instruction. Some students will improve rapidly and lack the patience to train at the same level as some of the slower runners. With all young participants it is important that you stress the value and benefit of running as a way of improving overall fitness and maintaining a healthy lifestyle.

The running plan can also be altered to include other forms of running, but make it fun! Design your program to include games that incorporate running, such as forms of tag or "capture the flag" types of team games. Design incentives to get children moving and running. If possible, avoid games that develop competition; rather, structure play such that children work as a group to reach a goal. One method is to have children set goals for some form of running every day in class. Develop a reward system for use when they do not miss a day. Note that the program and periodization plan presented on pages 161-162 can be applied to developing cardiovascular fitness lesson plans or training programs for other activities such as swimming, cycling, and rowing.

Another unique way to teach cardiovascular fitness is to include a unit on walking and hiking. A sample 10-week walking and hiking program follows. This can become either a teaching unit or physical preparation for a unit on jogging and running.

Walking and hiking can provide relatively low-impact exercise for students who want to remain active, maintain or gain healthy body composition, and enjoy the outdoors. While running and jogging generally lead more quickly to greater levels of aerobic fitness, walking and hiking can substantially raise one's level of physical health or fitness.

WALKING-HIKING PROGRAM

Here we describe a 10-week plan for walking or hiking (see table 9.5). Notice that the volume of training is measured according to total miles walked. Students who do not know the distance they have walked can monitor the duration.

On most days, walking or hiking should consist of relatively low-intensity workouts. People should not feel out of breath while walking or be unable to hold a conversation with a workout partner. Later in the training plan, one day of each week is marked with an asterisk. On these days, increase the intensity of the walk for one-third of the distance or time. For example, students walk 1 easy mile, then slightly increase the pace for the next mile, then recover with a slower pace for the third mile.

Never increase the total weekly volume by more than 10 percent. A student who walked 10 miles throughout a week should add no more than 1 additional mile the following week. Notice that the total weekly volume decreases during week 5. After four weeks of increasing total volume, drop the total volume to a lower level before beginning to increase it again. This will allow the body adequate time for recovery.

Table 9.5 10-Week Walking Program

	Sunday	Monday	Tuesday	Wednesday	Thursday	Friday	Saturday
1	3-mile walk		2-mile walk	4-mile walk		3-mile walk	
2	3-mile walk	2-mile walk		5-mile walk		3-mile walk	
3	4-mile walk		5-mile walk	2-mile walk		3-mile walk	
4	4.5-mile walk	3-mile walk		5-mile walk		3-mile walk	
5	3-mile walk		2-mile walk	5-mile walk		2-mile walk	
6	4-mile walk	2-mile walk		4-mile walk	2-mile walk	3-mile walk	
7	4-mile walk	2-mile walk	5-mile walk		2-mile walk	4-mile walk	
8	4-mile walk	2-mile walk		2-mile walk*	2-mile walk	3-mile walk	

(continued)

Table 9.5 *(continued)*

	Sunday	Monday	Tuesday	Wednesday	Thursday	Friday	Saturday
9	5-mile walk		2-mile walk	2-mile walk*	3-mile walk	3-mile walk	
10	6-mile walk	2-mile walk		3-mile walk*	2-mile walk	3-mile walk	

* Increase intensity

Weight Training The strength training program presented on pages 154-159 can be adjusted to form the basis for a teaching unit on weight training including both Stage I structural and postural strength and work capacity and Stage II skill and maximal strength and power development. When performed with proper technique and under appropriate supervision, weight training can and should be incorporated into the physical education curriculum. The risk of injury during weight training is the same as or less than for other exercise and sport involvement (Hamill, 1994; Pierce, Byrd, & Stone, 2006). Weight training can begin in the intermediate grades (4th-7th grades) with an exclusive Stage I focus. From 8th grade through high school there should be continued emphasis on Stage I development, progressing in intensity and loading (as appropriate to the technical proficiency and the goals of the student) to Stage II development. Developing strength as part of Stage I is paramount; but it is important to understand the definitions of the various types of muscular strength and the differences between them, as discussed earlier, and to know which type of strength you are developing in your program.

Weight training performed during Stage I should have a clear focus on structural and postural strength development that promotes work capacity, functional flexibility, and muscular strength, in this specific order. Training for structural and postural strength leads to overall gains in muscular strength, although unintended; muscular strength can (and usually does) develop ahead of physical function and skill. A common mistake with junior high school and high school athletes is training for muscular and skill strength to the detriment of structural and postural strength. For example, students might have great bench press strength but not be able to support body weight to perform push-ups, pull-ups, dips, or heavy squats because of low torso strength, resulting in injury to the back and knees. This inappropriate development of muscular strength promotes structural and postural weakness, reinforces bad technique, leads to dynamic compensations and a propensity for inferior performance, and ultimately injury.

When preparing teaching and training plans for younger students, adjust exercise intensity according to repetitions accomplished with correct technique rather than a percentage of the 1-RM. Incrementing training volume and intensity based on technique, not load lifted, will minimize inappropriate attempts at maximal lifts and reduce dynamic compensations. Likewise, reduce training loads when there are technical breakdowns.

Assessment

Assessment is a planned process for evaluating need, outcome, and value. In physical education, assessment includes evaluation of the program and the student. In assessing the physical development and skill competency of students, one evaluates both the effectiveness and the value of the program through the progress made by the students. The efficacy of a program can be confirmed or the program modified based on apparent deficiencies revealed through testing.

Diagnostic testing is important in monitoring individual progress. A sound assessment package can reinforce the value of physical education, physical activity, and health and fitness to students. It can serve to motivate individuals to begin or continue in a physical education program. On the other hand, administering assessments too often can decrease motivation and waste precious instructional time in the classroom.

Commanders in the Army ensure that fitness training is designed to assist soldiers in meeting the physical task demands specific to their mission, and not just to help them do well on the Army Physical Fitness Test. Physical educators at all levels must take this idea into consideration when developing assessment packages. Chapter 3 provides a detailed discussion of the function and principles of assessment.

West Point Physical Assessment

Four tests employed by the DPE to assess physical fitness are the Physical Aptitude Exam (PAE), the Army Physical Fitness Test (APFT), the Cadet Fitness Challenge (CFC), and the Indoor Obstacle Course Test (IOCT). With slight modifications, each of these tests is suitable for assessing the fitness levels of students in elementary school through college.

Stage I development is evaluated from the Physical Aptitude Exam and the Army Physical Fitness Test.

Physical Aptitude Exam A satisfactory score on the PAE is one of the requirements for admission to West Point. The PAE is a test of explosive power, muscular endurance, agility, coordination, and speed. It is useful in predicting a candidate's aptitude for successfully completing the challenging West Point Physical Program. The examination consists of five events: pull-ups (men) or flexed-arm hang (women), standing long jump, modified basketball throw, and 300-yard shuttle run. The entire PAE is administered indoors. Thus students should wear a shirt and shorts suitable for athletic activity and rubber-soled court shoes or cross-training shoes with good traction. The following sections present details of the tests and scoring scales.

PHYSICAL APTITUDE EXAM

PULL-UP

For both the pull-up and the flexed-arm hang, a bar 1 1/4 inches in diameter is suspended horizontally at least 8 feet (2.4 meters) above the ground. The bar must be fixed at both ends and should be immovable. During the pull-up (figure 9.2), students

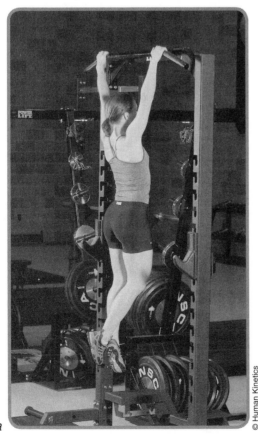

a *b* © Human Kinetics

FIGURE 9.2 Proper performance of the Physical Aptitude Exam pull-up.

begin by hanging from the bar with straight arms and palms facing away. The feet should not touch the ground in the fully suspended position. The test starts at the scorer's command "Up." At this command, students pull upward until the chin is above the bar and the jawline is parallel to the ground. At the scorer's command "Down," students lower themselves under control to the fully suspended position. Repetitions do not count if students fail to achieve the fully suspended position with arms straight, or fail to raise themselves so that the jawline is parallel to the ground, or use any type of kicking motion to raise themselves. No rest is permitted between repetitions. The mean pull-up score for a recent West Point class was 8.8 repetitions.

FLEXED-ARM HANG

Women begin the flexed-arm hang by ascending a ladder or using other means to raise the head above the bar with elbows fully flexed (figure 9.3). The hands are approximately shoulder-width apart, and the jawline is parallel to the ground. On the command "Go," the student steps off the support and maintains the fully flexed elbow position for as long as possible. The scorer keeps the time and stops the event when the student rests her chin on the bar, tilts her head backward such that her chin is no longer parallel to the ground, or begins to kick to maintain her position. The mean flexed-arm hang score for candidates from a recent class was 28 seconds.

STANDING LONG JUMP

The standing long jump is performed in a gymnasium with markings for a start line and at every 2 inches (5 centimeters) along the direction of flight. Students begin the test by placing their toes immediately behind the start line (figure 9.4). They jump as far forward as possible. Students may swing their arms and bend their knees before takeoff but may not take a preliminary hop in preparation for the jump. Students must jump and land using both feet simultaneously. The scorer records a foul if the student violates any of these conditions. At the conclusion of the jump, the scorer measures the distance from the start line to the body part that

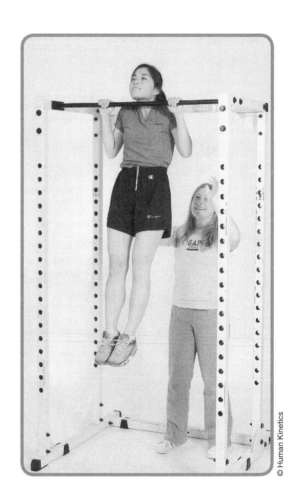

FIGURE 9.3 Proper performance of the Physical Aptitude Exam flexed-arm hang.

© Human Kinetics

is closest to the start line. Students are encouraged to take one practice jump. They are permitted three correctly executed jumps for score, with the longest counting for record. The mean scores for candidates from a recent West Point class were 7 feet 10 inches (2.4 meters) for men and 6 feet 2 inches (1.9 meters) for women.

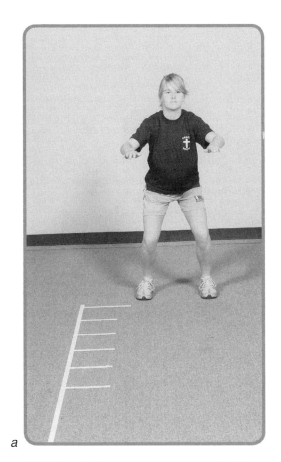
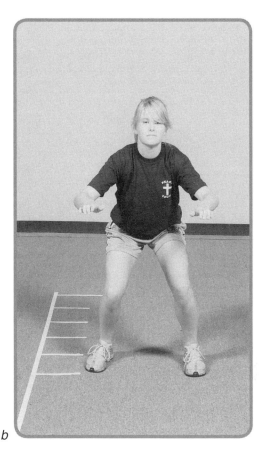

FIGURE 9.4   Proper performance of the Physical Aptitude Exam standing long jump.

MODIFIED BASKETBALL THROW

The modified basketball throw requires a regulation basketball, a 2-inch-thick mat placed behind the start line, and a measurement line marked on the gymnasium floor at 1-foot (.3-meter) intervals and extending a minimum of 90 feet (27 meters). A ceiling height of at least 22 feet (6.7 meters) is also recommended. The test begins with the student kneeling with both knees on the mat, immediately behind the start line (figure 9.5). The knees and shoulders must remain basically parallel to the start line during each attempt. For the attempt to count, neither knee may slide along or leave the mat during the throw. The student must throw the basketball as far as possible along the marked line using an overhand throw. Underhand or sidearm throws are discouraged. The nonthrowing hand may be used to steady the ball in preparation for the throw, but the student may not touch the floor or mat with either hand throughout the throw. Two scorers administer the test. One scorer controls activity at the start line, and the other measures the distance traveled. All throws are measured to the center of ball impact to the nearest 1 foot. Balls landing to either side of the scale are measured via visual estimation of a perpendicular line from impact to the scale. Any ball that hits the ceiling or a side wall or is not correctly thrown is not scored, and the student is given another attempt. Students receive one practice throw and three correctly executed throws for record. The best record throw counts for the score. The mean scores for candidates from a recent class were 67 feet (20 meters) for men and 39 feet (12 meters) for women.

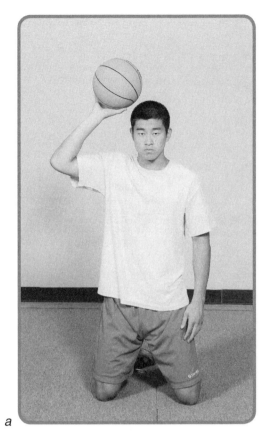
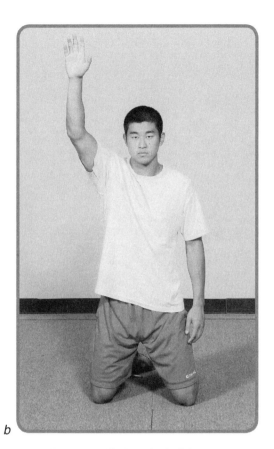

a   b

FIGURE 9.5 Proper performance of the Physical Aptitude Exam modified basketball throw.

300-YARD SHUTTLE RUN

The 300-yard shuttle run requires a gymnasium that measures at least 25 yards (23 meters) in length and a stopwatch for every scorer at the start/finish line. A start line and a turnaround line are established 25 yards apart and marked in a very visible way, for example with traffic cones. There are at least two lanes. Students may use a sprint, crouch, or standing start position as long as both feet are behind the line at the start. The start line also serves as the finish line. At the command "Go," students run six round trips as quickly as possible. Students must place at least one foot on or over the line at each turn. On the final lap, students sprint past the finish line. The score is recorded to a tenth of a second. If a student falls or is hindered by another student in an adjoining lane, he or she must stop. After a sufficient rest period, the student is given another attempt. The mean scores for candidates from a recent West Point class were 60.0 seconds for men and 69.1 seconds for women.

The score sheet for the PAE is shown on page 177. Both the scale and the events can be modified to meet your unique requirements. Certainly for younger populations such as elementary and middle school children, the scales should be adjusted. Moreover, it would probably be a good idea to substitute a smaller basketball for the modified basketball throw. However, the PAE should not require any adjustment for high school and college age students.

PHYSICAL APTITUDE EXAM SCORE SHEET

Name of candidate: _____

Home phone: _____

Address: _____

City: _____ State: _____ Zip: _____

SSN: _____

Signature: _____ Date: _____

Name of examiner: _____

Home phone: _____

Position: _____

Signature: _____ Date: _____

SCORES

Pull-ups (men) _____ (number of repetitions)

Standing long jump _____ (feet, inches)

Flexed-arm hang (women) _____ (seconds)

Kneeling basketball throw _____ (feet)

Push-ups _____ (number of repetitions)

300-yard shuttle run _____ (seconds)

Height _____ (inches)

Weight _____ (pounds)

Comments by examiner: _____

_____

_____

_____

_____

_____

Comments by candidate: _____

_____

_____

_____

_____

_____

From M. LeBoeuf and L. Butler, eds., 2008, *Fit & active* (Champaign, IL: Human Kinetics).

Army Physical Fitness Test Once students are at West Point, the APFT is the Army's evaluation of physical competency and basically represents the base level of fitness required to "wear the uniform." All soldiers in the U.S. Army, as well as USMA and Reserve Officers Training Corps (ROTC) students, must take and pass the APFT semiannually. The APFT events assess muscular endurance and cardiorespiratory fitness; they consist of repetition maximums in 2 minutes of the push-up and sit-up and a 2-mile run for minimum time. Alternatives for the 2-mile run include an 800-yard swim, a 10-kilometer cycle ergometer test, a 10-kilometer bicycle ride, or a 2.5-mile walk. Details on administering the APFT and standards of evaluation follow. A performance scale for each event is used to determine the student's score out of 100 points. Thus, there are 300 possible total points on the test. A sample scoring sheet is provided on page 180. Performance on the APFT is strongly linked to a student's fitness level and his or her ability to do fitness-related tasks.

Failure on the APFT, or on any of the physical testing performed during Cadet Basic Training or Cadet Field Training, places the cadet into the remediation program. This may include the Fitness Foundations course described earlier or one of the following programs:

- Commandant's Physical Remediation Program (CPRP): Cadets who record 60 points or less on an APFT event or have general failure are enrolled in CPRP, which is a daily physical development program administered by military staff from DPE.
- Commandant's Zone of Concern Program (CZCP): Cadets who record 70 points or less on an APFT event are enrolled in a remediation program administered by company tactical officers.

Cadets must accomplish a minimum of six weeks of remediation before retaking the APFT.

ARMY PHYSICAL FITNESS TEST

This section describes the push-up, sit-up, and cardiovascular fitness events that make up the APFT and presents the scoring scales and an APFT scoring sheet.

PUSH-UP

For the push-up (figure 9.6), the body must be kept in a generally straight line from the ankles to the shoulders throughout the entire exercise. The feet may be spread up to 12 inches (30 centimeters) apart. The starting position is the "up" position, in which the arms are fully extended and the balls of the feet are in contact with the ground.

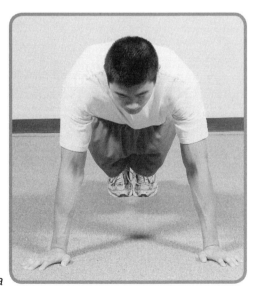
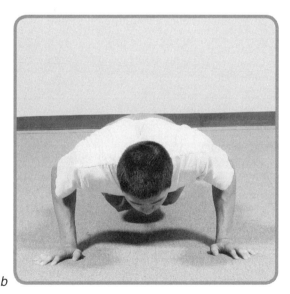

a *b*

FIGURE 9.6 The two positions involved in the push-up.

The hands may be positioned close together or wide apart. At the command to begin, the performer lowers the entire body toward the ground at least until the upper arm is parallel to the ground. Then the performer returns to the starting position by fully extending the arms. Students may sag at the waist or raise the buttocks in order to rest, but must return to the straight-body position before proceeding further. Students may not rest on the ground or use the ground to bounce off during the push-up. The hands may be repositioned during the event as long as they remain in contact with the ground at all times. Repetitions do not count for failure to (1) maintain the body in a generally straight line, (2) lower the body until the upper arms are at least parallel to the ground, or (3) extend the arms completely. The test is terminated if the performer remains on the ground and does not try to push up, or if the performer raises either hand or foot off the ground during the test. As long as students have not performed more than 10 repetitions, the grader stops those who perform the push-up incorrectly and provides instruction on the proper technique before sending them to a different grader.

SIT-UP

After finishing the push-up, students are permitted to rest for 10 minutes before performing the sit-up. The starting position for the sit-up is the "down" position (figure 9.7). Another student holds the performer's feet. The holder may use his or her hands to anchor the performer's feet. The performer's knees must be bent at about a 90-degree angle with the legs spread no wider than 12 inches (30 centimeters) apart. At the command to begin, the performer raises the torso off the ground to the "up" position. In this position the base of the neck must be raised vertically at least above the base of the spine. The fingers must remain interlocked behind the head, and the buttocks and heels must remain in contact with the ground throughout the event. The up position is the only authorized rest position, which performers can take as long as they do not brace the elbows against the knees to remain upright. After attaining the up position, the performer descends to the down position until at least the scapulae make contact with the ground. Repetitions are not counted for (1) failure to reach the vertical position, (2) failure to keep the fingers interlocked behind the head, (3) bucking off the ground by bouncing the buttocks, or (4) failure to keep the knee angle at less than 90 degrees. The test is terminated if the performer is in the down position and does not continue to attempt to sit up. As with the push-up, as long as students have not performed more than 10 repetitions, the grader stops those who perform incorrectly and provides instruction on the proper technique before sending them to another grader.

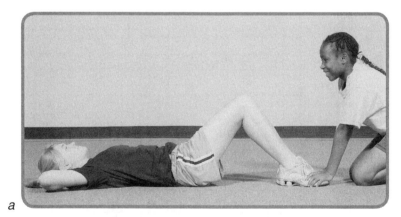

a

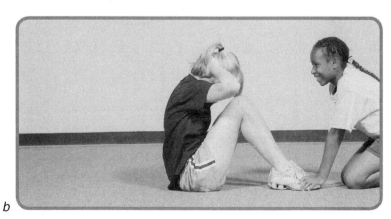

b

FIGURE 9.7　**The two positions involved in the sit-up.**

2-MILE RUN

Upon completing the sit-up, students are given a 10-minute rest before beginning the 2-mile run. The course must be relatively flat, with no more than a 3 percent grade. Additionally, the course must pose no significant hazards to the runners such as heavy pollution, obstacles to movement, and slippery surfaces. A 400-meter track is suitable in place of a quarter-mile (440-yard) track; however, one lap on a 400-meter track is 92 inches shorter than one lap on a 440-yard track. Therefore, students who run the 2-mile event on a 400-meter track must run eight laps plus an additional 61 feet 4 inches. If the test is not administered on a track, the grader must be careful to select a route that minimizes exposure to vehicular traffic. Students attempt to finish the 2-mile course in the shortest time possible. Walking is permitted but highly discouraged. Students must finish the run without any physical assistance. Encouragement and pacing from another person are permitted.

A sample scorecard for the APFT is shown in figure 9.8. The lowest passing APFT standards reflect the minimum acceptable fitness level for all soldiers in the Army. Standards for each gender are listed in the fitness testing information booklet, which can be accessed at www.usma.edu/dpe/testing/fm21-20/14ch.pdf. When applied to an Army unit, APFT results provide commanders with an assessment of the overall general fitness level of their units. As with Army units, the APFT may be used to promote competition between students to motivate them to improve their physical fitness levels.

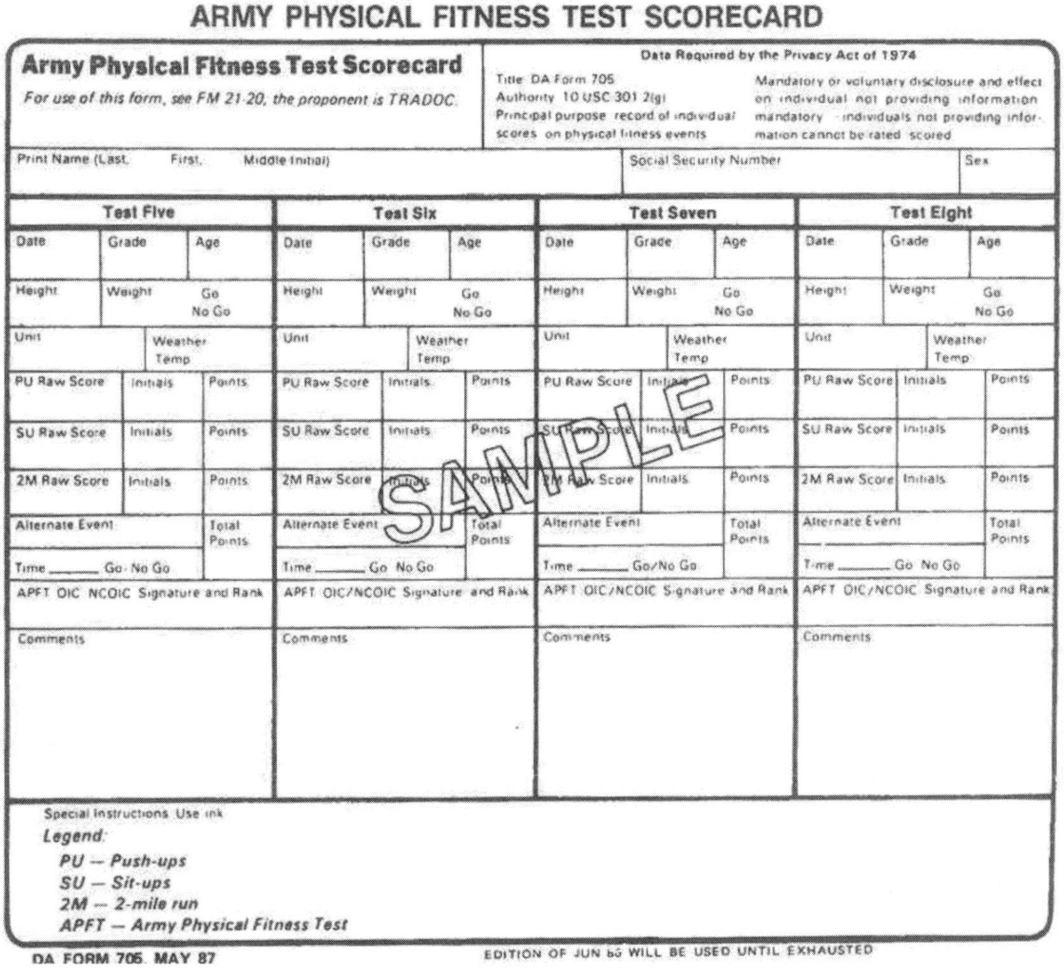

ARMY PHYSICAL FITNESS TEST SCORECARD

Army Physical Fitness Test Scorecard
For use of this form, see FM 21-20, the proponent is TRADOC.

Data Required by the Privacy Act of 1974
Title: DA Form 705
Authority: 10 USC 301 2(g)
Principal purpose: record of individual scores on physical fitness events
Mandatory or voluntary disclosure and effect on individual not providing information: mandatory - individuals not providing information cannot be rated scored

Print Name (Last, First, Middle Initial) | Social Security Number | Sex

Test Five	Test Six	Test Seven	Test Eight
Date / Grade / Age	Date / Grade / Age	Date / Grade / Age	Date / Grade / Age
Height / Weight / Go No Go	Height / Weight / Go No Go	Height / Weight / Go No Go	Height / Weight / Go No Go
Unit / Weather Temp	Unit / Weather Temp	Unit / Weather Temp	Unit / Weather Temp
PU Raw Score / Initials / Points	PU Raw Score / Initials / Points	PU Raw Score / Initials / Points	PU Raw Score / Initials / Points
SU Raw Score / Initials / Points	SU Raw Score / Initials / Points	SU Raw Score / Initials / Points	SU Raw Score / Initials / Points
2M Raw Score / Initials / Points	2M Raw Score / Initials / Points	2M Raw Score / Initials / Points	2M Raw Score / Initials / Points
Alternate Event / Total Points	Alternate Event / Total Points	Alternate Event / Total Points	Alternate Event / Total Points
Time ____ Go No Go	Time ____ Go No Go	Time ____ Go/No Go	Time ____ Go No Go
APFT OIC/NCOIC Signature and Rank	APFT OIC/NCOIC Signature and Rank	APFT OIC/NCOIC Signature and Rank	APFT OIC/NCOIC Signature and Rank
Comments	Comments	Comments	Comments

SAMPLE

Special Instructions: Use ink
Legend:
PU — Push-ups
SU — Sit-ups
2M — 2-mile run
APFT — Army Physical Fitness Test

DA FORM 705, MAY 87 EDITION OF JUN 80 WILL BE USED UNTIL EXHAUSTED

FIGURE 9.8 Sample Army Physical Fitness Test scorecard.

ALTERNATE ARMY PHYSICAL FITNESS TEST EVENTS

Students who cannot perform the 2-mile run may perform one of several alternate events designed to assess cardiorespiratory endurance. These tests include the 800-yard swim, the 10-kilometer (6.2-mile) stationary bike, the 10-kilometer bicycle ride, and the 2.5-mile (4-kilometer) walk. These events are graded on a pass/fail basis. The standards are presented in the following subsections. There are no alternate events for the push-up and the sit-up. The APFT counts for record as long as the student is able to perform any of the cardiorespiratory assessments.

800-Yard Swim Test

A swimming pool at least 25 yards (23 meters) long and 3 feet (.9 meters) deep is required for administering the 800-yard swim test. If the pool dimensions are metric, the scorer converts the distance traveled to yards by multiplying the number of meters by 39.37 and dividing the product by 36. That is, meters traveled × 39.37 / 36 = yards traveled. The student begins the test in the water by pushing off the pool wall. Students may use any stroke or combination of strokes to complete the 800-yard distance. Swimming goggles are the only equipment permitted. Students must touch the wall of the pool at each turn. The score is awarded based on the student's ability to complete the swim in a time equal to or less than that listed for his or her age and gender (see table 9.6).

10-Kilometer Stationary Bike Test

The 10-kilometer (6.2-mile) stationary bicycle ergometer test requires a bicycle ergometer and a level, firm base of support that measures at least 12 feet (3.6 meters) long by 6 feet (1.8 meters) wide. Before beginning the test, the student may adjust the seat height and handlebars for comfort. The scorer maintains the resistance setting on the ergometer flywheel at 2 kiloponds (20 Newtons) throughout the test. The student's score is based on the time required to complete the 10-kilometer distance.

6.2-Mile Bicycle Test

The 6.2-mile (10-kilometer) bicycle test is administered on a relatively flat course with a uniform surface and no obstacles to movement, including runners and walkers. The course must be clearly marked. The scorer should be able to see the student for the duration of the test; however, conducting the test on a 400-meter track is not advised. Although one-gear bicycles are preferred for this event, multigear bicycles may be used. If a multigear bicycle is used, the scorer must ensure that only one gear is used during the test. Taping the gear shifters at the appropriate settings is an acceptable way to do this. Students pedal at their own pace to complete the 6.2-mile course. The score is based on the student's ability to complete the distance in a time equal to or less than that listed for his or her age and gender (see table 9.6). The student is disqualified for leaving the course at any time during the test.

2.5-Mile Walk

The final alternate cardiorespiratory event is the 2.5-mile (4-kilometer) walk. This test can be administered on the same course as the 2-mile run. The student must walk throughout the entire test, with walking defined as having one foot in contact with the ground at all times. The score is based on the student's ability to complete the distance in a time equal to or less than that listed for his or her age and gender (see table 9.6).

Table 9.6 Alternate Test Standards by Event, Gender, and Age

Event	Gender	AGE							
		17-21	22-26	27-31	32-36	37-41	42-46	47-51	52+
800-yard swim	Men	20:00	20:30	21:00	21:30	22:00	22:30	23:00	24:00
	Women	21:00	21:30	22:00	22:30	23:00	23:30	24:00	24:30
6.2-mile bike	Men	24:00	24:30	25:00	25:30	26:00	27:00	28:00	30:00
(stationary and track)	Women	25:00	25:30	26:00	26:30	27:00	28:00	30:00	32:00
2.5-mile walk	Men	34:00	34:30	35:00	35:30	36:00	36:30	37:00	37:30
	Women	37:00	37:30	38:00	38:30	39:00	39:30	40:00	40:30

Evaluation of Stage II Physical Development

The Indoor Obstacle Course Test (IOCT) was developed at West Point and is unique to West Point. The IOCT is administered once per year to cadets, and the results are included in the cadet's physical grade. The IOCT is an evaluation of Stage I and II attributes, a combination of work capacity, muscular strength, agility, and gymnastics skills. The test includes running (with and without an external load), rope and apparatus climbing to move between the first and second levels of the gymnasium, vaulting, balancing, wall climbing, crawling, and other skills. Each of these skills is initially taught and developed in the Military Movement course during the plebe year. The Military Movement course and the IOCT are described in detail in chapters 4 and 8.

Evaluations conducted by DPE indicate that results from the combination of APFT and IOCT give a general indication of fitness and readiness for military performance. However, the specific definition of military fitness is not completely clear, and the physical attributes that preclude physical preparation for and prediction of military readiness and performance are not completely understood. For this reason, other assessments have been developed, and research is ongoing in an effort to understand the physical factors that predict military readiness and performance.

One such test is the Cadet Fitness Challenge. In the mid- to late 1990s, DPE created the CFC in an attempt to provide cadets with a fun, competitive fitness assessment designed to inspire them to achieve greater levels of personal physical fitness. The CFC addresses physical fitness through tests of work capacity, cardiorespiratory fitness, muscular strength, and flexibility. The CFC is grouped into five broad sections according to the fitness component addressed. These are cardiovascular or aerobic fitness, cardiovascular or high-intensity fitness, upper body muscular fitness, lower body and shoulder and midsection muscular fitness, and flexibility. The scales are criterion referenced and gender based. A particularly appealing aspect of the CFC is that students are permitted to choose from among a menu of activities within each grouping. Rationale for event inclusion focuses on availability of equipment, popularity of events based on cadet input, and use of existing national protocols. See page 183 for a score sheet for the CFC.

Cardiovascular fitness is evaluated with either a 3-mile run, a 6,000-meter row, a 22-minute cycle ergometer test, a 1,500-yard swim, or a 2.3-mile (3.7-kilometer) uphill run. High-intensity cardiovascular fitness is evaluated using either a 400-meter run, a 60-second rowing test, a 60-second cycle ergometer sprint test, a 100-yard swim, or a 300-yard shuttle run. Upper body muscular fitness is evaluated with a cadence pull-up test and one of the following: a chest press for repetitions test, a 1-RM chest press, or a hammer incline press. Lower body fitness is determined by either a leg press repetitions test, a 1-RM back squat, or a squat maximum repetitions test. Abdominal fitness is evaluated using an ankles-to-the-bar test, and flexibility is evaluated using the sit and reach test. Specific instructions for performing each test and scoring scales are presented on pages 183-197. Data from the CFC can be used to evaluate cadet physical development and in relation to the APFT and IOCT, leading to a better understanding of physical development and military readiness.

Score Sheet for Cadet Fitness Challenge

Aerobic cardiovascular fitness *(choose one event)*

Event	Date	Duration or kilogram meters	Points	Witness (verified by another person)
3-mile run				
6,000-meter row				
22-minute bike				
1,500-yard swim				
2.3-mile uphill run				
Anaerobic cardiovascular fitness *(choose one event)*				
400-meter run				
60-second row				
60-second bike				
100-yard swim				
300-yard shuttle run				
Upper body muscular fitness *(choose one event plus cadence pull-ups)*				
Chest press repetitions				
1-repetition chest press				
Hammer incline press				
Cadence pull-ups				
Lower body and shoulder/midsection muscular fitness *(choose one event plus ankles-to-the-bar)*				
Hammer independent leg press				
1-repetition back squat				
Ankles-to-the-bar				
Flexibility				
Sit and reach				

From M. LeBoeuf and L. Butler, eds., 2008, *Fit & active* (Champaign, IL: Human Kinetics).

CADET FITNESS CHALLENGE

Next we describe the events and scoring for the CFC.

AEROBIC CARDIOVASCULAR FITNESS

3-Mile Run

The 3-mile run is administered on a relatively flat course with no obstructions to movement. Students must complete the run in the fastest possible time. The scoring scale is shown in the following table.

3-Mile Run

MEN			WOMEN	
Mile pace	Time	Total points	Mile pace	Time
6:00	18:00	50	7:00	21:00
6:07	18:21	49	7:07	21:21
6:15	18:45	48	7:15	21:45
6:22	19:06	46	7:22	22:06
6:30	19:30	45	7:30	22:30
6:45	20:15	44	7:45	23:15
6:55	20:45	42.5	7:55	23:45
7:30	22:30	41	8:30	25:30
7:37	22:51	40	8:37	25:51
7:44	23:12	37	8:44	26:12
7:51	23:33	35	8:51	26:33
8:00	24:00	32	9:00	27:00
>8:00	>24:00	0	>9:00	>27:00

6,000-Meter Row

We use a Concept rowing machine for the 6,000-meter row. The damper setting for men and women is 3 and 2, respectively. Before the test begins, the distance indicator is set to 6,000 meters. Each student must row until the distance indicator reads 0 meters. At the conclusion of the test the scorer records the total time elapsed. The scoring scale is shown in the following table.

6,000-Meter Row

MEN			WOMEN	
500-meter pace	Time	Total points	500-meter pace	Time
1:50+	22:30	50	2:05+	25:30
1:55	23:00	49	2:10	26:00
	23:30	48		26:30

MEN		Total points	WOMEN	
500-meter pace	Time		500-meter pace	Time
2:00	24:00	46	2:15	27:00
	24:30	44		27:30
2:05	25:00	42.5	2:20	28:00
2:10	26:00	41	2:25	29:00
2:15	27:00	40	2:30	30:00
	27:30	38		30:30
2:20	28:00	37	2:35	31:00
2:25	29:00	35	2:40	32:00
2:30	30:00	32	2:45	33:00
>2:30	>30:00	0	>2:45	>33:00

22-Minute Bike Test

The 22-minute bike test is administered using a Stairmaster Upright Spinnaker 3000 machine set on self-pace. Students enter their weight and "22" for time. At the test's completion, the scorer records the total work performed, expressed in kilogram meters. The scoring scale is shown in the following table.

22-Minute Bike

MEN	Total points	WOMEN
Work (kgm)		Work (kgm)
31,000	50	25,730
30,500	49	25,315
30,000	48	24,900
29,500	46	24,485
29,000	45	24,070
28,250	44	23,448
27,500	42.5	22,825
25,500	41	21,165
24,500	40	20,335
24,000	38	19,920
23,500	37	19,505
22,500	35	18,675
21,000	32	17,430
<21,000	0	<17,430

1,500-Yard Swim

The 1,500-yard swim test can be administered in a 25-yard or 50-yard pool. If the pool you use is metric, use the following equation to convert to yards traveled: meters traveled × 39.37 / 36 = yards traveled. Students begin the test in the pool. At the command "Go," the student pushes off the pool wall and uses any stroke or combination of strokes to swim the prescribed distance. Students must touch the pool wall each time they make a turn, and must not touch the wall for longer than 2 seconds. The scorer counts the laps to ensure that the student swims 1,500 yards, and records the total time required to complete the distance. The scoring scale is shown in the following table.

1,500-Yard Swim

MEN		WOMEN
Time	Total points	Time
23	50	25:04
24:30	49	26:34
26	48	28:20
26:30	46	28:53
27	45	29:26
27:30	44	30:00
28	42.5	30:31
29	41	31:37
30	40	32:42
30:30	38	33:12
31	37	33:47
32	35	34:53
33	32	35:58
>33	0	>35:58

2.3-Mile Uphill Run

The course for the 2.3-mile (3.7-kilometer) uphill run begins at a point along the Hudson River and ends at the top of a small mountain at West Point. This route has been popular with students who want to tackle a real challenge. You can establish a course wherever you wish as long as you have a strategy to minimize safety hazards such as heavy traffic. The scorer records the total time required for the student to complete the course. The scoring scale is shown in the following table.

2.3-Mile Uphill Run

MEN		WOMEN
Time	Total points	Time
17:00	50	20:00
17:15	49	20:15
17:30	48	20:30
17:45	46	20:45
18:15	45	21:00
18:35	44	21:20
18:45	42.5	21:30
19:15	41	22:00
19:45	40	22:30
20:15	38	23:00
21:15	35	24:00
22:15	32	25:00
>22:15	0	>25:00

HIGH-INTENSITY CARDIOVASCULAR FITNESS

400-Meter Run

We administer the 400-meter run on a standard athletic track that measures 400 meters in length. However, you can establish this course anywhere you like as long as the surface is relatively level and vehicular traffic is minimal. Students may wear spikes and use starting blocks according to their personal preferences. The scorer records the time it takes the student to run one complete lap. The scoring scale is shown in the following following table.

400-Meter Run

MEN		WOMEN
Time (s)	Total points	Time (s)
62	50	68
63	49	69
64	48	70
65	46	71
66	45	72
67	44	73
68	42.5	74

(continued)

400-Meter Run *(continued)*

| MEN | | WOMEN |
Time (s)	Total points	Time (s)
78	41	84
83	40	89
85	38	91
88	37	94
93	35	99
98	32	104
>98	0	>104

60-Second Row

Students use a Concept rowing machine when performing the 60-second row. The damper must be set to 2 for women and 3 for men. Students set the time at 1 minute and row until the time has elapsed. The scorer records the number of meters rowed. The scoring scale is shown in the following table.

60-Second Row

| MEN | | WOMEN |
Distance (m)	Total points	Distance (m)
333	50	306
330	49	303
328	48	301
326	46	299
323	45	297
322	44	296
320	42.5	294
317	41	292
309	40	284
305	38	281
302	37	278
294	35	271
286	32	263
<286	0	<263

60-Second Bike

We use a Stairmaster Spinnaker 3000 machine for the 60-second bike test. Before starting the test, students set the machine for self-pace and enter their weight and 5 minutes for time. This is the lowest time setting the machine will accept. However, the scorer must ensure that the student pedals for only 1 minute. At the conclusion of the test, the scorer records the total work performed in kilogram meters. The scoring scale is shown in the following table.

60-Second Bike

MEN		WOMEN
Work (kgm)	Total points	Work (kgm)
3,200	50	2,790
3,100	49	2,700
3,000	48	2,610
2,900	46	2,523
2,800	45	2,430
2,700	44	2,349
2,600	42.5	2,250
2,400	41	2,070
2,200	40	1,890
2,100	38	1,827
2,000	37	1,710
1,800	35	1,530
1,600	32	1,350
<1,600	0	<1,350

100-Yard Swim

As with the 1,500-yard swim, the 100-yard swim can be administered in a 25-yard or 50-yard pool. Except for distance traveled, the rules for this event are similar to those for the 1,500-yard swim. The scoring scale is shown in the following table.

100-Yard Swim

MEN		WOMEN
Time (s)	Total points	Time (s)
68	50	75
69	49	76
70	48	77
71	46	78
72	45	79
73	44	80
74	42.5	81

(continued)

100-Yard Swim *(continued)*

MEN	Total points	WOMEN
Time (s)		Time (s)
76	41	83
78	40	85
79	38	86
80	37	87
82	35	89
84	32	91
>84	0	>91

300-Yard Shuttle Run

The 300-yard shuttle run can be administered indoors or outdoors as long as the course is established properly. The scorer marks a start line and a turnaround line 25 yards away. Students must complete six round trips as fast as possible. At least one foot must touch or cross the line at each turn. The scorer records the time required to complete the course. The scoring scale is shown in the following table.

300-Yard Shuttle Run

MEN	Total points	WOMEN
Time (s)		Time (s)
60	50	66
61	49	67
62	48	68
63	46	69
64	45	70
65	44	71
66	42.5	72
68	41	74
70	40	76
71	38	77
72	37	78
74	35	80
76	32	82
>76	0	>82

UPPER BODY MUSCULAR FITNESS

Chest Press Repetitions

We conduct the chest press repetitions event with a barbell and weight plates and a flat bench. Regardless of body weight, men lift 175 pounds (79 kilograms) and women lift 90 pounds (41 kilograms) for as many repetitions as possible until they reach momentary muscular failure. The head, shoulders, and buttocks must remain in contact with the bench throughout the entire test. The feet must remain in contact with the floor. The student's hands must grip the bar with a "thumbs-around" grip, locking the bar safely in the palms of the hands. The student's partner serves as both scorer and spotter. As spotter, the partner ensures that the student moves the weight through a full range of motion. Once the spotter touches the bar, no more repetitions are counted. Note that this test correlates well with a 1-RM lift strength test (r = 0.96). The scoring scale is shown in the following table.

Chest Press Repetitions

MEN		WOMEN
Repetitions	Total points	Repetitions
24	25	18
22	24	17
20	23.5	16
18	23	15
16	22.5	14
14	22	13
12	21.25	12
10	20.5	10
8	20	8
7	19.5	7
6	19	6
4	17.5	4
2	16	2
<2	0	<2

1-Repetition Chest Press

The 1-repetition chest press is also performed on a flat bench with a barbell and weight plates. The role of the partner and the basic lifting techniques and rules are similar to those for the chest press repetitions event. Additionally, after receiving a "lift" from the spotter, the student must hold the bar motionless for 1 second before lowering it to the chest. The bar must touch the chest in a brief pause in the lowered phase, and then must be held motionless again for 1 second before the student returns it to the rack. The student may not stop, bounce, shift the feet, change the position of the hands, or unevenly extend the bar during the lift. The goal is to achieve a valid maximum effort within three attempts. Students may wear a weight belt, but no other gear is permitted.

The spotter must remain vigilant throughout the lift. Attempts do not count if the spotter touches the bar before the 1-second pause at the conclusion of the lift. The scoring scale is shown in the following table.

1-Repetition Chest Press

MEN		WOMEN
Weight (lb)	Total points	Weight (lb)
300	25	155
285	24	150
275	23.5	140
255	23	135
245	22.5	125
235	22	120
225	21.25	115
215	20.5	110
205	20	105
200	19.5	100
195	19	
185	17.5	95
180	16	
<180	0	<95

Hammer Incline Press

We conduct the hammer incline press on a Hammer Strength inclined press machine. Before beginning the test, students adjust the seat height so that the handles are at the nipple line of the chest. The goal is to perform as many repetitions as possible. Men lift 105 pounds (48 kilograms) and women lift 60 pounds (27 kilograms), regardless of body weight. Students must use a full range of motion during the test. They may not allow the bar pads to touch the machine. The scorer ends the test when the student achieves momentary muscular failure and is unable to perform another correct repetition. The scoring scale is shown in the following table.

Hammer Incline Press

MEN		WOMEN
Repetitions	Total points	Repetitions
24	25	12
22	24	11
20	23.5	10
18	23	

MEN		WOMEN
Repetitions	**Total points**	**Repetitions**
16	22.5	9
14	22	
12	21.25	8
10	20.5	7
8	20	6
7	19.5	
6	19	5
4	17.5	4
2	16	3
<2	0	<3

Cadence Pull-Up

Students perform cadence pull-ups on a 1 1/4-inch bar suspended horizontally at least 8 feet (2.4 meters) from the ground and fixed at both ends. The feet should not touch the ground in the fully suspended position. The student begins the test by hanging from the bar with arms fully extended and palms facing away. When the student begins the hang, the scorer starts a chronograph. At the 5-second mark the scorer announces "up" and the student performs a pull-up until the jawline is parallel to the ground and the chin is above the bar. Once the student achieves this position, he or she returns to the fully suspended position and awaits the next command to pull. The scorer announces "up" every 5 seconds. The student must keep pace with the cadence during the test. Repetitions do not count if the student fails to get the chin above the bar or the jawline parallel to the ground, or kicks to raise the body. The scorer ends the test when the student can no longer correctly perform pull-ups to the cadence. The scoring scale is shown in the following table.

Cadence Pull-Up

MEN		WOMEN
Repetitions	**Total points**	**Repetitions**
17	25	7
16	23.5	6
15	22.5	5
14	21.25	4
13	20.75	
12	20.5	
11	20.25	

(continued)

Cadence Pull-Up (continued)

MEN		WOMEN
Repetitions	Total points	Repetitions
10	20	3
9	19.5	
8	19	2
7	18	
6	17.5	1
5	17	
4	16.5	
3	16	
<3	0	<1

LOWER BODY AND SHOULDER AND MIDSECTION MUSCULAR FITNESS

Hammer Independent Leg Press

We use a Hammer Strength machine to perform the hammer independent leg press. Men lift 180 pounds (82 kilograms) per leg (four 45-pound plates), and women lift 135 pounds (61 kilograms) per leg (three 45-pound plates). Before beginning, students must adjust the seat height such that the hamstrings are perpendicular to the floor when the foot is on the footpad. The entire foot must be in contact with the footpad throughout the exercise. The student presses with both legs simultaneously, and the scorer ensures that the student maintains a full range of motion. The machine must not hit the bumper guard at the end of the eccentric movement. If contact is made, the scorer stops the test. The scoring scale is shown in the following table.

Hammer Independent Leg Press

MEN		WOMEN
Repetitions	Total points	Repetitions
24	25	20
22	24	19
20	23.5	18
18	23	17
16	22.5	16
14	22	14
12	21.25	12
10	20.5	10
8	20	8
7	19.5	7

6	19	6
4	18	4
2	17.5	2
1	16	1
<1	0	<1

1-Repetition Back Squat

Students perform the 1-RM back squat using a barbell with weight plates and a squat rack. As a strength assessment, the goal is to lift as much weight as possible in one repetition. Students may wear a weight belt for support, but no other equipment is permitted. To mitigate risk to novice weightlifters, we stress that only experienced lifters should attempt this test. The scorer must also serve as the spotter. Once the barbell is positioned in the weight rack, the student assumes an upright position under the bar with the bar held horizontally across the shoulders. The thumbs must fully wrap around the bar. The student lifts the bar off the rack and takes a half-step backward to the starting position. He or she must remain motionless with knees locked in the starting position for 1 second. The student bends the knees until the top surface of the thighs at the hip joint is lower than the top of the knees. Students may not stop, bounce, shift the feet, or change the position of the bar on the shoulders during the attempt. To finish the lift, the student recovers to the starting position and holds this position for 1 second before returning the load to the weight rack. The spotter may assist in returning the load to the rack. The scoring scale is shown in the following table.

1-Repetition Back Squat

MEN		WOMEN
Weight (lb)	Total points	Weight (lb)
405	25	265
395	24	255
385	23.5	245
375	23	240
365	22.5	235
355	22	230
345	21.25	225
335	20.5	215
325	20	210
315	19.5	200
305	19	195
295	17.5	190
285	16	185
<285	0	<185

Ankles-to-the-Bar

Students perform the ankles-to-the-bar event by hanging from a 1 1/4-inch bar suspended horizontally above the ground. To begin the test, the student hangs from the bar with arms fully extended. The feet should not touch the ground. The palms should face away from the body, and the arms should be positioned approximately shoulder-width apart. The student flexes at the hip and rocks back until the ankles touch the bar and the hips are elevated higher than the shoulders. The student returns to the start position with arms fully extended before attempting another repetition. The outside of the legs may not rest against the inside of the arms in the up position. The scorer does not count incorrectly performed repetitions. The scoring scale is shown in the following table.

Ankles-to-the-Bar

MEN		WOMEN
Repetitions	Total points	Repetitions
17	25	7
16	23.5	6
15	22.5	5
14	21.25	4
13	20.75	
12	20.5	
11	20.25	
10	20	3
9	19.5	
8	19	2
7	18	
6	17.5	1
5	17	
4	16.5	
3	16	
<3	0	<1

FLEXIBILITY

Sit and Reach

The sit and reach test assesses lower back and hamstring flexibility. We use an Accuflex sit and reach box to perform this assessment. Before beginning, students should perform a thorough warm-up to increase muscle temperature. The scorer ensures that the 23-centimeter mark on the index scale is positioned at the soles of the performer's feet and braces the box by standing opposite the performer. The performer sits on the ground with legs fully extended and the soles of the feet flat against the box. He or she exhales and slowly reaches forward with both hands in an attempt to slide the index tab as far as possible past the toes. The knees must remain fully extended throughout the movement. The performer must momentarily hold the reach before returning to the sitting position. The student performs three attempts, and the scorer counts the farthest distance reached for record. The scoring scale is shown in the following table.

Sit and Reach

MEN		WOMEN
Distance (cm)	Total points	Distance (cm)
39	50	40
38.5	48	39.5
38	47	39.25
37.5	46	39
37	45	38.5
36.5	44	38.25
36	42.5	38
35.5	41	37.5
35	40	37
34	39	36
33.5	38	35.5
33	35	35
30	32	33
<30	0	<33

Evaluation of Stage III and Stage IV Physical Development Assessments also come by way of grading in Lifetime Activity classes and participation in athletics. Every cadet gets an athletic grade based on Core-, Club-, or Company-level athletics, and this is factored into their overall physical grade.

Adapting Assessments for Your Program

While it is relatively easy to adapt assessments, the biggest issue becomes developing tests to meet the needs and requirements of a particular curriculum. Assessments should be designed to evaluate and understand the impact of your program while pro-

viding an accurate assessment of student development. There are many packaged fitness and skills tests, including those utilized at West Point, that you can use to assess your program and students. Many of these assessments include normative data, scoring scales, or both. The scoring scales used at West Point are included at the end of each test. These can provide a model for determining scoring scales specific to your program. However, these scales and normative data are merely a good place to begin; ideally both should be specifically developed within your program.

The APFT can be modified to accommodate elementary and middle school children. First, the scoring scales can be norm referenced to your unique setting to provide a more valid assessment.

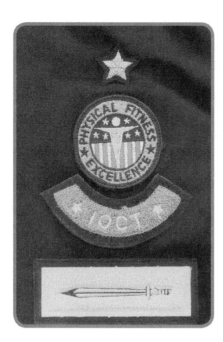

FIGURE 9.9 Some West Point incentives toward physical fitness excellence.

Second, the push-up is much easier to perform with the knees rather than the feet touching the ground. This technique might be considered for elementary school children. Third, although the sit-up is contraindicated in most situations, it is still the event the Army uses to measure hip flexor and abdominal muscular endurance. To prevent cervical strain, you can substitute another assessment such as the curl-up, or instruct children to place their hands on their hips or fold their arms across their chests while performing the sit-up. For young college-aged students there should be no requirement for adjustment of the APFT other than modifications to the sit-up event.

Developing a fitness challenge at your school can be quite easy. All it takes is a fundamental knowledge of exercise science, creativity, and a desire to make the experience fun. There is practically no end to the types of events that can be incorporated. Likewise, obstacle courses provide a unique, challenging, and enjoyable tool for evaluating the physical education program and student development. See chapters 4 and 8 for discussion of obstacle courses and how to adapt them for teaching and evaluation.

Consider motivational challenges, present fitness levels, and realistically challenging criterion levels specific to your population of students. Inspect the area around your school. Perhaps there is a prominent piece of terrain such as a hill or wide expanse of field that you can incorpo-

rate as a challenge. Even if you have a constrained budget, there is virtually no end to the types of events you can include in your evaluation package.

Incentive Programs

Incentive programs are a great way to extrinsically motivate students toward increased fitness. Be careful not to link all incentives exclusively to being a top performer (the "best" or the "fastest"). Incentives should reward improvement or excellent class participation, or encourage weaker performers to participate without feeling threatened about poor performance or finishing last. Be creative when developing incentives, which should depend on the student population and what they value. Pizza parties, banners, fitness badges, and public praise are examples of incentives that might work well. Aside from the grade, West Point cadets can earn badges for outstanding performance in our program. These badges (figure 9.9), worn on the physical education uniform, serve as a constant visual reminder of physical excellence.

Together, fitness development and assessment play a vital role in a well-rounded program that has the objective of increasing students' personal physical fitness. We recognize that West Point has a unique mission and purpose for developing fitness excellence in our students. Furthermore, our resources for accomplishing this goal are much more robust than in most school settings at any level. However, regardless of your situation, you can modify the information presented in this chapter not only to improve the fitness levels of your students, but also to increase the likelihood that they will adhere to a lifetime commitment to physical fitness.

References

American College of Sports Medicine. (2000). *ACSM's guidelines for exercise training and prescription.* (6th ed.). Baltimore: Lippincott, Williams & Wilkins.

American Heart Association. (2002). Guidelines for primary prevention of cardiovascular disease and stroke: 2002 update: Consensus panel guide to comprehensive risk reduction for adult patients without coronary or other atherosclerotic vascular diseases. *Circulation, 106,* 388-391.

Brechue, W.F. (1995). New guidelines for exercise training the middle-aged and elderly for fitness and health. *Science of Training, 7,* 59-65.

Daniels, J. (1998). *Daniels' running formula.* Champaign, IL: Human Kinetics.

Department of the Army. (2000). *Physical fitness training.* Field Manual No. 21-20. Washington, DC: Headquarters, U.S. Army.

Hamill, B.P. (1994). Relative safety of weightlifting and weight training. *Journal of Strength and Conditioning Research, 8,* 53-57.

Noakes, T.D. (1991). *The lore of running.* Champaign, IL: Leisure Press.

Pate, R.R., Pratt, M., Blair, S.N., et al. (1995). Physical activity and public health: A recommendation from the Centers for Disease Control and the American College of Sports Medicine. *Journal of the American Medical Association, 273,* 402-407.

Pierce, K.K.C., Byrd, R.J., & Stone, M.H. (2006). Position statement and literature review: Youth weightlifting. *Olympic Coach, 18,* 10-13.

Pollock, M.L., Feigenbaum, M.S., & Brechue, W.F. (1995). Exercise prescription for physical fitness. *Quest, 47,* 319-337.

Selye, H. (1951). General Adaptation Syndrome and diseases of adaptation. *Southern Medical Journal, 113,* 315-323.

U.S. Army. 1992. *U.S. Army field manual 21-20: Physical fitness training.* Washington, DC: Department of Defense.

Suggested Readings

Bompa, T., & Cornacchia, L. (1998). *Serious strength training: Periodization for building muscle power and mass.* Champaign, IL: Human Kinetics.

Cavanagh, P.R. (1980). *The running shoe book.* Mountain View, CA: Anderson World.

Fahey, T. (1996). *Basic weight training for men and women.* Mountain View, CA: Mayfield.

Fleck, S., & Kraemer, W.J. (1997). *Designing resistance training programs.* Champaign, IL: Human Kinetics.

Henderson, J. (1969). *Long slow distance—the humane way to train.* Mountain View, CA: World.

McKenzie, D.C., Clement, D.B., & Taunton, J.E. (1985). Running shoes, orthotics, and injuries. *Sports Medicine, 2,* 334-347.

Pretorius, D.M., Noakes, T.D., Irving, G.A., & Allerton, K.E. (1986). Runner's knee: What is it and how effective is conservative treatment. *Physician and Sportsmedicine, 14,* 71-81.

National Governing Organizations

American College of Sports Medicine (ACSM)
401 West Michigan Street
Indianapolis, IN 46202-3233
317-637-9200
Fax: 317-634-7817
www.acsm.org

National Strength and Conditioning Association (NSCA)
1885 Bob Johnson Drive
Colorado Springs, CO 80906
800-815-6826
Fax: 719-632-6367
www.ncsa-lift.org

USA Weightlifting
1 Olympic Plaza
Colorado Springs, CO 80909
719-866-4508
www.usaweightlifting.org

Wellness

Ralph Pim and Whitfield East

The goal of this chapter is to provide the public school and higher education teacher with a resource guide for the development of a health-related wellness course. This chapter is not intended to be a content resource. We offer some foundational statements, which we use to frame our Wellness course at West Point; however, the majority of this chapter focuses on lesson outlines and active learning activities.

Defining Wellness

Hoeger and Hoeger (2004) identified seven components of well-being—physical, mental, emotional, social, environmental, occupational, and spiritual—that affect our quality of life. The process of being well requires our selective attention to all the components of wellness. The critical or operative word in the previous sentence is "process." The act of well-being is a continuous, lifelong journey that requires a commitment to learning and adapting personal behaviors to changing physical, social, and emotional circumstances in order to optimize quality of life. Only when we teach our students to embrace well-being as a journey, rather than a destination, do we truly effect change in their lives.

Teaching Wellness

Throughout our life span, there are many cycles or periods that garner our primary attention. These cycles depend on our age and social circumstances. During the formative years, children are primarily focused on cognitive and psychomotor development and on building social relationships. Mortality is an irrelevant term for most youth, who show little concern for long-term health-related risks. Upon entering young adulthood, our personal focus shifts to career and family. Most individuals find themselves relatively healthy, as the effects of chronic lifestyle diseases are not yet manifest. Then quite suddenly we awaken as adults to the reality of being 30 pounds overfat with significant knee and back pain and showing signs of stage I hypertension with initial onset of coronary heart disease—and seemingly dumbfounded and incredulous at the gradual and often imperceptible way in which these physiological and emotional changes have occurred.

Human beings are predisposed to focus on the present and dwell on the past. Few in our society have the ability and the will to appreciate the long-term deleterious effects of certain lifestyle behaviors. A simple example of this fact is the percentage of adults engaging in vigorous leisure-time physical activity three or more times per week. Fewer than 26 percent of the adult population exercise regularly based upon the American College of Sports Medicine guidelines. There are certain iconic examples of the longitudinal effects of lifestyle behaviors that seem to resonate with students. The story of Wayne McLaren is just such a cautionary tale. McLaren portrayed the "Marlboro Man" in cigarette advertisements for almost 15 years. A rugged and handsome rodeo rider and Hollywood stunt man, he smoked a pack and a half of cigarettes every day for about 25 years until he was diagnosed with lung cancer in 1990. During his last months McLaren fought actively to educate the public about the hazards of smoking. Some of his last words were, "Tobacco will kill you, and I'm living proof of it. I've spent the last month of my life in an incubator and I'm telling you, it's just not worth it" ("Marlboro Man," 1992). He died at the age of 51.

The inability of most students to appreciate the long-term deleterious effects of lifestyle behaviors on quality of life truly defines the instructional dilemma for teaching wellness. Needs for immediate gratification often outweigh people's sense of health-related preservation. During the late 1980s, a television commercial for a popular oil filter used the premise that you can pay for regular maintenance now (i.e., good nutrition, regular exercise, etc.) or can pay later to repair the ensuing damage from engine neglect (i.e., clinical obesity, adult-onset diabetes, chronic pulmonary obstructive disease, etc.). Our inability to envision the long-term deleterious effects of a poor diet, lack of exercise, unprotected sex, and the use of tobacco or illicit drugs creates a downward spiral of health and well-being that significantly decreases the quality and quantity of life. The oil company's slogan, "You can pay me now, or pay me later" appropriately summarizes the conceptual framework that defines our instructional challenge. It is our mission to educate students about the effects of harmful lifestyle behaviors and then to motivate and inspire them to mitigate these risky behaviors.

Leading Health Problems in the United States

Through scientific advances, the lifestyle of Americans has changed drastically over the past 100 years. The rise in technology and automation has created an age of convenience characterized by sedentary living and diets high in simple sugars and saturated fat. The National Health and Nutrition Examination Survey (2005) indicates that Americans are becoming more obese and more unfit each year.

The U.S. Department of Health and Human Services (2000) reported that more people are at risk due to physical inactivity than to any of the other risk factors. The U.S. Department of Health and Human Services' Surgeon General's hallmark report, *Physical Activity and Health* (1996), estimated that less than 10 percent of the U.S. adult population participated in regular, vigorous physical activity for 20 minutes or longer three or more days per week. Only about 25 percent of adults reported physical activity on five or more days per week for 30 minutes or longer, and another 25 percent of adults did not participate in any regular physical activity.

Regular physical activity is important for the primary and secondary prevention of many chronic diseases (e.g., coronary heart disease, non-insulin-dependent diabetes mellitus, obesity), disabling conditions (e.g., osteoporosis, arthritis), and chronic disease risk factors (e.g., high blood pressure, high cholesterol).

The U.S. Department of Health and Human Services (2006) reported that nearly 50 percent of all deaths in the United States were caused by cardiovascular disease and cancer. Making healthy lifestyle changes could have prevented approximately 80 percent of these deaths. Adopting behaviors such as eating nutritious foods, being physically active, and avoiding tobacco can prevent or control the devastating effects of many of the nation's leading causes of death regardless of one's age.

Staying healthy is a lifelong process that requires individuals to accept responsibility for their personal well-being. Improving happiness, quality of life, and longevity is a matter of personal choice.

Purpose of the Course

The purpose of the Wellness course taught in the Department of Physical Education (DPE) is to introduce students to the dimensions of wellness that define a healthy lifestyle and to help cadets become good problem solvers and decision makers with regard to their own personal wellness. Empowering students with the knowledge and tools to shape their personal well-being enables them to assume responsibility, make good decisions, and adhere to a healthy lifestyle.

Students are encouraged to accept personal responsibility for their health and well-being. Lessons are generally formatted to provide content information and active learning scenarios to assist students in making informed choices. Students assess their current lifestyle behaviors to determine if these are contributing positively to their health and well-being. Strategies are provided to help students make behavioral changes. To facilitate this developmental process, we have established the following wellness competency goals. At the conclusion of this course, students will be able to do the following:

- Understand the dimensions of wellness and how they interact to improve the quality of life

- Though personal assessments identify health risks for themselves and others and establish ways to mitigate these risky behaviors

- Demonstrate communication skills and apply conflict resolution techniques to the promotion of health and the prevention of risk

- Demonstrate an understanding of and respect for differences among people

- Exhibit responsible personal and social behavior

- Understand the application of stress management techniques for the prevention of serious health risks

- Apply behavior management skills to nutrition-related health concerns

- Choose not to participate in substance abuse

- Participate in regular physical activity and gain competence toward lifetime physical activities

- Understand the behavior change process and the difficulties in changing health-related behaviors

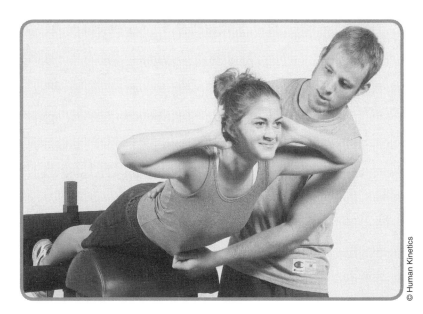

© Human Kinetics

Having friends who encourage you is an important part of achieving your fitness goals.

Course Overview

Due to the credit-hour limitations at the U.S. Military Academy, the DPE Wellness course is limited to 20 lessons (see table 10.1). In a public school setting, where this type of course may last for an entire term, we encourage teachers to expand the pertinent lessons to provide more opportunities for student learning. Cadets also enroll in an 18-lesson Personal Fitness course that focuses on the foundations of personal and unit fitness (chapter 11).

Sample Lesson Plans

The DPE Wellness course is a core requirement for all cadets at the Academy; therefore we teach approximately 1,000 cadets per academic year. This means that we utilize approximately 20 different instructors throughout the school year. Due to the skills and abilities of our instructors, we provide them with a sample "lesson format" rather than a specified "lesson plan." We believe the sample lesson formats provide sufficient structure for the instructors and the cadets to achieve the course objectives. Teachers may use the following lesson formats to develop specific lesson plans. The sample formats include objectives, key terminology, suggested questions to facilitate class discussion, activities for behavior change, and health and wellness resources on the Internet.

Table 10.1 Overview of Wellness Lessons

Lesson	Topic
1	Understanding wellness and fitness for life
2	Spiritual and emotional health
3	Managing stress: coping with life's challenges
4	Social support: creating healthy relationships
5	Communication and conflict resolution
6	Eating for wellness: basic nutrition
7	Making healthy nutritional choices
8	Nutritional supplements: is your health at risk?
9	Body composition and weight management
10	Eating disorders
11	Physical activity for health and wellness
12	Preventing cardiovascular disease
13	Advanced coronary risk factors
14	Reducing your risk of cancer
15	Understanding addictive behaviors
16	Taking responsibility for alcohol use
17	Preventing sexually transmitted diseases
18	Current events and special topics
19	Current events and special topics
20	Final exam

LESSON 1

Understanding Wellness and Fitness for Life

OBJECTIVES

- Recognize the importance of fitness and wellness in quality of life
- Explain the meaning and interrelationship of health and wellness
- Identify and explain the dimensions of wellness
- Explain the importance of personal decision making and behavior change in achieving a wellness lifestyle

KEY TERMS

chronic diseases—Illnesses that linger over time and may get progressively worse.

emotional wellness—The ability to understand your own feelings, accept your limitations, and achieve emotional stability.

health—A state of complete well-being and not just the absence of disease or infirmity.

mental wellness—A state in which your mind is engaged in lively interaction with the world around you.

physical wellness—Flexibility, endurance, strength, and optimism about your ability to take care of physical problems.

social wellness—The ability to relate well to others, both within and outside the family unit.

spiritual wellness—The sense that life is meaningful and that life has purpose.

wellness—Full integration of physical, mental, emotional, social, environmental, occupational, and spiritual well-being into a quality life.

DISCUSSION QUESTIONS

- Are the different wellness dimensions balanced in your life? Assign a score for yourself in each dimension of wellness. Rate yourself on a scale from 1 to 5, with 1 being the lowest score. Assess your strengths and weaknesses.

- Describe one lifestyle behavior that you routinely engage in that you regard as destructive to your health. Discuss your reasons for continuing to engage in this behavior. List the steps that you would take in order to change this unhealthy behavior.

- Why are young people at high risk for accidents, homicide, and suicide? Why do these risks decline with age? What programs, services, or policies are in place in your school or community to reduce the risk from these types of problems?

- Imagine you are the Surgeon General of the United States and that one of your responsibilities is to formulate national health policy. Describe what you believe is the primary health problem in the United States today. Discuss the steps you would take to correct this health problem.

- Explain how you would respond to a friend who says, "What's the point of adopting all these 'healthy habits' at my age? I eat a lot of fast foods, don't exercise, and smoke cigarettes to relieve stress, but I feel fine and have no symptoms of disease."

ACTIVITIES FOR BEHAVIORAL CHANGE

See Behavior Change Project on page 228.

WEB RESOURCES

- Healthy People 2010: www.healthypeople.gov
- Hooah 4 Health: http://hooah4health.com
- Healthfinder: www.healthfinder.org
- Mayo Clinic Web site: www.mayohealth.org
- Centers for Disease Control and Prevention (CDC): www.cdc.gov
- American Diabetes Association: www.diabetes.org

LESSON 2

Spiritual and Emotional Health

OBJECTIVES

- Define emotional wellness
- Discuss how anger, hostility, worry, anxiety, and perfectionism affect health
- Describe the connection between self-esteem and health
- Define explanatory style and explain the differences between a pessimistic style and an optimistic style, as well as their effects on health
- Explain the differences between internal and external health locus of control
- Define spiritual wellness
- Compare spirituality and religion
- Describe the connection between spirituality and health, including the power of prayer, forgiveness, and faith
- Describe the altruistic personality
- Contrast the health effects of hope and hopelessness

KEY TERMS

altruism—The act of giving of oneself out of a genuine concern for other people; unselfish devotion to the interests and welfare of others.

explanatory style—The way people perceive the events in their lives, from an optimistic or a pessimistic perspective.

external locus of control—One's prevailing belief that the things that happen are unrelated to one's own behavior.

health locus of control—The extent to which people believe that their behavior affects their health status.

internal locus of control—One's prevailing belief that events are a consequence of one's own actions and thus potentially can be controlled.

self-esteem—A sense of positive self-regard and self-respect.

DISCUSSION QUESTIONS

- Do you regard yourself as a "glass half empty" or a "glass half full"? Evaluate your explanatory style and discuss how it might affect your wellness.
- People over 65 years of age have a high rate of depression. What could you do to enhance the health and wellness of an elderly person?
- During your childhood, how did your interaction with your family members influence the development of your self-esteem? Which people were the most influential in the development of your self-esteem?
- How would you help a friend who suffers from low self-esteem?
- Have you ever thought about hurting yourself or others?
- What actions would you recommend for someone trying to be more positive, less hostile, and less critical of others?
- What does spiritual wellness mean to you? List ways in which you can incorporate spirituality into your daily life.

WEB RESOURCES

Spirituality and Health: www.spiritualityhealth.com

LESSON 3

Managing Stress: Coping With Life's Challenges

OBJECTIVES

- Define "stress" and "stressor" and use the General Adaptation Syndrome to explain how stress is related to health
- Explain the biology of stress and its relationship to heart disease, high blood pressure, the immune system, and digestive disorders
- List some personal causes of stress and discuss how their effects can be prevented or minimized
- Describe techniques to help manage stress

KEY TERMS

autogenics—A relaxation technique in which the person is trained, with the aid of specialized equipment, to relax all major muscle groups through a form of self-hypnosis, followed by imagery.

biofeedback—A relaxation technique that involves measuring and controlling physiological functions.

distress—Negative stress, usually consisting of too much stress in a short time, chronic stress over a prolonged time, or a combination of stressors.

eustress—Positive, desirable stress.

General Adaptation Syndrome—A three-stage attempt of the body to react and adapt to stressors that disrupt its normal balance.

homeostasis—A stable sense of physiological balance in which all of the body's systems are functioning normally.

meditation—A mental exercise to help gain control over thoughts.

progressive relaxation—A method of reducing stress that consists of tensing, then relaxing, small muscle groups.

stress—An automatic biological response to stressors.

stressor—Any situation or event that causes us to adapt or adjust.

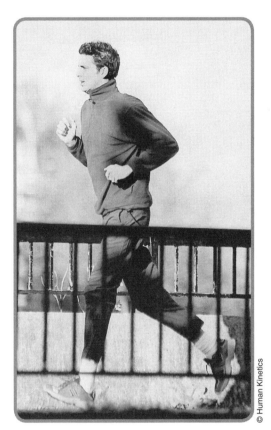

© Human Kinetics

Strenuous activities like running can help to manage and reduce stress.

DISCUSSION QUESTIONS

- Why are some students more susceptible to stress than others? What services are available in your school to help you deal with excessive stress?
- What are the greatest sources of distress in your life? What can you do to reduce your level of stress and keep yourself from becoming run down?
- Develop a personal stress reduction program that can be incorporated into your daily schedule.

- Have you noticed that you tend to get sick more often during certain times? Why might this occur?
- Explain how social support may make you more or less susceptible to stress.
- Describe any experiences that you have had with meditation, yoga, hypnosis, visualization, or any other form of relaxation. Describe how you became involved with this activity and for what purpose you used it. Would you recommend this technique to others?
- Suppose that you have two final exams scheduled for the same day. Describe a positive coping strategy that you could use to reduce your stress.

WEB RESOURCES

- Center for Anxiety and Stress Treatment: http://stressrelease.com
- Mind Tools: www.psychwww.com/mtsite/smpage.html
- American Institute of Stress: www.stress.org

LESSON 4

Social Support: Creating Healthy Relationships

OBJECTIVES

- Define social support and list four types of social support
- Discuss how social support systems contribute to health and well-being
- Define loneliness and discuss the relationship between loneliness and health
- Discuss the prevalence of loneliness among adolescents
- List the health hazards of divorce
- Explain the health benefits of marriage
- Contrast the health of divorced people with the health of those who are unhappily married
- Define grief and bereavement

KEY TERMS

appraisal support—Support that comes in the form of advice and direction.

bereavement—The process of "disbanding" from someone who played an important role in one's life and is now gone.

emotional support—Support from others that helps you understand your own feelings, accept your limitations, and achieve emotional stability.

grief—The overwhelming sorrow that follows a loss.

information support—Support that comes in the form of direct information, such as which classes to take.

instrumental support—Support that comes in the form of tangible aid, such as lending money, running an errand, or providing a ride to class.

loneliness—A condition that occurs when a person's network of social relationships is significantly deficient in either quality or quantity.

social support—The network of support that people provide to each other, including instrumental, emotional, informational, and appraisal support.

DISCUSSION QUESTIONS

- What factors do you consider the most important in choosing a friend?
- What people are your social support? Diagram your social support network. What type of support does each person provide?
- How does the environment at your school affect your social support? Discuss both positive and negative influences.
- How prevalent is loneliness at your school? What services are available to help someone who is suffering from loneliness?
- What characteristics are most important to you in a potential partner? If your parents or friends didn't like a potential partner, how important would their opinion be to you? What would you do in this situation?
- Do you know people who stay in unhealthy relationships? Why do you think they stay in those relationships?
- Although there are advantages and disadvantages in marriage, most people feel that marriage is a desirable option. Are there any advantages in remaining single? What are potential disadvantages?
- If your close friend showed some of the signs of suicide, what action would you take? Who would you contact first?
- Who are the people with whom you feel most comfortable talking about very personal issues? Do you talk with both males and females about these issues, or do you gravitate toward just one sex? Why do you think this is?

LESSON 5

Communication and Conflict Resolution

OBJECTIVES

- Define interpersonal communication and discuss the basic components of communication
- Explain the difference between hearing and listening
- Discuss ways to improve listening skills
- Discuss the difference between assertive behavior and aggressive behavior
- Discuss barriers to effective communication
- Define conflict and discuss how it can affect wellness
- Define conflict resolution and employ the problem-solving method for conflict resolution

KEY TERMS

conflict—A state of unresolved difference between two individuals, between an individual and a group, or between two groups.

decoding—The act of understanding messages.

encoding—The act of producing messages.

hearing—A physiological sensory process in which auditory sensations are received by the ears and transmitted to the brain.

interpersonal communication—The successful exchange of information between individuals.

listening—The psychological process of interpreting and understanding the significance of what someone says.

noise—Environmental, physiological, and psychological factors that decrease the likelihood that a message will be accurately expressed or understood.

nonverbal communication—Messages that are transmitted from one person to another by other than linguistic means.

DISCUSSION QUESTIONS

* How would you describe your communication style? Do you tend to be nonassertive, assertive, or aggressive? Should you alter your communication style in any way? If so, why?

* Think about the nature of communication that you have with someone who is important to you such as a parent or a close friend. How could you communicate more effectively with that person?

* When you have conflicts, does the content of your language accurately represent what you want to convey? How could you improve your conflict resolution skills?

* Do you think that males and females communicate in different styles? Why or why not? Are you more or less comfortable talking with women or men? Why? What can you do to improve your communication with members of the opposite sex?

* How does communication improve self-esteem and reduce stress?

* What are the most important communication skills for an effective teacher? Give specific examples based on personal experiences.

LESSON 6

Eating for Wellness: Basic Nutrition

OBJECTIVES

* Explain the concept of energy balance
* List the essential nutrients and define their functions and sources
* Describe the Food Guide Pyramid and explain its significance
* Explain current recommendations for healthy eating, and use the nutritional information provided on food labels to make healthy choices
* Differentiate the types of carbohydrate and describe the role of fiber
* Identify sources of antioxidants and explain how antioxidants work within the body
* Describe cholesterol and its functions

KEY TERMS

amino acids—Building blocks of protein.

antioxidant—A compound that protects other compounds from oxidation by being oxidized itself.

calories—Units used to measure energy; determined from the heat food releases when burned.

carbohydrate—Compound composed of carbon, oxygen, and hydrogen atoms, and the preferred fuel for the brain and nervous system.

cholesterol—A waxy substance found only in animal fat and oil.

essential fat—A group of fatty acids that are essential to human health. There are two types, the omega-3 (w3) and omega-6 (w6) families. Essential fat is made from the essential fatty acids linoleic and linolenic acid.

fat—Lipids in food or in the body that provide the body with a continuous fuel supply, protect it from mechanical shock, and carry fat-soluble vitamins.

hydrogenation—A chemical process by which hydrogens are added to monounsaturated or polyunsaturated fat to reduce the number of double bonds and make the product more saturated (solid) and more resistant to spoilage.

minerals—Inorganic elements found in the body and in food that are essential for normal body functions.

monounsaturated fat—Fatty acid that lacks two hydrogen atoms and has one double bond between carbons; found in olive oil, canola oil, and peanut oil.

nutrients—Substances obtained from food and used in the body to promote growth, maintenance, and repair.

polyunsaturated fat—Fatty acid that lacks four hydrogen atoms and has two or more bonds between carbons; found in sunflower, corn, soybean, and cottonseed oil.

protein—Compound composed of amino acids necessary for growth or tissue repair.

saturated fat—Fat carrying the maximum possible number of hydrogen atoms; usually found in animal products such as butter and lard.

vitamins—Organic, essential nutrients required in small amounts to perform specific functions that promote growth, maintenance, or repair; vitamins do not provide energy, but are necessary in energy-yielding reactions.

DISCUSSION QUESTIONS

- Discuss the major types of nutrients that your body needs. What happens if you fail to get enough of some of them?
- What factors influence your food choices? Do you read nutrition labels? If you do, which information do you think is the most important?
- Analyze the nutrition label from one of your favorite snack foods. What is your overall assessment of this food?

ACTIVITIES FOR BEHAVIORAL CHANGE

See the Nutrition Project and Food Label Analysis on page 234.

WEB RESOURCES

- USDA Center for Nutrition Policy and Promotion: www.usda.gov/cnpp
- National Cancer Institute's 5-a-Day Program: www.5aday.gov
- Berkeley Nutrition Services: www.nutritionquest.com

LESSON 7

Making Healthy Nutritional Choices

OBJECTIVES

- Identify the types of vitamins and describe their functions and nutrient sources
- Identify the minerals the body needs, their functions, and nutrient sources

- Explain how to make healthy choices when eating in the school cafeteria
- Develop a personal plan for healthy nutritional choices

KEY TERMS

adequate intakes (AI)—The average amount of a nutrient that appears sufficient to maintain a specific criterion.

dietary reference intakes (DRI)—A set of nutrient values for the dietary nutrient intakes of healthy people.

recommended dietary allowances (RDA)—The average daily amount of a nutrient considered adequate to meet the known nutrient needs of most healthy people.

tolerable upper intake level (TUIL)—The maximum amount of a nutrient that appears safe for most healthy people and beyond which there is an increased risk of adverse effects.

DISCUSSION QUESTIONS

- What are several factors that may influence the eating habits of the typical student?
- Which food groups from the Food Guide Pyramid are you most likely to eat adequate amounts of during the course of a typical day? Why is it more difficult for you to eat some of these food groups than others? What are some simple changes that you could make right now in your diet to help you comply with the Food Guide Pyramid recommendations?
- Which nutrient is most lacking in your diet? Why should this lack concern you? Are you planning to take action to correct this situation? What steps will you take?
- What problems cause you the most difficulty when you try to eat more healthful foods? Are these problems typical in your family, or are they unique to your current situation as a student?

WEB RESOURCES

- American Dietetic Association: www.eatright.org
- USDA Food and Nutrition Information Center: www.nal.usda.gov/fnic/
- Sports, Cardiovascular and Wellness Nutritionists: www.nutrifit.org

LESSON 8

Nutritional Supplements: Is Your Health at Risk?

OBJECTIVES

- Define nutritional (dietary) supplement and ergogenic aid
- Discuss the Dietary Supplement Health Education Act (DSHEA) of 1994 and the role of the Food and Drug Administration (FDA) regarding the production, marketing, and regulation of supplements
- Discuss the latest research on ephedrine, creatine, and androstenedione
- Understand the difference between times when nutritional supplements are needed and helpful and times when they are unsound and pose health risks

KEY TERMS

anabolic steroids—Synthetic versions of the male sex hormone testosterone, which promotes muscle development and hypertrophy.

creatine—An organic compound derived from meat, fish, and amino acids that combines with inorganic phosphate to form creatine phosphate.

ephedrine—An herb that excites the central nervous system and cardiovascular system.

supplements—Tablets, pills, capsules, liquids, or powders containing vitamins, minerals, amino acids, herbs, or fiber that are taken to increase the intake of these nutrients.

DISCUSSION QUESTIONS

- Would you consider using supplements for the sole purpose of increasing your body build and potentially your performance?

- Do you think androstenedione should be declared illegal? Why or why not?

- Suppose you read an advertisement for a product that is said to eliminate body fat while you sleep. According to the ad, this product helps you lose weight quickly by increasing your metabolic rate. It claims that you do not need to exercise more often or eat less food. Explain why you think this ad is a source of reliable or unreliable health information.

- Studies show that the contents of some supplements vary greatly from the information displayed on the label. Many experts believe that because of product contamination, U.S. athletes are at risk for failing drug tests if they take any dietary supplement. What needs to be done to protect the health and safety of consumers?

WEB RESOURCES

- Food and Drug Administration: www.fda.gov
- Office of Dietary Supplements: http://dietary-supplements.info.nih.gov/
- Quackwatch: www.quackwatch.com
- Herb Research Foundation: www.herbs.org
- Center for Science in the Public Interest: www.cspinet.org

LESSON 9

Body Composition and Weight Management

OBJECTIVES

- Define body composition and explain various techniques used to assess body composition
- Identify the differences between essential and storage fat
- Assess body composition using the skinfold thickness technique and the Army Tape Test
- Understand the importance of waist-to-hip ratio and body mass index

KEY TERMS

anthropometric measurement techniques—Measures of skinfold thickness and body size and circumferences designed to estimate body composition.

body composition—The different components (fat, bone, muscle, etc.) that, when taken together, make up a person's body weight.

body mass index (BMI)—A number calculated from a person's weight and height, which provides an indicator of body fatness for most people and is used to screen for weight categories that may lead to health problems.

essential fat—Fat required for normal physiological functioning, consisting of fat stored in the marrow of bones, heart, lungs, liver, spleen, kidneys, intestines, muscles, and lipid-rich tissues of the central nervous system.

lean body mass—The percentage of your body composition that is composed of muscle, bone, and organ tissue.

percent body fat—The percentage of your body composition that is composed of essential and storage fat.

skinfold thickness—The thickness of your skin and the underlying layer of fat; used to estimate percent body fat.

storage fat—Fat stored by the body in adipose tissue as a function of resting metabolism, energy intake, and energy expenditure.

waist-to-hip ratio—A rudimentary estimate of body composition based upon the ratio of the circumference of the waist to the circumference of the hips.

DISCUSSION QUESTIONS

- What is the relationship between body composition and physical performance?
- What is the relationship between body composition and health-related diseases?
- How do measures of body composition relate to the onset of eating disorders?
- How do the media influence your satisfaction with your body size and shape?
- What are the metabolic advantages to lean tissue over adipose tissue?
- What are the different types of body fat, and how do your diet and level of exercise contribute to your potential of becoming obese?

WEB RESOURCES

- Body Composition Procedures Manual: www.cdc.gov/nchs/data/nhanes/nhanes_01_02/body_composition_year_3.pdf
- Body Composition Tests: www.americanheart.org/presenter.jhtml?identifier=4489
- Body Composition Fact Sheet: www.rowett.ac.uk/edu_web/sec_pup/body_comp.pdf

LESSON 10

Eating Disorders

OBJECTIVES

- Define anorexia nervosa, bulimia nervosa, and compulsive overeating
- List common symptoms of anorexia nervosa

- List common symptoms of bulimia nervosa
- Discuss how eating disorders compromise wellness
- Describe the risk factors associated with eating disorders
- Discuss ways to help an individual with an eating disorder and identify the professional points of contact

KEY TERMS

anorexia nervosa—An eating disorder characterized by self-imposed starvation to lose weight and maintain very low body weight.

bulimia nervosa—An eating disorder characterized by a pattern of binge eating and purging in an attempt to lose weight and maintain low body weight.

DISCUSSION QUESTIONS

- How have eating disorders touched your life?
- Which groups or individuals in your school appear to be at greatest risk for eating disorders? What social factors might encourage this? Why do you think society tends to overlook eating disorders in males? What programs are available in your school to help someone with an eating disorder?
- How do the media influence your satisfaction with your body size and shape?
- Discuss the pressures, if any, that you feel to improve your personal body image. Do these pressures come from the media, family, friends, or from concern for your personal health?

WEB RESOURCES

- McLean Hospital: www.mclean.harvard.edu/patient/child/edc.php
- Eating Disorders Shared Awareness: www.something-fishy.org
- National Eating Disorders Association: www.nationaleatingdisorders.org
- Sports, Cardiovascular and Wellness Nutritionists: www.nutrifit.org

LESSON 11

Physical Activity for Health and Wellness

OBJECTIVES

- List and explain the components of physical fitness
- Discuss the differences between sedentary and active lifestyles and develop strategies to become more active
- Explain the benefits of exercise as a strategy for enhancing wellness
- Discuss and understand the basic principles of physical training
- Discuss motivation techniques for maintaining a successful fitness program
- Understand the difference between overweight and obesity
- Understand the health consequences of obesity

KEY TERMS

aerobic exercise—Activity that requires oxygen to produce the necessary energy (adenosine triphosphate, ATP) to carry out the exercise.

anaerobic exercise—Activity that does not require oxygen to produce necessary energy (ATP) to carry out the activity.

atrophy—A decrease in the size of a cell.

body composition—The fat and nonfat components of the human body.

cardiorespiratory endurance—The ability of the lungs, heart, and blood vessels to deliver adequate amounts of oxygen to the cells to meet the demands of prolonged physical activity.

dynamic training—Strength training method referring to a muscle contraction with movement.

flexibility—The ability of a joint to move freely through its full range of motion.

hypertrophy—An increase in the size of the cell.

hypokinetic disease—A condition associated with a lack of physical activity.

isometric training—Strength training method that uses muscle contractions producing little or no movement, such as pushing or pulling against immovable objects.

maximal oxygen uptake ($\dot{V}O_2$max)—The maximum amount of oxygen the body is able to utilize per minute of physical activity.

muscular endurance—The ability of a muscle to exert submaximal force repeatedly over a period of time.

muscular strength—The ability to exert maximum force against resistance.

obesity—An excessive accumulation of body fat, usually at least 30 percent above recommended body weight.

overload principle—Training concept that the demands placed on a system must be increased systematically and progressively over time to cause physiological adaptation.

overweight—Excess weight according to a given standard, such as height or recommended body fat.

physical fitness—The ability to meet the ordinary as well as the unusual demands of daily life safely and effectively without being overly fatigued and still have energy left for leisure and recreational activities.

principle of specificity—Principle that training must be done with the specific muscle the person is attempting to improve.

progressive resistance—A gradual increase of resistance over a period of time.

recovery time—Amount of time the body takes to return to resting levels after exercise.

DISCUSSION QUESTIONS

- Which components of physical fitness would you like to improve or develop? What types of activities will you do to improve your fitness level?

- What benefits would you derive from adopting a more physically active lifestyle?

- What laborsaving devices would you be willing to eliminate from your daily routine so you could use your muscles more and improve your level of fitness?

- Why is it important to have good flexibility throughout life? What specific actions can you take to improve your flexibility?

- What specific actions can you take to increase your muscular strength? Muscular endurance? How would you measure your improvement?

WEB RESOURCES

- American Heart Association: Just Move: www.justmove.org
- President's Council on Physical Fitness: www.fitness.gov

- Shape Up America! Fitness Center: www.shapeup.org
- American College of Sports Medicine: www.acsm.org

LESSON 12

Preventing Cardiovascular Disease

OBJECTIVES

- Explain how the heart and lungs deliver oxygen and remove carbon dioxide
- List and explain the risk factors for cardiovascular disease
- Explain the relationship between cholesterol and the risk of heart attack
- Define hypertension, and list its common risk factors

KEY TERMS

cardiovascular disease (CVD)—The array of conditions that affect the heart and the blood vessels.

coronary heart disease (CHD)—Condition in which the arteries that supply the heart muscle with oxygen and nutrients are narrowed by fatty deposits, such as cholesterol and triglycerides.

diastolic pressure—Pressure exerted by the blood against the walls of the arteries during the relaxation phase of the heart.

HDL (high-density lipoprotein) cholesterol—Cholesterol-transporting molecules in the blood that help clear cholesterol from the blood.

hypertension—Chronically elevated blood pressure.

LDL (low-density lipoprotein) cholesterol—Cholesterol-transporting molecules in the blood that tend to increase blood cholesterol.

systolic pressure—Pressure exerted by the blood against the walls of the arteries during the forceful contraction of the heart.

DISCUSSION QUESTIONS

- What do you think is your biggest CVD risk factor right now? What is your second-biggest risk factor? List four actions that you can do this week to reduce these risk factors.
- One of your friends says that his father had a heart attack at age 50 and asks you, "What impact does genetics play in my future health and longevity?" Discuss your answer.
- Consider what happens when people who suffer a heart attack survive. What challenges do they face?
- Discuss the role that exercise, stress management, and dietary changes can play in reducing risk for CVD.

WEB RESOURCES

- American Heart Association: www.americanheart.org
- National Stroke Association: www.stroke.org

LESSON 13

Advanced Coronary Risk Factors

OBJECTIVES

* Explain the relationship between cholesterol and the risk of attack
* Explain the relationship between homocysteine and cardiovascular disease
* Define atherosclerosis and list effective treatments for it
* Explain what happens during a myocardial infarction (MI) and what can be done to prevent and treat such attacks
* Define stroke and transient ischemic attacks (TIAs) and explain their cause, prevention, and treatment

KEY TERMS

C-reactive protein—A test measuring the concentration of a protein in serum that indicates acute arterial inflammation.

diabetes mellitus—A disease in which the body doesn't produce or utilize insulin properly.

homocysteine—An amino acid that, when allowed to accumulate in the blood, may lead to plaque formation and blockage of arteries.

oxygen free radicals—Highly reactive molecules due to the presence of unpaired electron(s), which are thought to play an important role in the pathogenesis of coronary artery disease.

synthetic HDL—A synthesized form of high-density lipoprotein, derived from the ApoA-I Milano lipoprotein, which in preclinical studies showed rapid removal of plaques from diseased arteries.

triglyceride—Fat formed by glycerol and free fatty acids.

vascular inflammatory disease—Inflammation and vascular infection that contribute to endothelial dysfunction and are thought to play an important role in atherosclerosis.

DISCUSSION QUESTIONS

* What are some nutritional alternatives to help manage the body's production of homocysteine?
* How can vascular inflammatory disease be treated with a common over-the-counter drug?
* Discuss the paradox of increased physical activity and the body's production of free oxygen radicals.
* Discuss the role of antioxidants in the management of oxidative stress.

WEB RESOURCES

* Effect of Synthetic HDL: www.prnewswire.com/cgi-bin/stories.pl?ACCT= 104&STORY=/www/story/11-04-2003/0002051223&EDATE=
* The Role of C-Reactive Protein: www.americanheart.org/presenter.jhtml ?identifier=4648
* Oxidative Stress: www.bionutrition.org/OXidative-stress.asp
* Homocysteine information site: www.homocysteine.net/

LESSON 14

Reducing Your Risk of Cancer

OBJECTIVES

- Define cancer and list the seven warning signs
- List and explain the risk factors for cancer
- Identify the most prevalent cancers for men and women
- Identify ways of protecting against various cancers
- List the reasons people start using tobacco and why they continue to use it
- Explain the short-term and long-term health risks associated with tobacco use and exposure to environmental tobacco smoke
- List the health problems that people can prevent by quitting smoking and identify several recommended ways to quit

KEY TERMS

benign—Noncancerous.

cancer—A group of more than a hundred diseases in which cells grow at an uncontrolled rate, mature in an abnormal way, and invade nearby tissues.

carcinogens—Cancer-causing agents.

malignant—Cancerous.

metastasis—The process that occurs when cancer cells from one growth break off, enter the bloodstream or lymph system, and are carried to a distant part of the body, where they cause another cancerous growth to begin.

DISCUSSION QUESTIONS

- Make a list of all the factors that you think increase the risk of developing cancer. Rank the items on your list from highest risk to lowest risk. Are any of the risk factors relevant to your life? If so, describe how you can modify your lifestyle to reduce the risk of developing cancer.
- What types of cancers do you think you are at greatest risk for right now? Do you practice regular breast or testicular self-examinations?
- You have been asked to return to your middle school to discuss the negative consequences of tobacco. Identify your key points of emphasis on why a young person should not begin using tobacco products.
- Have you noticed an increase in the number of your friends who have become smokers or occasional smokers? What are their reasons for smoking?
- Do you think women and men begin smoking for the same reasons? Why are women smoking more than ever before? Should pregnant women be required to participate in a smoking cessation program?
- Because nicotine is so highly addictive, should it be regulated as a controlled substance?
- Do you think the United States could ever be smoke free? Should all public places, indoor and outdoor, be smoke free?

- Look at a popular magazine and count the number of cigarette ads. Study each ad and answer the following questions: Who is the ad targeting? How is the ad appealing to its target audience? Besides the warning label, which is required by law, does the ad mention any negative side effects of smoking?

ACTIVITIES FOR BEHAVIORAL CHANGE

See the Great American Smoke-Out Project on page 240.

WEB RESOURCES

- American Cancer Society: www.cancer.org
- American Lung Association: www.lungusa.org/
- Action on Smoking and Health: www.ash.org
- National Cancer Institute: http://cancer.gov
- National Cancer Institute's 5-a-Day Program: www.5aday.gov
- Skin Cancer Foundation: www.skincancer.org
- Harvard Center for Cancer Prevention: www.yourcancerrisk.harvard.edu

LESSON 15

Understanding Addictive Behaviors

OBJECTIVES

- Define addiction and differentiate it from a habit
- List characteristics of addictive behavior
- Delineate the difference between physiological addiction and psychological addiction
- Discuss the threats of addiction on all dimensions of wellness
- Discuss addictive personality traits
- List the major risk factors of addiction
- Discuss the physiological and psychological effects of MDMA (Ecstasy), GHB, Rohypnol, methamphetamine, ketamine, and LSD

KEY TERMS

addiction—Compulsive and uncontrollable behavior(s) or use of substance(s).

withdrawal—Response that occurs when the body begins to clear a substance (drug) from its system and the altered body chemistry disrupts normal functioning.

DISCUSSION QUESTIONS

- Have you ever seen signs of addiction in a friend or family member? What types of negative consequences have you witnessed? Is it possible for you to tell whether someone else is really addicted?
- Why do we tend to knowingly protect others from the consequences of their destructive behaviors? Have you ever confronted someone you were concerned about? What suggestions would you give someone who is going to confront a loved one about an addiction?

- Why do you think people with addictions resist treatment, even when they admit they have a problem? What could you do to help someone who is fighting a substance abuse problem?
- Can you think of any habits you have that could potentially become addictive?
- Plan an educational program for 6th grade students that discourages illicit drug use. What key points would you include in your presentation?
- Do you think Internet addiction could be a problem among your friends? What might be some potential problems of Internet addiction?
- Do you think any of our current laws governing drugs should be changed or eliminated? What criteria should be used to determine if use of a drug is legitimate or illegitimate?
- If you had unlimited power and resources, what would you do to solve the illegal drug problem?

WEB RESOURCES

- National Institute on Drug Abuse: www.clubdrugs.gov
- Habitsmart: www.habitsmart.com
- National Clearinghouse for Alcohol and Drug Information: www.ncadi.samhsa.gov
- Center for Online Addiction: www.netaddiction.com/

LESSON 16

Taking Responsibility for Alcohol Use

OBJECTIVES

- Discuss alcohol use and alcohol abuse in the United States
- Discuss the health risks associated with excessive or chronic alcohol consumption
- Define binge drinking
- Discuss the prevalence of binge drinking
- Understand the ramifications of underage drinking and supplying underage drinkers with alcohol
- Define fetal alcohol syndrome and discuss the risks of drinking during pregnancy
- Discuss strategies for responsible alcohol use
- Understand acceptable behavior with respect to alcohol use
- Discuss the responsibility of leaders and peers to be proactive in identifying alcohol problems instead of reactive

KEY TERMS

alcohol—A depressant drug that affects the brain and slows down central nervous system activity.

alcoholism—Disease in which an individual loses control over drinking alcoholic beverages.

binge drinking—Imbibing at least five alcoholic beverages in one sitting for men and four for women.

fetal alcohol syndrome—A set of mental and physical characteristics in a newborn caused by moderate-to-heavy alcohol consumption during pregnancy.

DISCUSSION QUESTIONS

- How is alcohol used in your family? How much do you think your family's attitudes and behaviors toward alcohol have shaped your behavior?

- As you watch television, count the number of beer advertisements. Study each ad and answer the following questions: Who is the ad targeting? How is the ad appealing to its target audience? Does the ad mention any negative side effects of alcohol?

- Have you thought that blood alcohol concentration (BAC) is based only on the amount of alcohol one drinks? What other factors contribute to BAC? Are these factors different for men and women?

- What do you think the legal BAC for drivers should be? Should all states lower the legal limit to .08?

- What should the penalty be for people arrested for driving under the influence of alcohol for the first offense? The second offense? The third offense?

- What are some of the most common negative consequences college students experience as a result of binge drinking? What are secondhand effects of binge drinking?

- Why do we hear so little about fetal alcohol syndrome in the United States when it is the second leading cause of mental retardation and the third most common birth defect? Is this a reflection of our society's denial of alcohol as a dangerous drug?

WEB RESOURCES

- College Alcohol Study. Harvard School of Public Health: www.hsph.harvard .edu/cas

- Phoenix House: www.factsontap.org

- Mothers Against Drunk Driving (MADD): www.madd.org

- Alcoholics Anonymous: www.alcoholics-anonymous.org

- National Clearinghouse for Alcohol and Drug Information: www.ncadi.samhsa.gov

- National Institute on Alcohol Abuse and Alcoholism: www.niaaa.nih.gov

LESSON 17

Preventing Sexually Transmitted Diseases

OBJECTIVES

- Define sexual health and sexually healthy relationships

- List the sexually transmitted diseases and describe the symptoms and treatment for each

- Discuss methods for preventing infection from sexually transmitted diseases

- Define HIV infection and describe its symptoms
- Identify the means of HIV transmission
- Explain some practical methods for preventing HIV infection

KEY TERMS

acquired immunodeficiency syndrome (AIDS)—The final stage of the HIV infection, characterized by opportunistic infections that are rare or harmless in people with normal immune function.

chlamydia—A sexually transmitted disease (STD) caused by bacteria that infect the mucous membranes lining the genitals, rectum, anus, mouth, and eyes; the most common bacterial STD in the United States.

genital warts—An STD caused by the human papilloma virus and characterized by warts around the genitals or mouth.

gonorrhea—An STD caused by bacteria that infect the cervix, rectum, urethra, or mouth.

hepatitis B—A form of hepatitis spread through exposure to the contaminated blood or body fluids of an infected person; can cause long-term liver damage.

herpes genitalis—An infection caused by the herpes simplex-2 virus and characterized by blistering sores on the genitals.

human immunodeficiency virus (HIV)—The virus that weakens and destroys the immune system and gradually leads to AIDS.

human papilloma virus (HPV)—The virus that causes genital warts; some strains of the virus also have been linked to cervical cancer.

pelvic inflammatory disease (PID)—A severe infection of the lining of the abdominal cavity, usually caused by bacterial STDs.

pubic lice—Commonly called "crabs"; tiny parasites that feed on the small blood vessels of the skin beneath the pubic hair.

scabies—Tiny mites that burrow under the skin at night; may be spread by nonsexual contact.

sexually transmitted disease (STD)—A disease that is passed from one person to another through sexual contact.

syphilis—An STD caused by bacteria, occurring in four stages; untreated, it is fatal.

DISCUSSION QUESTIONS

- Analyze your behaviors regarding your risk for contracting STDs. What can you do to lower your risk of contracting a sexually transmitted disease?
- Should the names of individuals who test positive for HIV be reported to public health officials?
- Do you think that sexually transmitted diseases are a threat to our national security? Why or why not?

ACTIVITIES FOR BEHAVIORAL CHANGE

See STD Learning Activity—Party Time on page 241.

WEB RESOURCES

- American Social Health Association: www.ashastd.org
- The Body: A Multimedia AIDS and HIV Information Resource: www.thebody.com
- CDC Center for STD Prevention: www.cdc.gov/nchstp/od/nchstp.html

LESSONS 18 AND 19

Current Events and Special Topics

OBJECTIVES

- Students bring in wellness issues that are in the news and discuss relevance to the course.
- Class discusses the Behavior Change Project.
- Instructor facilitates class discussion.
- Discussion questions will be based on the topics the students present during these class sessions.
- Instructor answers questions to assist students in reviewing for the final exam.

LESSON 20

Final Exam

The Wellness course outlined in this chapter covers a wide variety of topics and health-related issues. The final exam, a comprehensive, 55-minute exam with 100 questions, is used to assess how much knowledge the students have gained. The best test method for a final assessment in this type of course is the multiple-choice exam with some true-and-false questions.

Adapting This Course for Your School

When developing your wellness lesson outline, it is important to consider the demographic and socio-graphic makeup of your students and any requirements of your district or state. We thought it might be helpful for you as you develop your lesson outline to review the extensive list of competency goals for grades 6 through 12 provided by the North Carolina Department of Public Instruction (DPI) (2000). We suggest that you contact the corresponding agency in your state to obtain a list of state-specific competency goals. If no comprehensive goals are provided, perhaps these goals may serve as a framework for your age-specific lesson outline and competency goals.

Grade 6

At the conclusion of this course, students will be able to do the following:

- Explain health risks for age group
- Describe the incidence of high-risk behaviors for age group
- Appraise their health behaviors
- Explain sources of self-concept
- Project behavioral consequences as a means of anticipating problems
- Cope with failure appropriately
- Initiate requests for help or assistance from another
- Demonstrate stress management through breathing patterns, muscular relaxation, and directing thoughts
- Use the problem-solving method to make decisions
- Describe individual behaviors that can harm or help the healthfulness of the environment
- Identify sources of noise pollution and preventive measures for hearing impairment

- Differentiate between positive and negative effects of peer pressure
- Communicate their feelings
- Demonstrate attention to and interest in expressions of others
- Enact nonviolent conflict resolution strategies
- Assess health claims on food labels
- Explain that obesity is a disease as well as a risk factor for diabetes and cardiovascular disease
- Evaluate advertising for tobacco and alcohol
- Explain the immediate social and physical consequences of tobacco use
- Identify short-term and long-term benefits of resistance to substance abuse
- Describe how one might encourage a friend not to be involved in substance abuse
- Complete a health-related personal fitness test
- Participate daily in some form of health-enhancing physical activity
- Acknowledge differences in the behaviors of people of different gender, culture, ethnicity, and disability and seek to learn more about both similarities and differences
- Work cooperatively and productively in a group to accomplish a set goal

Grade 7

At the conclusion of this course, students will be able to do the following:

- Differentiate between objective and subjective perceptions of personal health risk
- Explain the concept of cumulative risk in regard to disease and injury
- Recognize and manage habits
- Recognize the incidence of high-risk behaviors
- Use imagery to maintain self-esteem
- Anticipate and monitor personal stressors
- Explain the risks of premarital sexual intercourse
- Demonstrate techniques and strategies for becoming or remaining abstinent by dealing with peer pressure

- Understand that a mutually faithful monogamous relationship is the best lifelong means of avoiding sexually transmitted diseases
- Analyze messages in the media targeting teenagers
- Identify feelings in communications with others
- Define tolerance and explain its importance to a healthy society respectful of differences and diversity
- Plan, select, and prepare healthful meals that emphasize the principles of the Dietary Guidelines for Americans
- Determine the benefits of vitamins and minerals
- Define conditions under which nutrient supplementation may be appropriate
- Identify risks of megadoses of specific nutrients
- Define eating disorders and resources for treatment
- Describe health risks involved with harmful substances
- Quantify the contribution of alcohol to death and injury
- Demonstrate refusal skills that refute persuasion to abuse substances
- Complete a health-related personal fitness test and achieve fitness scores at an acceptable level
- Establish personal physical fitness goals
- Engage in fair play and sportsmanship behaviors during physical activity
- Demonstrate competence in skills needed for individual physical activity and team games

Grade 8

At the conclusion of this course, students will be able to do the following:

- Predict the potential for health risks in a variety of situations
- Identify automobiles, alcohol, and handguns as three factors associated with the majority of fatal and serious injuries
- Accept responsibility for their own behaviors
- Recognize and seek help for self-destructive thoughts and behaviors

- Identify the signs of suicide and develop a plan for seeking help
- Demonstrate basic cardiopulmonary resuscitation (CPR) techniques and procedures
- Demonstrate skills and strategies for remaining or becoming abstinent from sexual intercourse and avoiding sexually transmitted diseases
- Explain methods of contraception, their effectiveness, and failure rates
- Project potential personal health consequences of global environmental problems
- Select personal behavior goals and strategies contributing to environmental improvement
- Develop and maintain confidential relationships
- Describe constructive and risky means of expressing independence
- Analyze barriers to healthful eating patterns and describe strategies for overcoming these barriers
- Demonstrate how to balance caloric intake with caloric expenditure to maintain, gain, or reduce weight
- Identify media and peer pressures toward unhealthy weight control through eating disorders, fad dieting, excessive exercise, and smoking
- Relate the potential impact—social, emotional, physical, mental, and spiritual—of harmful substance use on themselves
- Explain the relationship between physical activity, nutrition, adequate sleep, and weight management
- Establish personal physical fitness goals and monitor progress toward goals
- Express the value and importance of regular physical activity
- Work cooperatively with peers of differing skill
- Display sensitivity to the feelings of others during physical activities
- Consistently engage in fair play and sportsmanship behaviors during physical activity

Grades 9 Through 12

At the conclusion of this course, students will be able to do the following:

- Identify the value of personal outcomes acquired from lifelong learning about health education
- Determine individual control over health risks
- Discern the relationship of health to quality of life
- Develop awareness of their own control over stress
- Associate behaviors with personal, family, and cultural values
- Cope with losses appropriately
- Explain activities undertaken for disaster preparedness
- Prioritize their own health risks and construct a model health risk behavior self-management plan
- Explain the importance of early detection, including medical examination and self-examination
- Assess behavior and decisions as to their likelihood of resulting in infant morbidity and mortality
- Refine skills and strategies for remaining or becoming abstinent from sexual intercourse and avoiding sexually transmitted diseases
- Analyze problems resulting from unhealthy relationships
- Utilize anger management skills
- Demonstrate conflict resolution skills
- Provide detailed examples of how nutrition and physical activity can reduce the risk for chronic diseases
- Develop a personal healthful eating plan that incorporates food choices outside the home
- Design a plan for personal weight management based on realistic and healthful body image
- Describe the potential effects on others of substance abuse by individuals
- Delineate the risks involved in binge drinking
- Complete a health-related fitness test and assess personal level of physical fitness, including monitoring of the heart
- Recognize the implications of cardiovascular disease on healthy living
- Participate regularly in health-enhancing and personally rewarding physical activity outside the physical education class setting

- Appreciate and value the importance of regular physical activity
- Work productively as a member of a team and contribute to the team's success through the assumption of a variety of noncompetitive duties
- Apply cooperative social skills to partner and group activities such as dance, outdoor activities, team building, problem solving, and cooperation games
- Practice acceptable sportsmanship and fair play behaviors in physical activity settings

References

Hoeger, W.K., & Hoeger, S.A. (2004). *Principles and labs for fitness and wellness.* (7th ed.). Belmont, CA: Wadsworth/Thomson Learning.

"Marlboro Man" dies at age 51 of lung cancer. (1992, July 25). *Associated Press.* www.worldsfastestclown.com/man_dies.html.

National Health and Nutrition Examination Survey (NHANES). (2005). *2003–2004 public data general release file documentation; years of coverage: 2003–2004.* Atlanta: U.S. Department of Health and Human Services, Centers for Disease Control and Prevention.

North Carolina Department of Public Instruction. (2000). Healthful living standard course of study and grade level competencies, K-12. Raleigh, NC: Author.

Prochaska, J.L., & DiClemente, C.C. (1992). Stages of change in the modification of problem behavior. In *Progress in behavior modification,* vol. 28, ed. M. Hersen, R. Eisler, & P.M. Miller. Sycamore, IL: Sycamore.

U.S. Department of Health and Human Services. (1996). *Physical activity and health: A report of the Surgeon General.* Atlanta: U.S. Department of Health and Human Services, Centers for Disease Control and Prevention.

U.S. Department of Health and Human Services. (2000). *Promoting better health for young people through physical activity and sports.* Washington, DC.

Suggested Reading

Corbin, C.B., Lindsey, R., Welk, G., & Corbin, W.R. (2002). *Concepts of fitness and wellness.* (4th ed.). Boston: McGraw-Hill.

Miniño, A.M., Heron, M., Smith, B.L., & Kochanek, K.D. Deaths: Final data for 2004. Health E-Stats. Released November 24, 2006 at www.cdc.gov/nchs/products/pubs/pubd/hestats/finaldeaths04/finaldeaths04.htm.

ACTIVITIES FOR BEHAVIORAL CHANGE

The following provides instructions and the necessary forms for students to successfully complete the behavior change project.

PART 1. BEHAVIOR CHANGE PROJECT

Overview: As part of the Wellness course you will participate in a behavior change project. Select a health-related and wellness behavior from one of the dimensions of wellness (physical, emotional, mental, social, and spiritual) in which you would like to experience personal growth during the course. You must select a specific behavior in which you can experience personal growth. The following are some examples:

- Investigate the prevalence of cancer or coronary heart disease in your family—how could you alter your lifestyle to avoid becoming a victim?
- Quitting or modifying smoking or dipping behavior.
- Dietary intervention, improving your diet by reducing cholesterol and saturated fat.
- Reducing stress through increased sleep and sleep awareness.
- Reducing stress by improving time management skills.
- Proper use of ergogenic or nutritional supplements.
- Improving self-efficacy and self-esteem through spiritual development.
- Building better relationships and communications skills to build a social support network.
- Using support groups as a coping strategy for lifestyle change and social support.
- Using meditation or prayer to reduce daily stress.
- Helping myself by helping others to realize the benefits of altruistic giving.

The expectation is that you will commit to changing some health-related wellness behavior. The following is a brief summary of some of the literature on lifestyle change. Ultimately you will need to justify why you selected your health-related behavior, relative to overall wellness, and how you arrived at the plan to change your behavior.

Transtheoretical Model of Change (Prochaska & DiClemente, 1992)

1. Precontemplation
    a. The person does not intend, or is not ready, to change.
    b. The person may not understand the consequences of the behavior or the advantages of making the change.
    c. The person may be resistant to change.
    d. The person may view the pros of the negative behavior as greater than the cons.
2. Contemplation
    a. The person has some knowledge of the consequences or advantages of the change.
    b. Pros and cons of change are judged about equal.
    c. The person intends to change or is thinking about change, but may not know how to get started.

From M. LeBoeuf and L. Butler, eds., 2008, *Fit & active* (Champaign, IL: Human Kinetics).

3. Preparation

   a. The person has determined that the pros outweigh the cons.

   b. The person intends to make a change.

   c. The person has a plan of action for change within six months.

4. Action

   a. The person takes action on a regular basis (e.g., attending a class, eating nutritiously).

   b. He or she tends to feel empowered and in control of life.

   c. This is the time of greatest risk for relapse.

5. Maintenance

   a. The person has sustained the change for at least six months (e.g., walked daily, quit smoking).

   b. The old behavior has terminated, and prevention of relapse is important.

   c. Behavior change becomes part of the person's lifestyle.

Personal Log

You will keep a brief log associated with the behavior change project. The log can be hand written and will be turned in after the reflective presentation. The log will chronicle your personal feelings concerning the behavior change process, both positive and negative, and both successes and failures. The expectation is that you will have several entries each week.

Presentation

Your presentation will provide an overview of your behavior change experience. The behavior you choose to modify should involve one of the five dimensions of wellness, as it relates to your life as a student. Support your plan with reliable, refereed sources and materials.

Presentation and Reflection Format

You will have 5 minutes to present the results of your behavior change project. The format is up to you; PowerPoint, active learning, discussion, and so on are all acceptable as long as you get your message across.

1. *Introduction:* A discussion of the behavior you selected to modify.

2. *Change Process:* A review of the behavior change process and the foundation information you used as a basis for your behavior change process. You should support your statements with credible sources. You should be sure to critically analyze your sources and provide your own insight where appropriate.

3. *Results:* This section should summarize the results of your behavior change efforts, both successes and failures. Make specific recommendations on how the other students in the class might benefit from what you have learned and how your experience might be applicable to cadets and soldiers.

4. *References:* You should have sources and references to support your project. You may use references from the Internet, textbooks, or journals.

From M. LeBoeuf and L. Butler, eds., 2008, *Fit & active* (Champaign, IL: Human Kinetics).

(continued)

Behavior Change Timeline

Part 1A and 1B	Behavior identification	Lessons 1-3
Behavior change contract	Finalize behavior, goals, and process	Lesson 5
Begin project	Initiate project—begin record log	Lesson 7
Reflection	Written reflection on project	Lesson 17
Presentation	Oral reflection on project	Lessons 18 and 19

WELLNESS INVENTORY: GOAL SETTING (PART 1A)

Directions: Write a brief operational definition for each wellness dimension and list one of your strengths and one of your weaknesses for each dimension.

Wellness dimension	Definition	Strength	Weakness
Physical			
Emotional			
Mental			
Social			
Spiritual			

BEHAVIOR CHANGE PROJECT (PART 1B)

Identify Three Behaviors You Would Like to Change

Attach the Wellness Inventory and Goal Setting worksheet (Part 1A) that you did for Lesson 1. Use your knowledge of yourself and the results of the worksheet to identify five behaviors you could change (one from each of the five domains) to improve your wellness. The following are some examples:

- Quit or modify smoking or dipping behavior
- Reduce my stress level
- Feel better about myself
- Not be so cynical
- Reduce my anger level
- Develop a stronger relationship with God
- Reduce my social isolation

1. _____
2. _____
3. _____
4. _____
5. _____

Select One Behavior

Review the list of behaviors that you made and select one to pursue for your behavior change project. Circle a behavior from your list that is important to you and that you are strongly motivated to change.

Using table 1, follow the directions as you begin to reflect on the behavior you want to change.

Table 1 Current Behavior

Description of current behavior	
Negative consequences of current behavior	1. 2. 3. 4.

From M. LeBoeuf and L. Butler, eds., 2008, *Fit & active* (Champaign, IL: Human Kinetics).

(continued)

Using table 2, follow the directions as you begin to think about the positive effects of your new behavior.

Table 2   New Behavior

Description of new behavior	
Positive consequences of new behavior	1. 2. 3. 4.

Identify two *actions* you might select that will result in a change in *behavior*, that will in turn result in an improvement in a wellness *dimension*. Discuss how these *actions* will bring about these changes.

1. _____

   _____

   _____

   _____

2. _____

   _____

   _____

   _____

PART 2. BEHAVIOR CHANGE CONTRACT

Your next step in creating a successful behavior change plan is to complete and sign a behavior change contract. Your contract should include details of your program and indicate your commitment to changing your behavior. Use the information from Part 1 to complete the contract.

1. I, _____, agree to work on the following wellness dimension for the next four (4) weeks: _____.

From M. LeBoeuf and L. Butler, eds., 2008, *Fit & active* (Champaign, IL: Human Kinetics).

2. I will improve the following component of that wellness dimension: _____

_____.

3. I will execute my behavior change plan during the four-week period from

_____ to _____.

4. I will record my progress during the behavior change project by keeping a log, diary, or journal throughout the four weeks.

Circle one of the following: log   diary   journal

5. I have developed a systematic and progressive four-week action plan to accomplish my short-term goals.

	Weekly plan	Indicators of success
Week #1		
Week #2		
Week #3		
Week #4		

6. Upon faithfully executing the action plan for four weeks, I expect to achieve the following results.

_____

_____

_____.

7. I have identified the two most significant obstacles I expect to face as I work toward my short-term goals and how I will overcome them.

1. _____

2. _____

_____   _____
                Signature   Date

From M. LeBoeuf and L. Butler, eds., 2008, *Fit & active* (Champaign, IL: Human Kinetics).

NUTRITION PROJECT: DIET ANALYSIS

STUDENT INSTRUCTIONS

Overview: The nutrition project is a two-part project. There are two separate due dates. Do not begin Part 2 until Part 1 has been graded and returned.

Purpose: The purpose of the project is to increase your knowledge of nutrition and improve your healthy eating practices.

Part 1: Part 1 requires you to record your nutritional intake for five consecutive days. Input your daily information into a nutritional analysis software program similar to the MyPyramid.gov Web site. Once you have completed the five days, analyze your food intake data. From this information, identify the areas that need improvement and establish two goals and strategies to accomplish the goals. Remember, a goal must be measurable, observable, and achievable.

Part 2: Using the strategies outlined in Part 1, record your nutritional intake for another five consecutive days. Once again, analyze your food intake to determine if you have accomplished your goals.

Computer Printouts: After you have finished entering your foods for a particular day,

1. print out "Dietary Guidelines,"
2. print out "Nutrient Intakes," and
3. print out "MyPyramid."

NUTRITION PROJECT PART 1: REQUIREMENTS (130 POINTS)

Required Printouts (20 points)

1. Provide the following printouts:
   - Profile Daily Recommended Intake (DRI) Goals
   - Macronutrient Ranges
   - Fat Breakdown
   - Intake vs. Goals
   - Food Pyramid Analysis
   - Energy Balance
2. Select the One Day Option for a day of your choice and provide the following printouts:
   - Nutrient Intakes
   - Dietary Fiber
   - Saturated Fat

3. Printout of the "Intake Spreadsheet" report
4. Printout of the "Activities Spreadsheet" report

Caloric Intake and Requirement (20 points)

Complete these questions:

1. In the following chart, enter your five-day average caloric intake from the printouts, your daily energy requirement, and your daily energy requirement (as recommended by the Diet Analysis program—refer to the report "Energy Balance"). Discuss which of the recommended energy requirements is correct for you and whether you are over or under these daily energy requirements. Discuss the consequences of being significantly over or under your daily energy needs. How many calories should you consume per day?

	Caloric intake	Computed energy need	Diet Analysis recommendation
Five-day average total intake (Kcal)			

2. Examine the Intake vs. Goals report. In the following chart, enter your five-day average caloric intake (in grams) for carbohydrate, protein, and fat and the DRI recommended by the Diet Analysis program. Compare your individual intake (in grams) to the recommended Diet Analysis DRI in grams. Insert your Actual Diet Analysis % from the "Energy Nutrient Intake" box. Discuss your macronutrient balance (%) relative to the 55/15/30 percentages proposed in class.

Average intake	Intake (gms)	Diet Analysis DRI (gms)	Actual DA %	Recommended DRI
Carbs (grams)				55%
Protein (grams)				15%
Fat (grams)				30%

Saturated Fat and Cholesterol Intake (20 points)

1. Examine your "Fat Breakdown" report. Enter your five-day average intake of saturated, polyunsaturated, and monounsaturated fat as a percentage of your total caloric intake: Sat: _____; Poly: _____; Mono: _____. How did your three values compare to the DRIs discussed in class (i.e., what are the DRIs)?

2. Examine the "Source Analysis." For each day on the following chart, list your total saturated fat, the food that was highest in saturated fat, and a specific lower-fat alternative choice you could have made for those high saturated fat foods. Do *not* repeat alternative choices.

Saturated fat	Monday	Friday	Sunday
Total saturated fat			
Highest saturated fat food			
Healthy alternative			

From M. LeBoeuf and L. Butler, eds., 2008, *Fit & active* (Champaign, IL: Human Kinetics).

(continued)

3. Examine the "Intake vs Goals" report. Compare your five-day average intake of cholesterol in milligrams with the recommended DRI in milligrams:

   Your intake: _____   Recommended: _____

4. Coronary Heart Disease (CHD) is the leading killer in the United States. Discuss how a diet high in cholesterol contributes to the CHD process. What are two changes you can make in your diet that will help you lower cholesterol intake and better protect you against possible stroke or heart attack?

Fiber Intake (20 points)

1. Discuss two significant benefits of a high-fiber diet relative to long-term health.

2. Examine the "Intake vs Goals" report for "Dietary Fiber." Compare the "Intake" column for your five-day average intake of dietary fiber in grams with the DRI for dietary fiber:

   Your intake: _____   Recommended: _____

3. Refer to the "Source Analysis" chart for "Dietary Fiber, Total" for Thursday, Friday, and Saturday. List the two foods that were the highest in fiber for *each* day. In the following chart, list two different foods that were available (1) in the cafeteria and (2) when ordering out that would also increase fiber in your diet. Do not repeat options from day to day:

Dietary fiber sources	Thursday	Grams	Friday	Grams	Saturday	Grams
Highest fiber						
Next-highest fiber						
Cafeteria fiber source	–		–		–	
Order-out fiber source	–		–		–	

4. List two sources of fiber that are readily available in the mess hall or commissary that would help improve your fiber intake.

Vitamin and Mineral Intake (20 points)

1. Based on information from the "Intake vs Goals" report in the Diet Analysis program, enter the two vitamins and two minerals (micronutrients) you are most deficient in, and give the percentage of the recommended amount that you consumed (if you did not have any deficiencies, select two that were the lowest). Use the five-day average.

   For each of the deficiencies, list the (1) important dietary sources, (2) major functions, and (3) signs of prolonged deficiency.

From M. LeBoeuf and L. Butler, eds., 2008, *Fit & active* (Champaign, IL: Human Kinetics).

Deficient areas	Name	% of recommended amount	Dietary sources	Major functions	Signs of deficiency
Vitamin #1					
Vitamin #2					
Mineral #1					
Mineral #2					

2. Select your highest vitamin and mineral intake levels. Complete the following chart.

    a. Enter your five-day average in grams, milligrams, or micrograms.

    b. Enter the Tolerable Upper Intake Levels (UL) for each of those micronutrients (do an Internet search for selected nutrients).

    c. Enter both the major functions and the toxic effects of megadoses for the micronutrients that you selected (do an Internet search).

Highest intake	Avg. grams consumed	Tolerable Upper Intake Level (UL)	Major functions	Toxic effects
Vitamin: _____				
Mineral: _____				

Improvement Areas and Goal (10 points)

1. Describe three major areas of weakness in your diet based upon your diet analysis.

2. Select two specific areas that you would like to improve during Part 2 of the nutrition project and write a specific, measurable goal. (Example: I will increase my daily intake of fiber from _____ to _____ grams.)

Action Plan (20 points)

1. Discuss specific strategies you will use to achieve each of your two dietary goals. (Consider strategies for eating in the cafeteria, buying snack foods, ordering out, eating on weekends, etc.)

2. Discuss obstacles that might hinder your ability to reach your desired goals. Discuss ways in which you can overcome these obstacles.

From M. LeBoeuf and L. Butler, eds., 2008, *Fit & active* (Champaign, IL: Human Kinetics).

(continued)

NUTRITION PROJECT PART 2: REQUIREMENTS (70 POINTS)

1. Attach Part 1, your nutrition project.
2. Results (40 points)

   Your discussion should include but not be limited to the following:

   a. List your specific and measurable goals for Part 2 of the nutrition project.

   b. Evaluate your strategies for achieving each goal and give specific reasons why they worked or why they didn't work.

   c. Discuss your success in reaching your nutritional goals; list the values for support.

   d. Compare your five-day average caloric intake for carbohydrate, protein, and fat (in grams) to your daily recommended intake (DRI) estimated by the Diet Analysis. List the % intake by macronutrient; are your macronutrients in better balance than in Part 1?

3. Personal Application (30 points)

   a. After completing 10 days of dietary analysis, what are your *two* biggest dietary weaknesses? What acute or chronic health or performance issues may arise from your current dietary weaknesses?

   b. Discuss your two greatest dietary strengths.

NUTRITION PROJECT PART 3: FOOD LABEL ANALYSIS

Select a Nutrition Facts label from any food that you commonly eat. *The container must have more than one serving.* Attach the label to this form. Analyze the food as follows:

Food: _____ Manufacturer: _____

Serving size: _____ Servings per container: _____ Serving volume: _____

In your opinion, is this an appropriate portion size (why or why not)? _____

Total calories per serving: _____

Total fat (grams) in three servings: _____

Percentage of calories from total fat: _____

Total carbohydrate (grams) in two servings: _____

Percentage of calories from saturated fat: _____

Total protein (grams) in four servings: _____

Percentage of calories from protein: _____

Relative to the RDA, comment on the amount of cholesterol in this food if you ate two

servings: _____

_____

From M. LeBoeuf and L. Butler, eds., 2008, *Fit & active* (Champaign, IL: Human Kinetics).

Relative to the RDA, comment on the amount of sodium in this food if you ate the entire box, carton, or bag: _____

_____

Relative to the RDA, comment on the amount of fiber in this food: _____

_____

What is the ratio of simple to total carbohydrate in one serving? _____

_____

What is your overall assessment of this food? (i.e., nutritional value, nutritional density)?

_____

_____

_____

_____

_____

_____

_____

_____

_____

_____

_____

_____

_____

Name: _____

From M. LeBoeuf and L. Butler, eds., 2008, *Fit & active* (Champaign, IL: Human Kinetics).

GREAT AMERICAN SMOKE-OUT PROJECT

To participate in the Great American Smoke-Out (GAS) project, students are required to print up note cards with the 10 smoking facts listed below. Students carry the cards and a recording sheet (see the following sample) with them for two weeks prior to the Great American Smoke-Out (traditionally the third Thursday in November). Students must approach smokers and dippers, present the Smoking Facts card (for them to keep), and tell them about the GAS. To receive additional points, students must follow up on any individual to whom they gave a Smoking Facts card to see who quits for the day.

SMOKING FACTS

- There are 4,000 known chemicals in tobacco. Forty-three of these are proven to cause cancer.
- About half the people who smoke will die as a direct result of their habit.
- In the United States alone, 419,000 people die each year as a result of smoking.
- Smokers live at least 15 years less than nonsmokers.
- People who smoke cause 30% of all cancer-related deaths.
- Three out of every 10 people between the ages of 35 and 69 die because of cigarettes.
- Three thousand nonsmokers die each year of lung cancer as a direct result of second-hand smoke.
- If you smoke, you have twice the risk of dying of a heart attack, 10 times the risk of dying of lung cancer, and five times the risk of developing emphysema or chronic bronchitis compared to someone who does not smoke.
- By inhaling hot toxic fumes you are burning the linings of your air passages thus reducing the ability to ward off airborne diseases.
- Smoking causes a narrowing of blood vessels that carry blood to the arms and legs. If you get a blood clot and it blocks the arteries, it can result in the loss of an arm or leg.

The following is an example of a Great American Smoke-Out Recording Sheet that the students can carry to record the names of those who received the GAS facts and are committed to quit.

Told About GAS   Committed to Quit

1. _____   _____
2. _____   _____
3. _____   _____
4. _____   _____
5. _____   _____
6. _____   _____
7. _____   _____
8. _____   _____
9. _____   _____
10. _____   _____

From M. LeBoeuf and L. Butler, eds., 2008, *Fit & active* (Champaign, IL: Human Kinetics).

STD LEARNING ACTIVITY—PARTY TIME

Before class, the teacher randomly places self-stick notes under two to four seats or desks, then displays the following instructions for the Party Time exercise.

PARTY TIME

- Circulate throughout the room introducing yourself to each student you meet. Tell them your name and your favorite sport.
- On the second "pass," select two students to "party" with you on Saturday night.
- Record their names on a piece of paper.
- You cannot mutually select, that is, if you select a student, that student cannot select you back.
- Return to your seat when you have selected two students for your "party."

Prior to the students entering the classroom, the teacher will place four self-stick notes which will be numbered 1, 2, 3, 4 under four seats selected at random. The teacher will have four envelopes numbered 1, 2, 3, 4 which will contain the following notice from the doctor stating that they are either positive (2 each) or negative (2 each) for the HIV virus.

From the county health nurse: Your blood test has come back and you are HIV – Please continue to use precautions if you are sexually active.	**POSITIVE**
From the county health nurse: Your blood test has come back and you are HIV – Please continue to use precautions if you are sexually active.	**NEGATIVE**

After the students have gone through the selection process and returned to their seats, the teacher informs them that blood samples were obtained during their last physical and that she has the reports for some of the students. The students are told to look under their seats to see who has the numbered self-stick notes. Those students then come to the front of the room and the teacher gives them the corresponding numbered envelope. The students open the envelopes and read the information to the class that they either are or are not infected with the HIV virus. After they have read the report, they read the names of people they "partied" with, and those individuals stand up. Those standing then read the names of those they "partied" with, and so on. Normally, by the conclusion of the exercise almost everyone in the class is standing (infected).

From M. LeBoeuf and L. Butler, eds., 2008, *Fit & active* (Champaign, IL: Human Kinetics).

11

Personal Fitness

Matthew Beekley and Jason Lehmbeck

Personal fitness encompasses muscular strength and endurance, cardiorespiratory fitness, flexibility, and body composition, which is affected by nutrition. The idea of personal fitness suggests that individuals take responsibility for their own fitness and requires knowledge about exercise principles.

An obesity epidemic is occurring in America today, among adolescents (12-19 years) as well as other age groups. According to work comparing the National Health and Nutrition Examination Survey (NHANES) III (1988-1994) and the 1999-2000 NHANES study findings, the overweight levels of adolescents ages 12 to 19 increased from 10.5 to 14.8 percent. The most recent statistics from 2003-2004 suggest that 17.4 percent of adolescents aged 12 to 19 are overweight (National Center for Health Statistics). It is clear that obesity, with all its negative health effects, is increasing in the U.S. adolescent population.

What can be done to combat the obesity epidemic? Virtually all authorities are recommending an increase in school-directed exercise programs. The Centers for Disease Control and Prevention released a study in 2000 titled *Promoting better health for young people through physical activity and sport,* recommending that school programs "include daily physical education that helps students develop the knowledge, attitudes, skills, behaviors, and confidence to maintain physically active lifestyles." However, the percentage of students that participate in daily physical education has been dropping; for instance, the percentage of high school students participating in daily physical education classes dropped from 42 percent in 1991 to 27 percent in 1997. In addition to providing students with an academic education, schools are charged with educating students about how to exercise. Therefore, a personal fitness course is a necessary and crucial element in educating and empowering high school students regarding the "how-tos" of exercise.

In this chapter we outline how the Personal Fitness course is taught at West Point. Because the course consists of only 18 lessons, this outline could be adapted for use at the collegiate level as a half-semester course, as at West Point, or used over a full semester as part of a combined health-wellness and fitness class. We also provide some modifications of the course at the end of the chapter for use as part of a three-week unit in a high school level health-wellness and fitness course.

Purpose of the Course

The purpose of the Personal Fitness course is to build upon concepts from the Wellness course, as well as to learn and apply the principles required for developing a lifetime habit of personal fitness. The course emphasizes the human physiology of exercise and the mechanisms by which the body adapts to and benefits from physical training. Students participate in a variety of active learning labs in which they learn how to assess, monitor, develop, and maintain fitness in all five components of fitness: cardiorespiratory, muscular strength, muscular endurance, flexibility, and body composition.

Instructional Area

The instructional area for this course includes both classroom and out-of-classroom spaces. Classrooms should typically be outfitted with chalkboards, overhead projectors, or PowerPoint slide projectors, since some concepts will need illustration. Out-of-classroom areas used include a 400-meter–1/4 mile track, a weight or resistance training room, a cardiovascular exercise room, and a changing and locker room for students to change clothes and shower in.

Risk Management

In general, risk management for this class should entail careful consideration of fitness levels of all participants. Note also, however, that cardiovascular risk among entering college freshman is gener-

ally very low. Table 11.1 presents risk identification and risk reduction strategies to be used in the entering undergraduate college population.

Teaching Personal Fitness at the College Level

The Personal Fitness course as taught at West Point assumes that students have some previous knowledge of basic nutrition (a subject taught in the Wellness class). Since cadets are required to maintain a base level of fitness, a basic level of physical fitness is assumed. A standard collegiate-level introductory fitness text is also used. The Personal Fitness course provides education in nutrition and energy sources, cardiovascular exercise, resistance training exercise, and flexibility (see table 11.2). Also embedded in the course are labs that allow students to assess their own fitness, flexibility, and body composition. Finally, there are two projects: the Personal Fitness Plan, which allows students to tailor a fitness plan directly to their personal needs, and the Cadet Fitness Challenge, which challenges all aspects of a student's fitness. The Cadet Fitness Challenge (CFC) tests all of the health-related components of fitness. A fitness challenge could be used for a collegiate-level course. Chapter 9 presents more details on the CFC.

Course Overview

The Personal Fitness Plan (PFP) is a report required of each student in order to complete the Personal Fitness class. Students construct a physical fit-

Table 11.1 Possible Risks in the Personal Fitness Course

Risk identification	Reduction strategies
General falling injuries	• Avoid horseplay; provide proper supervision.
Muscle strains, ligament and tendon strains	• Always use proper warm-up prior to physical activity; provide proper supervision.
Angina (chest pain)	• Allow students to perform all exercises within their comfort zone. • Carefully monitor students for symptoms; have students cleared by physician for exercise.
Muscle soreness	• Warn students that nonexercisers will experience soreness and that this is a normal response to exercise.

ness plan in which they are encouraged to use the concept of periodization. Periodization is the concept of "back planning" and of using a calendar to train for a specific athletic event. A calendar with specific events of the student's own choos-ing is required, and students must show how their particular program plan will achieve their goals. A rubric for the PFP is presented at the end of the chapter. See table 11.2 for an overview of the Personal Fitness lessons.

Table 11.2 Overview of Personal Fitness Lessons

Lesson	Topic	Activities
1	Introduction to personal fitness	
2	Variables and principles of training; periodization	
3	Energy systems	
4	Sport nutrition and body composition	
5	Body composition lab	Lab activity
6	Cardiorespiratory I	
7	Cardiorespiratory I lab	Lab activity
8	Cardiorespiratory II	
9	Cardiorespiratory II lab	Lab activity
10	Midterm exam	
11	Muscular strength and endurance I	
12	Muscular strength and endurance lab	Lab activity
13	Muscular strength and endurance II	
14	Flexibility lab	Lab activity
15	Exercising in extreme environments	
16	Classroom work on personal fitness plan and fitness challenge	
17	Review for final exam and turn in personal fitness plan and fitness challenge	
18	Final exam	

Sample Lesson Plans

The following are examples of lesson plans typically used at West Point, but modified for "civilian" schools.

LESSON 1

Introduction to Personal Fitness

OBJECTIVES

* Identify the scope and purpose of personal fitness.
* Discuss the Personal Fitness Plan assessment rubric (see p. 264).
* Discuss the exercises and the scoring of the Fitness Challenge.
* Understand and define the health-related components of fitness (muscular strength, muscular endurance, cardiorespiratory fitness, flexibility, and body composition).

KEY TERMS

body composition—The relative percentages of muscle, fat, bone, and other tissues of the body.

cardiorespiratory fitness—Arguably the most important part of physical fitness; requires delivery and utilization of oxygen, thus involving the capability of the lungs, heart, muscle, and circulatory system; improved through aerobic exercise.

flexibility—The ability to perform range of motion in daily life or exercise; stretching is the primary technique used to improve flexibility.

muscular endurance—The ability of muscle to produce a submaximal force many times.

muscular strength—The force a muscle can produce one time (1-repetition maximum or 1-RM).

periodization—General principles for planning variations in training, discussed in "Principles of Periodization."

DISCUSSION QUESTIONS

* What role does fitness play in your life?
* Where is fitness on your list of life priorities?
* Which are your strongest health-related components of fitness? Which are your weakest?

LESSON 2

Variables and Principles of Exercise Training and the Concept of Periodization

CORE CONCEPTS

In this section we discuss the variables of training, which are used for exercise prescription, and the principles of exercise training, which guide application of the prescription. Then we address the concept of periodization, or conscious, deliberate variations in training over a given time period.

Variables of Exercise Training

The variables of training provide the prescription for exercise training. The acronym FITT (for frequency, intensity, time, and type) refers to the variables of exercise training and is an aid to learning and remembering these variables.

* Frequency: Frequency refers to the number of times per week exercise is performed. At least two or three exercise sessions for cardiorespiratory fitness, muscle endurance, muscle strength, and flexibility should be performed each week to improve fitness levels.

* Intensity: Intensity refers to how hard one trains. Training at the right intensity may be the most important consideration in personal fitness gains. Intensity is typically inversely proportional to time or volume. Intensity related to strength training is typically based on the percentage of 1-repetition maximum (1-RM) lifted. Intensity related to cardiorespiratory training is typically based on the percent of heart rate maximum or percent of heart rate reserve.

* Time or duration: The time spent exercising depends on the type of exercise being done. Time is usually inversely proportional to intensity. Some intense cardiorespiratory fitness training sessions may last only 8 minutes (six 400-meter [1/4-mile] intervals at 80 seconds each is a good example). Resistance training can also be short and intense. A full-body exercise program utilizing push and pull exercises may take only 20 minutes.

* Type (mode): Type refers to the specific exercise performed or the exercise modality. Running, biking, swimming, resistance training, and stretching exercises are all examples of exercise modality or type. Exercises should be chosen based on one's goals.

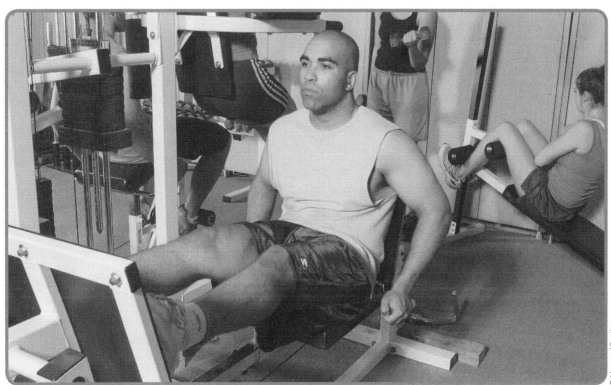

© Human Kinetics

Resistance training is an important part of personal fitness.

Principles of Exercise Training

The principles of exercise training form the foundation for applying the dose (FITT) of exercise. They assist us in regulating the dose, resulting in an appropriate or optimal level of response. The acronym PROVIRRBS is a good way to learn and remember the principles of exercise training.

- Progression: The intensity or the duration (time) of exercise, or both, must gradually increase to improve the level of fitness. The workload must systematically increase.

- Regularity: Regularity refers to the number of times one exercises per week. To achieve a training effect, a person must exercise often and at repeatable intervals. The regularity tends to be inversely related to the intensity.

- Overload: The workload of each exercise session must exceed the normal daily demands placed on the body in order to bring about a training effect.

- Variety of equipment or activities: Providing a variety of activities or training on different types of exercise equipment reduces boredom, increases motivation and progress, and enhances adherence. Further, a program using a variety of equipment or activities will ensure adequate or improved training of all components of health-related fitness and the motor skill–related abilities.

- Individuality: People must understand their own body type, how much training experience they have, and which physical exercises work for them and which do not.

- Recovery: A hard day of training for a given component of fitness should be followed by an easier training day or a rest day for that component or those muscle groups to help facilitate recovery.

- Realism: Training must be accomplished with the time and resources available. Setting realistic goals is critical to a fitness program. Some locations may not have the best or the most appropriate equipment. It is important to be realistic about what can be achieved within a given set of limitations.

- Balance: To effectively increase overall fitness, a program should include activities that address all five physical fitness components, since overemphasizing any one of them may hinder the development of the others. The concept of incorporating and undertaking exercises that push and pull, and that alternate upper and lower body movement, is important to remember in relation to building up the muscular strength and endurance component.

- Specificity: Specificity refers to utilizing specific training for specific performance goals, for instance, doing running to specifically improve your running time. Swimming may improve your general aerobic fitness but may not improve your running time.

Principles of Periodization

Periodization is the concept of "back planning" and of using a calendar to train for a specific athletic event. Periodization is commonly used by elite and amateur athletes in virtually every sport.

One should incorporate base, build, peak, and recovery weeks into one's training calendar. The base period typically lasts anywhere from 4 to 8 weeks, during which one gradually builds training volume, exercises at a lower intensity, and incorporates a variety of exercises. The build period can last from 4 to 10 weeks, during which one gradually increases intensity or volume and focuses on exercise specificity and proper form. During the base and build periods, intensity and volume should not be increased simultaneously in any one week. Typical increases in intensity or volume should not exceed about 10 percent per week. Approximately every third or fourth week during the base and build weeks, you should incorporate a lighter training week to allow for recovery and rest. Resistance training athletes may have a transition period during which they focus on hypertrophy or power training.

The peak period (also known as taper or precompetition) usually lasts only one to two weeks and should occur immediately preceding a competition. During the peak period, training volume is reduced (typically a 40-60 percent reduction) but training intensity increases. A rule of thumb for organizing exercise peak time is 14 days for running, 10 days for cycling, and 7 days for swimming. The recovery period usually lasts one to three weeks, during which volume and intensity of the exercise are reduced. This is a period of "active" rest and should include a variety of exercises.

OBJECTIVES

- Identify the variables of training (FITT: frequency, intensity, time, and type).
- Identify the principles of training (PROVIRRBS: progression, regularity, overload, variety, individuality, recovery, realism, balance, specificity).
- Explain the general concept of periodization.
- Apply the concept of periodization to both endurance and resistance training, using FITT and PROVIRRBS.
- Define and explain why recovery and recovery periods are important.

KEY TERMS

base period—The initial phase of training in the periodization cycle.

build period—The heavy training (increased volume and intensity) phase of the periodization cycle.

peak or taper or precompetition period—The period before competition in the periodization training cycle, typically a time of reduced volume.

recovery—Allows the body to rebuild from intense training and prevents burnout and overtraining.

transition period—The period between periodization cycles.

volume—Hours per week, mileage, or other quantity of physical training.

DISCUSSION QUESTIONS

- What training programs have you used in the past two years, and how successful have they been?
- Does doing the same exercise(s) day after day allow one to progress? Why or why not?
- Why are there some days when physical exercise seems very difficult while at other times the same workout seems easy?
- Do you have a plan when you study? When you work? Is there a plan for your life? What are the benefits of having a plan for exercise?

LESSON 3

Energy Systems

OBJECTIVES

- Understand the final common energy source for the body. Adenosine triphosphate (ATP) is the final common energy source for muscular work, and all foodstuffs are finally converted to this high-energy molecule.

- Identify the energy source, response time, limitations, and trainability of the *immediate* energy system. The immediate energy source, besides the small amount of ATP in the muscle, is the creatine-phosphate system.
- Identify the energy source, response time, limitations, and trainability of the *intermediate* energy system. The intermediate energy source is oxygen-independent glycolysis, which converts glycogen or glucose to lactate.
- Identify the energy source, response time, limitations, and trainability of the *long-term* energy system. The long-term energy system is the oxygen-dependent system, utilizing glycogen and glucose and fat as energy (converting to ATP).
- Identify the locations of glucose and glycogen in the body. Glucose is found in blood sugar and glycogen is found in skeletal muscle and the liver.
- Define the "crossover" concept of fuel use and exercise intensity, and identify how it changes with training. The crossover concept refers to the fact that at lower exercise intensities (<60 percent of $\dot{V}O_2$max), fat predominates as the fuel source, while at higher exercise intensities (>60 percent of $\dot{V}O_2$max), carbohydrate predominates. Thus, if you wish to exercise intensely, you must replace muscle glycogen regularly by eating a high-carbohydrate diet. At any particular workload, a higher percentage of fat is used as fuel after cardiorespiratory training, indicating that the crossover point has changed.

KEY TERMS

maximal oxygen uptake or $\dot{V}O_2$max—The maximal oxygen consumption of an individual; typically measured on a treadmill test. $\dot{V}O_2$max is only a fair predictor of exercise performance, but is closely related to mortality and morbidity.

peak oxygen uptake or $\dot{V}O_2$peak—The maximal oxygen consumption during a particular exercise modality; typically lower than a treadmill $\dot{V}O_2$max.

DISCUSSION QUESTIONS

- Theoretically speaking, how is the supplement creatine purported to work?
- Ms. Johnson, who desperately wants to lose weight, has complained to you that the high-intensity interval training you have prescribed for her "is not in the fat-burning range, and so it won't help me lose weight." What do you tell her and why?

LESSON 4

Sport Nutrition and Body Composition

OBJECTIVES

- Identify the requirement for calories, protein, and carbohydrate in sedentary people and in active athletes (both endurance and strength or power). (*Note:* This lesson assumes basic nutritional knowledge from a course such as Wellness, described in chapter 10.)
- Describe the recommended amount of fluid for hydration and rehydration during exercise. The American College of Sports Medicine recommends drinking ~500 milliliters (17 ounces) 2 hours before competition. During exercise, enough fluid should be consumed to equal weight or sweat loss or should be the maximal

amount tolerated. Rehydration should replace the weight lost at a rate of 16 ounces per pound of weight lost. Some sodium should be included in the postexercise diet.

• Describe a precompetition diet for a strength athlete and an endurance athlete. Because of the crossover concept, it is obvious that a precompetition diet should be high in complex carbohydrate for intense exercise.

Calculating Daily Protein and Carbohydrate Needs

Here we present a format for calculating daily protein and carbohydrate needs for students and athletes. These are easy calculations that simply require students to know their own current body weight in pounds (see table 11.3).

Table 11.3   Daily Protein and Carbohydrate Needs for Athletes

Athlete or diet plan	Protein need	Carbohydrate need
Sedentary student	0.36 grams per pound BW	At least 130 grams
Endurance athlete	0.6 grams per pound BW	4.0 grams per pound BW
Strength or power athlete	0.75 grams per pound BW	3.5 grams per pound BW

BW = current body weight.

Calculating your own protein needs:

_____ pounds × _____ = _____ grams of protein per day
(body weight)   (protein needs value from table 11.3)

Calculating your own carbohydrate needs:

_____ pounds × _____ = _____ grams of carbohydrate per day
(body weight)   (carbohydrate needs value from table 11.3)

Tables 11.4 and 11.5 show amounts of protein and carbohydrate content in various foods. Students can use the tables to "guesstimate" what they would have to eat to obtain their protein and carbohydrate requirements.

Table 11.4   Examples of Protein Sources

Food	Serving	Protein (g)
Turkey	3 oz (size of a deck of cards)	26
Chicken	3 oz	24
Lean beef	3 oz	20
Fish	3 oz	20
Peanut butter	2 tbsp	10
Milk	1-pint carton	8
Beans	1/2 cup	7

Table 11.5 Examples of Carbohydrate Sources

Food	Serving	Carbohydrate (g)
Bread	1 slice	12
One medium fruit	1	20
Beans	1/2 cup	24
Potato	1 large	50
Cold cereal	1 cup	24
Rice	1 cup	50
Pasta	1 cup	34

Calculating Daily Caloric Needs

The following information will allow you to calculate your daily caloric balance (your daily caloric need). First, calculate your resting metabolic rate using the formula. Then, multiply your resting metabolic rate by an appropriate activity factor. RMR = resting metabolic rate.

Men: RMR = 9.99 × weight in kilograms + 6.25 × height in centimeters − 4.92 × age in years + 5

Women: RMR = 9.99 × weight in kilograms + 6.25 × height in centimeters − 4.92 × age in years − 161

Activity factor (multiply the RMR results you obtained by the following activity factor based on your activity level):

Sedentary   1.0
Moderately active   1.1
Very active   1.3

DISCUSSION QUESTIONS

* For a marathon, do you think eating high-carbohydrate meals the day before would be beneficial? Why or why not?

* What supplements have you taken? Do you think they have "worked"? Why or why not?

* Mike is about 10 pounds (4.5 kilograms) overweight. Name three key strategies involving diet and exercise for him to use in the next two months to aid in safe weight loss.

* Kim will be participating in a long triathlon in high heat and humidity. She wants to make sure she is hydrated and drinks lots of water the day before the race and during the race. You also know that Kim is concerned about her health and follows a strict low-salt diet. On race day, midway through the race, Kim starts to act strangely and urinates frequently. What do you suspect is happening, and what do you do about it?

* James is participating in your weight training program, which is currently at its highest volume and intensity. James continues to insist on eating a high-protein

diet, since "all this exercise is breaking us down." You notice that his performance is suffering. Why is James' performance suffering and what do you do about it?

- Cheryl is also participating in your weight training program, which again is currently at its highest volume and intensity. Cheryl eats a high-carbohydrate vegetarian diet and has refused to eat any meat since you have known her. You notice that her performance is suffering. Why is Cheryl's performance suffering and what do you do about it?

- What are the approximate percentages of each macronutrient you should be consuming to enhance performance?

- How much protein does a typical American consume?

LESSON 5

Body Composition Lab

OBJECTIVES

- Perform a hip-to-waist measurement and compare the result to regularly published tables.

- Perform the skinfold method and calculate your percent body fat (see figure 11.1). Virtually all collegiate-level fitness texts have instructions and calculation materials for doing this lab. If your facilities allow, you may also perform alternative methods of body composition, such as underwater weighing.

- From your percent body fat, calculate how many pounds of you are lean tissue and fat tissue.

EQUIPMENT

- Tape measures
- Skinfold calipers
- Other equipment to measure body composition, such as underwater weighing tank (optional)

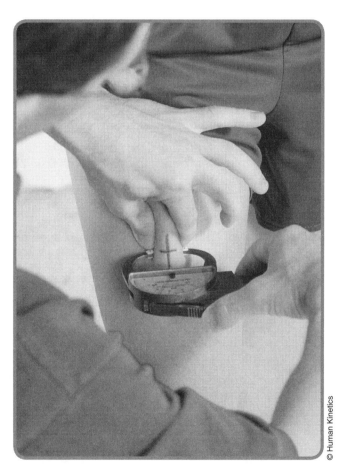

FIGURE 11.1   Skinfold test.

© Human Kinetics

LESSON 6

Cardiorespiratory I

OBJECTIVES

* Explain in general how the heart and lungs deliver oxygen and remove carbon dioxide.
* Understand the formula $CO = HR \times SV$ and its ramifications for training adaptation. Cardiac output (CO) is directly related to repetitive muscular work. At any given workload, adaptation to cardiorespiratory training results in an increased stroke volume (SV) and a decreased heart rate (HR).
* Explain how $\dot{V}O_2$max and $\dot{V}O_2$peak are related to performance. $\dot{V}O_2$max is only fairly closely related to performance; a high $\dot{V}O_2$max suggests a good competitor, but the highest $\dot{V}O_2$max in a group of athletes with high $\dot{V}O_2$max rarely wins the race.
* Explain what happens to resting submaximal and maximal HR, $\dot{V}O_2$max and $\dot{V}O_2$peak, blood pressure, blood lipids, and fat-burning enzymes, as well as the crossover point after chronic adaptation to cardiorespiratory training. In response to cardiorespiratory training, maximal HR remains unchanged; submaximal HR decreases; $\dot{V}O_2$max increases; blood pressure decreases; blood lipids decrease; fat-burning enzymes increase; and the crossover point shifts to the right, allowing a greater reliance on fat as fuel at the same workload.
* Understand the use of a heart rate monitor to monitor exercise intensity. Since exercise intensity during cardiorespiratory training is hard to gauge and is directly related to HR, a HR monitor is one of the most accurate ways to monitor exercise intensity.
* Understand the use of the Borg Rating of Perceived Exertion (RPE) scale to monitor exercise intensity. Because HR is also related to perception of exertion during exercise, the RPE can be a useful monitor of exercise intensity.
* Demonstrate how to calculate training heart rates at various exercise intensities.

KEY TERMS

barometric pressure—The atmospheric pressure, as measured by a barometer; important in calculating the partial pressure of oxygen.

cardiac output (CO)—The amount of blood (liters per minute) that the heart can output.

partial pressure of oxygen—The pressure of oxygen in the atmosphere; since oxygen is ~21 percent of atmospheric gas, other gas pressures also make up atmospheric (barometric) pressure.

stroke volume (SV)—The amount of blood pumped by the heart with each heartbeat.

DISCUSSION QUESTIONS

* Sally Mae is running a marathon on October 4. On October 3, she visits a "recommended" Mexican restaurant and develops diarrhea early in the evening before the race. It continues all night and into the morning of the race. How will this affect Sally's marathon performance? Explain using physiological reasons.

* Jerry went out binge drinking with his friends last night, and today he has 2-a-day football practices scheduled in high heat and humidity. What will likely happen to Jerry's performance during practice and, physiologically speaking, why?

LESSON 7

Cardiorespiratory I Lab

OBJECTIVE

Demonstrate how to use a heart rate monitor to determine various exercise intensities during a run. The students can then be asked to calculate their heart rates at various exercise intensities, and then alter their pace to keep their heart rate within the prescribed range. Note that this can be done with a different exercise modality, for example cycling, if desired.

EQUIPMENT

Heart rate monitors (*Note:* With younger populations, you can place the HR monitor directly on the students' T-shirts and wet the shirts with water from a spray bottle. This saves time in that students do not need to put the monitor directly on their chest in a changing area.)

LESSON 8

Cardiorespiratory II

OBJECTIVES

* Explain how FITT and PROVIRRBS apply to cardiorespiratory training.
* Explain the use of intervals in improving speed during cardiorespiratory training.
* Explain the use of fartlek training in improving speed during cardiorespiratory training. Interval and fartlek training have been shown to improve $\dot{V}O_2$max, exercise tolerance, and energy transitions, which can result in improved speed during exercise performance.
* Explain how to select and replace footgear for cardiorespiratory training.
* Explain the basics of good running form.

DISCUSSION QUESTIONS

* Billy needs to decrease his run time to be able to stay on the varsity team. What program would you suggest and why?
* The track coach takes the athletes to the golf course for a run. What could be the reason for this?
* Your friend comes to you and wants to implement interval training in her fitness program. How would you help her design this?

CARDIOVASCULAR CROSS-TRAINING EQUIPMENT

Often it is preferable to work out indoors because the weather is not suitable for training outdoors. Additionally, cross-training can help prevent injury and maintain aerobic fitness during periods of injury or boredom and burnout. Use this guide to become familiar with the advantages and disadvantages of using each machine for cross-training.

STAIR CLIMBER

Stair climbing machines give the exerciser benefits similar to those with climbing stadium stairs, without the hassle of searching for stairs to climb and with less impact on the legs. Stair climbing on the machine requires a consistent and continuous use of large muscle groups, resulting in a rhythmically aerobic workout. Since stair climbing on the machine is less weight bearing than climbing actual stairs, injured people can usually use this machine to help them maintain an aerobic base without the high impact associated with activities like running. People should always maintain optimal posture (upright posture, hips set and abdominal muscles tight) while on the machine. Some disadvantages of this machine are that it doesn't involve the upper extremity and requires body control (which may not be appropriate at some levels of injury) and that, secondary to fatigue, you cannot reach the high revolutions per minute that can be achieved on a stationary bike.

ELLIPTICAL TRAINER

This machine offers many of the same advantages as the stair climber. However, you can exercise at higher revolutions per minute on the elliptical trainer than you can on the stair climber. The very fluid motion attained on this machine more closely resembles running, but the level of weight bearing is similar to that with a cross-country ski machine. The elliptical trainer offers an excellent rehabilitation opportunity for people with foot or lower extremity injuries, as it limits weight bearing and does not require much ankle motion. The unique motion required of the body to use this machine is somewhat awkward and thus requires practice.

CROSS-COUNTRY SKI MACHINE

The cross-country ski machine involves the use of large muscle groups in both the upper and lower extremities to offer a balanced aerobic endurance workout. One slight disadvantage to its use is that the movements do not simulate running as well as the elliptical trainer. Also, the unique motion required of the body is somewhat awkward and thus requires practice.

TREADMILL

One of the main advantages to using the treadmill is its versatility. Just as with the stair climber, you can tailor your workout to your aerobic ability and preferred intensity. Many treadmills offer a feature that allows the exerciser to program a full workout with a warm-up, gradual increased pace, training pace, and then a cool-down. You can also set up an interval training session by adjusting the time and intensity of the workout. It's an excellent tool for teaching pace. Additionally, most treadmills have a height elevation feature for hill training. If you live on flat terrain, you can do your hill workout on the treadmill. To mimic trail running, you can program hills and a short, fast-tempo pace at regular or irregular intervals. Treadmills have a soft surface compared to concrete; but just as with running, this activity is full weight bearing. For people with lower body injuries, this activity is not the best choice for cross-training.

STATIONARY AND RECUMBENT BIKES

The bike is one of the most versatile types of endurance training equipment. You can maintain higher revolutions per minute on the bike than on other low-impact machines due to less fatigue from supporting your full body weight. At low settings, these bikes can also be used for a warm-up or cool-down before or after running, weight training, or other sports. They are ideal for people who require a reduction in weight-bearing activity. A disadvantage of cycling is that it can place stress on the knees in some people, especially those who already have knee pain. However, adjusting the seat height to accommodate full straightening of the knee (without locking the knee) on the downstroke can minimize knee injuries.

ROWING MACHINE

A major advantage to using the rowing machine for cross-training is that it works both the upper and lower body, allowing for a nearly full-body workout. The rowing motion promotes good posture of the upper back by toning the muscles that prevent forward rounding of the shoulders. A disadvantage is that the rowing motion requires constant attention to good form to prevent back strain.

LESSON 9

Cardiorespiratory II Lab

OBJECTIVES

Demonstrate how to use a heart rate monitor during intervals (at West Point, we use 1/4-mile [400-meter] intervals).

EQUIPMENT

Heart rate monitors

LESSON 10

Midterm Exam

In the past, the midterm exam at West Point was typically between 75 and 100 true-and-false and multiple-choice questions. It was given during one class period. Because of the number of classes taught concurrently, one exam was created and is used by all instructors.

LESSON 11

Muscular Strength and Endurance I

OBJECTIVES

- Define a motor unit. A motor unit is the nerve and all the muscle fibers the nerve innervates.
- Explain the characteristics of slow-twitch oxidative (SO) muscle fibers. These fibers have slow-twitch speed and are dependent on oxidative energy systems.
- Explain the characteristics of fast-twitch oxidative-glycolytic (FOG) muscle fibers. These fibers have fast-twitch speed and are dependent on both glycolytic and oxidative energy systems.
- Explain the characteristics of fast-twitch glycolytic (FG) muscle fibers. These fibers have fast-twitch speed and are dependent upon the glycolytic energy system.
- Identify athletes who have mostly SO muscle fibers and athletes who have mostly FG muscle fibers. Typically, sprint athletes have mostly FG, while marathoners have mostly SO.
- Describe the different types of skeletal muscle contractions. The different types of contractions are isometric, isotonic, isokinetic, eccentric, and concentric.
- Identify the major muscles of the muscular system and the major bones of the skeletal system, and be able to identify which muscles and bones are being worked during a particular exercise.

KEY TERMS

concentric—The phase of the muscle contraction in which muscle shortens.

eccentric or "negatives"—The phase of the muscle contraction in which muscle lengthens.

isokinetic—"Same speed"; muscle is held at a constant speed during contraction by a specialized machine. These machines are found at many colleges in research or athletic training or rehabilitation departments.

isometric—"Same length"; muscle contractions without movement.

isotonic—"Same weight"; muscle contractions against constant weight; typically what we are doing when lifting free weights.

DISCUSSION QUESTIONS

- Hypothesize about your own muscle fiber type.
- Why don't those "muscle-abdominal stimulators" you see advertised on TV work?
- Demonstrate for the class an example of an isotonic, an isometric, an isokinetic, a concentric, and an eccentric contraction.

LESSON 12

Muscular Strength and Endurance Lab

OBJECTIVES

- Demonstrate correct technique while performing various lifts. Demonstrating various "typical" exercises, for example bench press, in the school weight room or gym is suggested.
- Demonstrate correct spotting techniques.
- Demonstrate correct techniques for performing negatives.
- Explain safety procedures in the weight room.

LESSON 13

Muscular Strength and Endurance II

OBJECTIVES

- Explain how FITT and PROVIRRBS apply to muscle strength and muscle endurance training.
- Explain the blood pressure response during heavy lifts and thoroughly explain any implications. During very heavy weightlifting, blood pressure can rise enormously; thus, in some hypertensive populations, performing 1-RM or heavy lifting is contraindicated.
- Identify strengthening and stretching exercises for the abdomen and low back.
- Explain the benefits of improved flexibility. There is little scientific and epidemiological evidence that improved flexibility reduces risk of injury; however, flexibility should still be emphasized to improve range of motion, posture, and so on.
- Identify four types of stretches.

KEY TERMS

ballistic (dynamic) stretching—Stretching completed with jerky, rapid, and bouncy movements. Because numerous sports involve ballistic movements, many advocate that ballistic stretching be employed to assist in optimal performance in sport. Similar to a "high-intensity" strength or cardiorespiratory workout, these training programs are beneficial but must be performed under strict supervision by a coach or qualified individual. Ballistic stretching will increase flexibility but is *not* recommended for sedentary people or those with low fitness.

passive stretching—This type of stretch involves a force (other than an opposing muscle) imposed on the muscle. For example, a partner may push a body part through a range of motion. Another body part, weights, pulleys, or gravity may impose the force, which causes movement and a stretch to take place.

proprioceptive neuromuscular facilitation (PNF) stretching—A "contract–relax" sequence helps muscles relax, which results in greater muscle length. A partner *slowly* pushes the body part in the direction of the stretch until slight discomfort is felt. The person being stretched tells the partner when to stop applying pressure. The position is held for 8 to 10 seconds. (This first stretch does not cover the entire range of motion.) The person being stretched performs an isometric contraction, pushing back against the partner's resistance with about 25 percent of maximal effort. The isometric contraction is held for 4 to 5 seconds. The person being stretched relaxes the muscles, and the partner *slowly* pushes the body part a little farther in the direction of the stretch. This "contract, then relax" sequence is repeated two to five times.

slow, sustained (static) stretching—Muscles are lengthened gradually through a joint's complete range of motion and held for a period of time. This stretching is conducted slowly, causing the muscles to relax so that greater length can be achieved. This type of slow, sustained movement causes little pain and imposes a low risk of injury.

DISCUSSION QUESTIONS

- At the annual World's Strongest Man contest, do the former bodybuilders do well? Why or why not?
- Mary Ann needs to increase her upper body strength; she is unable to complete one pull-up. What program would you suggest and why?
- Which is more important for fitness—muscular strength or muscular endurance?

LESSON 14

Flexibility Lab

OBJECTIVES

- Perform a flexibility assessment using a sit and reach box. Obtain a standard sit and reach box. Have the student sit on the floor with legs together, knees extended, and the soles of the feet placed against the edge of the box (student should

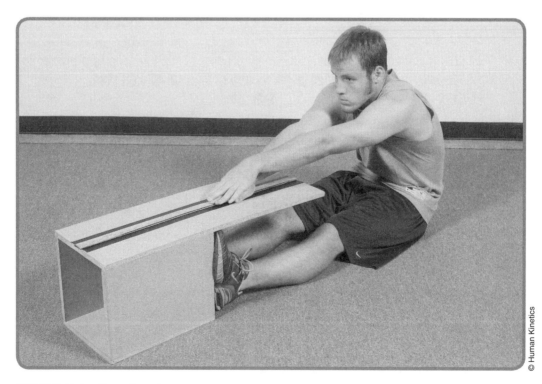

FIGURE 11.2 Sit and reach test.

© Human Kinetics

have shoes off). Most boxes have a zero point set at 23 centimeters. Instruct the student to reach forward slowly and as far as possible along the top of the box while keeping hands parallel, with overlapping fingers (see figure 11.2). Most boxes have a small metal latch to push forward. Make certain that the knees do not flex. The score is the most distant point to which the latch is moved or the fingertips make contact.

- Demonstrate correct technique for slow, passive, and PNF stretches.

EQUIPMENT

Sit and reach box: A number of commercial alternatives are available on the market.

LESSON 15

Exercising in Extreme Environments

OBJECTIVES

- Explain the performance differences between men and women and explain physiologically why there are some performance differences. Some of the differences are related to the increased testosterone in men versus women, which results in increased skeletal muscle mass, decreased body fat, increased aggression, increased blood and heart volume, and other effects. On the other hand, women tend to have increased flexibility compared to men.
- Explain the physiologic ramifications of exercising in high heat and humidity and what can be done to prevent these effects.
- Explain the physiologic ramifications of exercising in extreme cold and what can be done to prevent these effects.
- Explain the physiologic ramifications and adaptations of exercising at altitude during acute and chronic exposure and what can be done to prevent the ramifications. Virtually all of these conditions, at least acutely, lead to dehydration, loss of plasma volume, and thus decreased stroke volume and increased heart rate, adversely affecting exercise performance. Typically, the best way to combat this is acclimatization to the condition (usually ~10 days to two weeks) and use of good rehydration practices.
- Understand factors of exercise adherence and strategies of exercise adherence. Virtually all collegiate-level textbooks have a section on exercise adherence.
- Explain the psychological aspects of physical training.

DISCUSSION QUESTIONS

- Julie injures her knee on a run. She wishes to continue to train, however. What exercise modalities do you suggest?
- You are going on a camping trip with your friends, and all of you are going to be mountain climbing. What do you tell your friends about what to expect physically and what to eat and drink, and why?
- Several of your friends have bought "oxygenated water" to "aid" them in their trip to the mountains. What do you tell them about oxygenated water?

Teaching This Course at the Secondary Level

For high school students, some of the material we have presented must be altered. This course is likely taught as a three-week unit in health or physical education. Fitness challenges are typically discouraged at the high school level; use of fitness assessments, such as the Cooper Institute's Fitnessgram, seems more common.

The concept of periodization should be deemphasized; concentration instead should be on simple planning for personal fitness or seasons for various sports. High schools can use the concept of FITT discussed earlier, but simplifying the principles of training to overload, specificity, and progression is recommended.

Additionally, the concept of target heart rate should be used in place of measures like maximal oxygen consumption. Target heart rate, resting heart rate, and recovery heart rate can be used for high school students.

Getting students up and moving is critical if we are to reduce the incidence of obesity in our country. The key to doing this, and doing it successfully, is to help make students successful and show how they can improve, as well as making the experience fun and including variety.

It is very important to emphasize a variety of activity. In a personal fitness unit, it is critical that students experience a wide range of activity. Resistance training is one aspect of personal fitness. Consider using all five components of health-related fitness as your guide to developing a curriculum. For example, do a day of yoga, a day of hiking (or snowshoeing or cross-country skiing), a day of resistance training of some kind, a day of cardiovascular lab, and then mix in a team game. The number-one motivator is success, and second to that is fun. High school students probably will not respond well to daily weight room training, whereas collegiate-level students might.

The use of these concepts and terms for high school students is really a matter of consistent reinforcement of the principles. For example, throughout the year, discussion of the FITT principle on a weekly basis provides reminders and reinforcement. The following are some examples of ways to teach some of these concepts within a fitness unit.

Cardiovascular Laboratory

PURPOSE

To demonstrate the intensity of cardiovascular exercise by monitoring heart rate

SPACE

Gym or outdoors

ACTIVITY

1. Prepare a worksheet on which the students can record heart rates for different types of activities and the target heart rate (THR) formula. Decide what activities you will use. Simple activities like walking, jogging, and running are the easiest, but if you would like to use an activity like basketball you can adapt activities that have different levels of intensity.

2. When students arrive, have them sit down and rest immediately, hand out the worksheet, and then, after they have rested a few minutes, ask them to find their pulse. This will serve as the resting heart rate for the THR formula.

3. Calculate THR (see previous labs).

4. Proceed with the activities that you have planned. After each activity, stop and check HR, record, and move on to the next activity. Activities should model a warm-up, activity, and cool-down progression.

5. Proceed through the activities to show that different activities had different effects on individual students. Point out that cardiovascular health is different for each individual.

Resistance Laboratory With "Garage Sale" Workout Equipment

PURPOSE

To demonstrate the possibilities of resistance training without access to a fitness center or expensive equipment

EQUIPMENT

Variety of dumbbells, barbells, weighted plates, cans of paint, old milk jugs full of water (8 pounds [3.6 kilograms] per gallon)

SPACE

Gym or outdoors

ACTIVITY

Use a variety of items that may be found around the house, or a simple weight set obtained at a garage sale, to do a full-body resistance training workout. Incorporate each muscle group and variations of grips and techniques for different equipment.

Partner Training Assessment Laboratory

PURPOSE

To conduct a mock interview with a fitness center client, asking the requisite questions

SPACE

Classroom

ACTIVITY

Ask students to pair up (one is the trainer; the other is the client). Have the fitness trainer ask about background health risk information and fitness goals of the individual and then aid in developing a plan.

Fitness Plan Assessment

A rubric is a guideline for what to look for in a student's product (in this case the fitness plan) to determine its quality. The rubric (see table 11.6) aids the instructor by leading to more objective grading and at West Point is used to encourage consistent grading across instructors.

Table 11.6 Personal Fitness Plan Assessment Rubric

Component	Description of component and grading standards	Points earned
1. Personal analysis (5 points)	**Excellent:** List your top four or five life priorities, not necessarily all fitness related. **Sub-excellent:** Omitted or inadequately covered items	
2. Fitness assessment (20 points)	**Excellent:** (1) List objective measurements of your most recently performed physical fitness tests (by event). (2) List your current assessment of performance in all other areas cited as fitness objectives (most recent marathon time, 1-RM bench press, etc.). (3) Most important: Write a paragraph including a subjective assessment of fitness-related personal strengths and weaknesses. **Sub-excellent:** Omitted or inadequately covered items, unclear measurement standards	
3. Fitness objectives (20 points)	**Excellent:** (1) List specific long-term (>1 year), medium-term (3 months to 1 year), and short-term (<3 months) physical fitness goals. (2) List specific performance objectives by event. **Sub-excellent:** Omitted or inadequately covered items; not using the same, measurable standards for each event as in fitness assessment; unreasonable objectives (too high or too low)	
4. 52-week training schedule (30 points)	**Excellent:** A 52-week calendar that must include, at a minimum: (1) major events (races, etc.); (2) major time constraints; and (3) a logical plan of base, build, and peak weeks built around these events and constraints. Prioritize events and schedule your plans around the events. **Sub-excellent:** Omitted or inadequately covered items; an inappropriate periodization plan based on the fitness assessment and objectives	
5. Three detailed training weeks— planned exercises (50 points)	**Excellent:** Choose one event and, leading up to that event, detail three separate training weeks—one each from a base, build, and peak period. Include a list of appropriate frequency (number of times per week), intensity (percent maximal HR, rating of perceived exertion, interval pace and rest times, percent of 1-RM, etc.), time (total minutes of work, number of work intervals, and number or reps per set and number of sets per workout, etc.), and type (the actual exercises you are doing—e.g., bench press, 400 m intervals) for each day of the week. Describe the main objectives of each week and the total volume (hours of training) for each week. **Sub-excellent:** Inappropriate FITT values based on the fitness objectives, training requirements, and available time; failure to follow periodization principles	
6. Narrative (50 points)	**Excellent:** Describe how your overall plan will help you reach your fitness goals. Focus your discussion on the preparation for one event—the same one as in step 5. Describe in detail, using training principles (PROVIRRBS) and variables (FITT), how your three detailed training weeks fit into and contribute to the plan. Compare and contrast the three weeks, and explain how they fit into an overall plan to bring you to optimum performance for that "A"-level event. Emphasize the training required to improve *your* weaknesses, maintain *your* strengths, and achieve *your* objectives identified in steps 2 and 3 pertaining to that one event. (Do not generically explain PROVIRRBS and FITT.) **Sub-excellent:** Omitted or inadequately covered items; inappropriate FITT values based on the fitness objectives, available training time, and directed fitness events	
7. Adherence plan (15 points)	**Excellent:** Write a paragraph describing personal planned strategies for improving adherence to your plan. **Sub-excellent:** Omitted or inadequately covered items	
8. Reflective statement (10 points)	**Excellent:** Include a paragraph describing your thoughts on the personal fitness plan and a paragraph on the course in general. **Sub-excellent:** Omitted or inadequately covered items	
Total score (200 possible points)		_____ / 200

Key Terms

FITT—Frequency (how often), intensity (how hard), time (how long), type (what activity).

health-related fitness components—Cardiovascular endurance (aerobic conditioning), muscular strength, muscular endurance, flexibility, body composition.

overload—Doing more than you normally do.

physical fitness—The ability to carry out one's daily routine without stress and still have energy to pursue some recreational activity; the ability to handle emergency situations; the ability to go through a day without fatigue and in most cases with increased energy. Physical fitness is not necessarily related to being a good athlete.

progression—The increase of overload over time; must be done at a gradual, methodical pace.

specificity—Using an activity that matches the goals of training.

sport-related fitness components—Agility, speed, balance.

training principles—General concepts that are simple enough for planning an effective training program.

References

Centers for Disease Control and Prevention, National Center for Health Statistics. (Reviewed January 30, 2007). www.cdc.gov/nchs/products/pubs/pubd/hestats/overweight/overwght_child_03.htm.

U.S. Department of Health and Human Services. (2000). *Promoting better health for young people through physical activity and sports*. Washington, D.C.

Suggested Readings

Corbin, C.B., Lindsey, R., Welk, G., & Corbin, W.R. (2002). *Concepts of fitness and wellness*. (4th ed.). Boston: McGraw-Hill.

Prentice, W.E. (2001). *Get fit, stay fit*. (2nd ed.). Boston: McGraw-Hill.

Sharkey, B.J. (2002). *Fitness & health*. (5th ed.). Champaign, IL: Human Kinetics.

PART IV

Lifetime Activity Courses

12

Tennis

Karen Peck and Sandor Helfgott

Tennis is a sport that can be played by people of all ages and abilities, and for this reason it is often referred to as a lifetime sport. There are many formats in which tennis can be played. It can be played as "singles," with one player pitted against another; as "doubles," with competition between two teams of two; or even in a game called Canadian doubles in which three players can compete at once on a single court. Tennis can also be a team sport with teams composed of singles players and doubles teams, with the number of matches won determining the winning team.

The level of competition also varies. Some tennis clubs organize social tennis round robins. Players come to these parties and play a number of short matches interspersed with a lot of social time. The intent here is not the competition but the socialization. At the other end of the spectrum is the United States Tennis Association (USTA), which organizes individual tournaments and team play in which the competition can be extremely intense. Players compete at the local, regional, and national levels. The USTA also runs the U.S. Open Professional Tennis Tournament.

While players at any level can enjoy tennis, it is a game that requires years of practice to compete at an elite level. There is also a large mental component to the game, which people must learn in order to be successful. It is not always the best player who wins, but often the player who can adapt his or her playing style and use the most effective strategy.

Purpose of the Course

At West Point all seniors are required to take a "lifetime sport," and tennis is one of the options that they may choose. The purpose of the lifetime sport program is to promote a lifetime of fitness. In addition, tennis is unique in that it can also be considered a social sport. Tennis and other social sports, such as golf, are often a means of meeting others or an alternative to the office meeting for business associates. The ability to participate in these social sports at some level can benefit a player's career or social life.

As distant as it may seem to 22-year-olds, there is the possibility that many of them will be parents within five years. This class gives the students enough information that they could introduce their children to the sport and be able to provide them with the right opportunities should they be interested in becoming serious about tennis.

Lastly, it is important that students of tennis become educated spectators of the sport. They should know enough about the game that they can watch a higher-level match, understand the rules and the basic strategies that are being employed, and appreciate the skills that are being demonstrated.

Instructional Area

We are fortunate to have beautiful facilities at our disposal for tennis instruction, including 12 outdoor and seven indoor hard courts. Four students are assigned per court and two instructors are assigned to each class, which creates a low student-to-teacher ratio. This ratio is advantageous because it allows us to offer much individual feedback to the students.

While having access to great facilities is nice, it must be stressed that tennis can be taught in a variety of settings—even without the use of established tennis courts. Gymnasiums are excellent places for teaching beginner skills, as students can hit balls to themselves against the wall. Surfaces should not be a limiting factor. Professional tennis players play on all kinds of surfaces, including asphalt, clay, grass, and carpet; and students of the game should also learn to play on a variety of surfaces.

Equipment

As with any sport, it is important to carefully choose the equipment you use. It does not have to be expensive; however, to ensure the best learning experience possible, it must be in serviceable condition.

Balls

The equipment used in our tennis class includes two ball machines with 150 balls each and approximately 150 extra balls contained in several hoppers. Various other forms of equipment are used to enhance the drills, including hula hoops, cones, athletic tape, and court markers.

Shoes

The requirement for proper footwear is very important for both safety and court maintenance. If a student is wearing the wrong type of sneaker for tennis, the risk of ankle or knee injuries can increase. All students are required to have a court shoe or a cross-training shoe that is designed for lateral movement on a hard surface. Sneakers also must have a nonmarking, light-colored bottom. If the sneaker does not have a nonmarking bottom, it can leave scuff marks on the court.

Racket

Every student in tennis class is issued a racket to use both in class and outside of class for the entire term. This allows students some consistency when working on skills in class and also allows them to work on their game outside of class. Tennis is a game that requires much repetition in order to be successful, so it is important that the student get as many opportunities to practice as possible.

It is not necessary for a beginner to buy an expensive racket. It is important that the racket be comfortable for the player and that the grip be in good condition and the right size for the player's hand. If the player decides to pursue the game at a higher level after the introductory class, then it may be worthwhile to purchase a more expensive racket.

While having tennis rackets for every member of the class is ideal, it is not necessary. Drills can be modified to allow for the sharing of rackets. A creative teacher can even make this a challenging and fun part of the drill. For example, in a game called Around the World, players form one line at each end of the court. Players must hit the ball from one side of the court and then run to the other side of the court to receive a ball. The game becomes a little more exciting and challenging when there are only two rackets. In this case players must run to the other side of the court and pick up a racket before hitting the next ball. As many as 12 players can participate in this game with only one court, one ball, and two rackets!

Clothing

Clothing needs are very basic. Clothing should be comfortable and allow enough movement so that students can execute all skills. For students who are more advanced and involved in game situations, it is most convenient if they have shorts with pockets so that they can carry one or more extra balls. Other accessories such as hats and sweatbands may be used but are by no means necessary.

Risk Management

Tennis is a low-risk sport. It is noncontact, and many players enjoy the game well into their 70s and 80s. However, no sport is totally without risk. With a little bit of advanced thought and planning, the few risks that do exist can be eliminated or greatly diminished. Table 12.1 provides an example of some risk management strategies.

Course Overview

There are 18 lessons in this undergraduate tennis class (see table 12.2). Each lesson lasts approximately 45 minutes.

Skills and Techniques

There are basic skills and techniques that a beginner should learn in an introductory tennis class. It is important that these primary skills be learned correctly so the student does not have to correct bad habits later. It is much easier to build upon skills that have been learned correctly. If a student should decide to pursue tennis at a higher level, the foundation for success will already be in place.

Table 12.1   Possible Risks of Tennis

Risk identification	Reduction strategies
Lower extremity injuries	• Ensure that all students wear court shoes. • Ensure that all students have a basic level of fitness before enrolling in tennis.
Student hit with ball	• Design each new drill with safety in mind. • Provide clear instructions before each new drill. • Provide verbal and written warnings.
Student hit with racket	• Design each new drill with safety in mind. • Instruct students in proper grip technique. • Provide rackets with grips in good condition. • Regularly check the condition of the racket grips.
Student runs into fence	• Point out to students the locations of fences and the difference in court dimensions between singles and doubles courts. • Ensure that all gates are closed during class. • Design drills that are adequately spaced from the fences.
Ball machine injuries	• Regularly inspect ball machines to make sure they are in good working order. • Instruct entire class on safe use of ball machines before using machines in class. • Ensure that all electrical cords are away from drill areas.
Lightning injuries	• Educate students with regard to the lightning policy. • As the instructor, follow the lightning policy and change the class meeting place accordingly.

Table 12.2 Overview of Tennis Lessons

Lesson	Lesson topics	Assignments
1	• Introduction to tennis • Ball handling • Introduction to the volley	Read risk assessment page from the Web site.
2	• Forehand and backhand ground strokes • Areas of the court	
3	• Volley • Scoring	Read scoring page from the Web site.
4	• Serve • Singles play	Schedule a match observation.
5	• Lob • Overhead • Doubles play	
6	• Ground stroke skills testing • Etiquette	Read etiquette page from the Web site.
7	• Slice • Approach shot	
8	• Volley testing • Tiebreakers	Read rules page from the Web site.
9	• Serve testing • Serve return	
10	• Singles strategy	Read strategy page from the Web site.
11	• Singles tournament day 1	
12	• Singles tournament day 2	
13	• Skills testing • Canadian doubles	
14	• Doubles strategy	
15	• Doubles tournament day 1	
16	• Doubles tournament day 2	Observation paper due.
17	• Student evaluations • Skills testing	Study for the written exam.
18	• Written exam	Complete course evaluation on the Web.

Ground Strokes

The key to producing consistent ground strokes is to create topspin. Topspin causes the ball to drop down into the court, which allows the player to hit the ball higher over the net. Hitting the ball higher over the net creates a greater margin of error. Spin is created by combining the correct racket face angle with the correct stroke. Topspin requires a closed racket face and a low-to-high stroke. A closed racket face is one in which the hitting surface of the racket is angled toward the ground. The low-to-high stroke originates below the hips, makes contact with the ball at about the waist level, and follows through over the nondominant shoulder.

A closed racket face is produced through use of the Eastern forehand grip for the forehand ground stroke and the Eastern backhand grip for the backhand ground stroke. There are eight bevels, or flat surfaces, on the handle of the racket. A right-handed player places the "V" of the hand (created by the thumb and forefinger) on the first bevel to the right when the racket is held with the strings perpendicular to the ground. This forms an Eastern forehand grip and creates a closed racket face. Likewise, a right-handed player places the "V" of the hand on the first bevel to the left to form an Eastern backhand grip.

The forehand ground stroke is generally hit with one hand. However, the backhand can be a one-handed or a two-handed stroke. For a two-handed stroke, the dominant hand is placed on the racket as if one were executing a one-handed backhand, and the nondominant hand is then placed above the dominant hand on the racket handle. All other aspects of the stroke should be the same as for a one-handed stroke. The racket face should be closed on contact with the ball, and the stroke should be low to high.

TEACHING CUES

- Ready position.
- Eastern forehand or backhand grip.
- Pivot—racket back.
- Step out in front with nondominant foot.
- Shift weight to the front foot.
- Swing low to high.
- Make contact with the ball out in front of the body.
- Return to the ready position.

COMMON MISTAKES

One problem that many beginners have is making contact with the ball too close to the body. Some players may not be accustomed to making contact with a ball with anything but their hand, and a 27-inch (69-centimeter) racket can create some spacing challenges. Encourage these students to move their bodies into a position in which they feel as if they have to lean over and reach for the ball when making contact. You can also accomplish this by feeding balls to students far away until they are making contact at the correct distance.

Another common error is late preparation. Players are late in their backswing, which causes them to contact the ball late or to rush the stroke. Early preparation, which involves recognizing where the ball will land, moving the feet to position the body, and bringing the racket back early, is crucial when players are hitting ground strokes. Encourage players to bring the racket back as soon as they decide whether they will hit a forehand or backhand. They can then make adjustments with their feet with the racket already in the backswing position.

Ideally, contact should be made with the ball after the bounce, at or after the apex, and with the ball at about waist height. Instead of moving back so that contact can be made at waist height, beginners have a tendency to contact the ball too high or when the ball is still on the rise after the bounce. A drill that can correct this problem is a game played without rackets. Players throw the ball back and forth over the net. However, they may catch the ball only at waist height. They must move their feet and position their body in order to catch the ball at the correct height during the flight of the ball.

Volley

One of the most important aspects of the volley is footwork ensuring that the body is in the correct position to execute the stroke. With the exception of the net player in doubles, it is necessary for players to move from the baseline to the net in order to be in a position to volley. After moving toward the net and before executing the volley, the player should perform a split step. The split step is characterized by a slightly bent waist, bent knees, feet hip-width apart, and the chest facing the net (see figure 12.1). The racket should be held out in front of the body so that either a forehand or backhand can be easily used. The purpose of the split step is to control the player's momentum toward the net and to allow the player to quickly move right or left. The step following the split step is called the crossover step (see figure 12.2). When the player is performing the forehand volley, the nondominant foot should cross over in front of the dominant foot, which will create a sideways body position and allow for more reach on the forehand side. The crossover step for the backhand volley is the opposite, with the dominant foot crossing over in front of the nondominant foot. The crossover step allows for more lateral reach and allows the player to use the body to produce more power on the volley. The volley footwork should be introduced and practiced before the volley stroke is introduced.

The grip that should be used for the volley is the continental grip. The "V" of the hand should be placed on the top bevel when the racket is held with the strings perpendicular to the ground. This grip is the same for the forehand and the backhand volley.

The volley is different from the ground stroke in many ways. It is a much shorter stroke and can be described as a "punch" or a "block" rather than a long stroke. The backswing should not go behind the plane of the body, and the follow-through should only return the racket to the ready position out in front of the body. The racket head should remain above the wrist. The wrist should remain stiff, and most of the movement should originate from the shoulder and not from the elbow or wrist. Contact should be made out in front of the body, and most of the power for the shot should come from the opponent's ball and the correct footwork, not from the swing of the racket.

TEACHING CUES

Volley Footwork

- Split step
- Crossover step

Volley

- Ready position—split step.
- Continental grip.
- Crossover step.

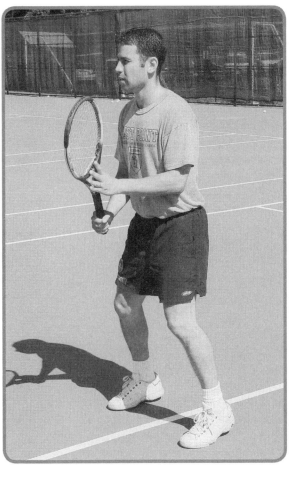

FIGURE 12.1   Split step.

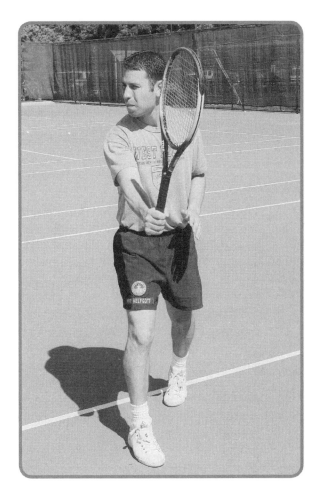

FIGURE 12.2   Crossover step.

- Very little backswing—pivot from the shoulder.
- Stiff wrist.
- Meet the ball out in front.
- Punch the ball.
- Return to the ready position.

COMMON MISTAKES

Many beginners attempt to swing at the ball in order to put the ball away. This causes them to hit the ball out of the court, mis-hit the ball, or miss the ball entirely. There are several drills to correct this problem. Have students stand with their back touching a fence or wall while a classmate tosses balls to either the forehand or the backhand side. If the racket touches the fence or wall, this is an indication that the backswing needs to be shortened. If students are following through too far instead of "punching" the ball, have them do the same drill standing close to and facing the net. Instruct them to end their follow-through before they touch or cross the plane of the net.

Another common flaw during volleying occurs when players wait for the ball to come to them rather than going to the ball. Most of the power on the volley originates from footwork and from the power of the opponent's shot. Be sure to emphasize the footwork skills before the upper body skills so that students understand where the power should originate. It may also help to instruct players to make contact with the ball out in front of the body. This forces them to use their feet to move to the ball.

Serve

There are three main types of serves—slice, flat, and topspin. The slice serve is the easiest to learn and, because it has spin, is a more reliable serve. It is probably the best serve to teach to beginners.

The most important part of the serve is the toss. A good toss will have no spin, will apex at an adequate height, and, if allowed to hit the ground, will land approximately 12 inches (30 centimeters) in front of the nondominant foot. The toss should apex at a height at least as high as the reach of the racket with the shoulder and elbow fully extended. After the toss, the nondominant arm should remain straight with the hand pointed upward toward the ball. The arm should remain in this position until the shoulders rotate to bring the racket up to make contact with the ball.

The continental grip should be used for the slice serve. The stroke of the serve looks very similar to the arm motion when a ball is being thrown. The motion of the serve begins in the back-scratch position, in which the bent elbow is close to the ear, the hand is behind the head, and the racket could be used to scratch the middle part of the player's back. Some players move to this position directly at the beginning of their motion, while others prefer to loop the racket up from behind before moving to the back-scratch position. Either motion can be used, although it may be easier to teach beginners to move directly to the back-scratch position.

From the back-scratch position, the arm should fully extend so that the racket makes contact with the ball at the highest point possible. When the ball is contacted high, a greater margin of error is created with a steeper angle down into the opposite service box. When players are executing the slice serve, there should be a snap of the wrist on contact and the racket should brush the back of the ball. For a right-handed player, the racket should brush from left to right across the back of the ball so that spin is applied to the ball. After contact with the ball, the follow-through will take the racket down and across to the nondominant side of the body.

TEACHING CUES

Ball Toss

- Straight arm.
- No spin.
- At least as high as the reach of the racket.
- Nondominant hand stays pointing toward the ball.

Service Motion

- Continental grip.
- Left foot 45 degrees to the baseline.
- Right foot parallel with the baseline.
- Backswing.
- Back scratch.
- Contact the ball high.
- Snap the wrist.
- Brush the back of the ball.
- Hit down into the court.

COMMON MISTAKES

Beginners often toss the ball too low, which causes them to make contact with the ball too low. This creates a very shallow angle into the court, which increases the chances for error. The fence drill may help to correct this problem. Students stand 1 foot (30 centimeters) away from the fence and face the fence at a 45-degree angle, with the nondominant shoulder closest to the fence. While in the back-scratch position, they execute the toss, which should be very close to the fence. They move their rackets as if they are serving from the back-scratch position and make contact with the ball against the fence, trapping the ball between the fence and the racket. If they are executing correctly, the dominant arm will be fully extended after trapping the ball.

When beginners do not hit down on the ball, they hit the ball long. To correct this, the instructor can have students serve from the service line or closer. This will force them to hit the ball down into the court. Then the instructor can gradually move them back so that they are eventually serving from the baseline.

Many beginners and even advanced players sometimes drop their nondominant arm too soon. This "drop" causes the entire body to drop and also causes premature shoulder rotation. This usually results in a serve that lands in the bottom of the net. Always remind students to keep their nondominant arm pointed toward the ball as long as possible before rotating the shoulders.

Lob

The lob is a ball that is hit high over the net for several reasons. It can be used to hit over a player who is standing at the net or to change the pace of the point. It can also be used defensively as a means of creating more time to recover from bad court positioning.

The technique for hitting a lob is very similar to that of the forehand and backhand ground stroke. The difference is that the player should open the racket face slightly and exaggerate the low-to-high motion of the stroke. This will allow the player to hit the ball high over the net and still apply some topspin so that the ball will drop down into the backcourt.

TEACHING CUES

- Ready position.
- Slightly open racket face.
- Pivot—racket back.
- Step out in front with nondominant foot.
- Shift weight to the front foot.
- Swing low to very high.
- Make contact with the ball out in front of the body.
- Return to the ready position.

COMMON MISTAKES

The most common mistake people make when hitting a lob is to hit it too low or too short, thereby making it an easy target for the opposing player. Encourage players to hit their lobs so that they land in the back 2 to 3 feet of the court. When playing indoors, players should aim for the ceiling.

Overhead

The overhead is a stroke that is used to return a lob, ideally with a lot of power and good placement so that the ball cannot be returned. Players are generally playing up at the net when they hit an overhead, and they are usually hitting a ball that the opponent has attempted to lob but has hit too low or too short.

The technique of the overhead is nearly identical to that of the serve. As soon as the player decides to hit an overhead, he or she should turn sideways to the net, point the nondominant hand toward the ball, and bring the racket to the back-scratch position. As the ball is approaching it is important that the player sidestep in order to place the body in the correct position to hit the overhead. Contact should be made in the same place as with the serve—slightly out in front of the body with the dominant shoulder and elbow fully extended.

TEACHING CUES

- Continental grip.
- Sideways body position.
- Nondominant arm pointed toward the ball.
- Racket in the back-scratch position.
- Sidestep to position the body underneath the ball.
- Contact the ball high.
- Snap the wrist.
- Hit down into the court.

COMMON MISTAKES

Probably the most common error when players are preparing to hit an overhead is the failure to move the feet during preparation for the shot. Because lobs are in the air longer than other shots, variables such as velocity, spin, and trajectory may change during the flight of the ball (Brown, 1976). Players should get the upper body set early and make constant corrections by sidestepping with the feet until contact with the ball is made.

Similar to what happens with the serve, some players may drop their nondominant arm too early, resulting in an overhead hit into the net. Remind players to keep their nondominant arm pointed toward the ball as long as possible before shoulder rotation.

Strategy

Two basic strategies are employed by advanced players. "Baseliners" tend to stay at the baseline and rely on their ground strokes to win points. "Serve and volleyers" will do everything they can to approach the net and win the point by volleying. It takes many years of practice and match play to develop these strategies of play. It is important to introduce the beginning student to more basic concepts of strategy, which can apply to all players. The following is a list of simple strategies that can help a beginning player be much more successful in match situations.

General Strategy

- The person who makes the least number of mistakes will win. Do not try to hit the ball too hard or try to hit impossible shots. Keep the ball in play and let your opponent make the mistakes.

- Know your opponent's weaknesses and attack them. For example, if an opponent has a weak backhand, hit more balls to his or her backhand.

- Hit more balls cross-court than down the line. The court is much longer from corner to corner than it is from end to end. The net is shorter in the middle of the court than it is at the sidelines (see figure 12.3). By hitting cross-court, you are dealing with a longer court and a shorter net, which will give you a greater margin of error.

- When serving, try to get approximately 70 percent of your first serves in the service box. Many players make the mistake of trying to annihilate the first serve. When they miss, they are forced to hit a very weak second serve, which can be exploited by their opponent.

Doubles Strategy

- Remember the saying "long to long, short to short." A player at the baseline (long) should hit the ball to the opponent at the baseline (long) and not to the net player (short). A player at the net (short) should hit the ball to the opponent at the net (short) and not to the player at the baseline (long).

- Try to position both players at the net as quickly as possible during the point. It is easier to win a point with an easy volley or overhead at the net than by hitting ground strokes from the baseline.

Scoring

Scoring in tennis is very different from that in any other game and often doesn't make much sense to those unfamiliar with it. It will probably require quite a bit of instructional time to teach the scoring system in tennis, especially for those students who have no previous knowledge in this area. It may be less confusing for younger students if scoring is introduced to them in small lessons. Teach them how to keep score in games and then let them play several games. Then teach them how to keep score in sets and have them play a set or two. When they are very comfortable with that, they are ready to learn tiebreakers. By introducing these concepts individually, you can avoid some of the confusion that is inevitable when you introduce them all at once.

The server will serve the entire first game. The winner of the first point is said to have "15" and the loser "love," with the server's score announced first. Therefore, if the server wins the first point, the score is "15-love." The second point is said to be "30," the third "40," and the fourth "game." Therefore, if the server has won 2 points and the receiver has won 3 points, the score is "30-40." If the receiver wins the next point, the receiver wins the game. The game must be won by at least 2 points. If the score becomes "40-40," it is called "deuce," and the winner of the next point is not the winner of the game. Instead, that player is said to have the "advantage." If that same player wins the next point, then he or she is the winner of the game. If that player loses the next point, the score returns to "deuce" and the game continues until a winner is determined.

Cross-court shot: Length of the court = 82.5 feet
                     Height of the net = 3 feet
Down-the-line shot: Length of the court = 78 feet
                     Height of the net = 3 1/2 feet

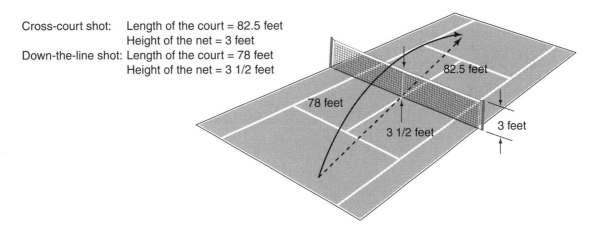

FIGURE 12.3   Court dimensions.

At the end of the first game, the score is 1-0, and the receiver becomes the server. Players continue to play games until a player wins six games by a margin of two. The winner of six games is the winner of the set.

If the set reaches the score of 6-5, another game will be played. If the score then becomes 7-5, the set is over, and the player with seven games is the winner of the set. If the score becomes 6-6, a tiebreaker is played.

The first player to serve in a tiebreaker is the player who received serve during the last game played. This player serves 1 point from the deuce court (right side). Numerical scoring is used in a tiebreaker so that the score following that point is called 1-0. The receiver now becomes the server and will serve two consecutive points starting from the ad court (left side). Play continues with each player serving two consecutive points until a player has reached 7 points with a winning margin of two. That player is then the winner of the tiebreaker and the winner of the set, and the score of the set is said to be 7-6.

Most tournaments utilize a "best of three" format, meaning that the first player to win two sets is declared the winner of the match. However, a men's tournament may have a "best of five" format, in which the first player to win three sets is declared the winner.

Rules of Play

Very few recreational tennis players know and understand all of the rules of tennis. However, it is important that beginning students know the basic rules so that they can enjoy match play outside of class. The following is a list of the most basic rules of tennis that should be understood by beginners.

1. The first step in match play is to determine who will serve first. Spinning the racket or tossing a coin can accomplish this. The winner chooses either the order of serve or the side of the court on which players will begin play.

2. If any part of the ball lands on the line, it is in play.

3. Players may not touch the net during the point.

4. Contact with the ball must be made on one's own side of the net, although the follow-through of the racket may pass over the net after contact is made.

5. The serve must be contacted out of the air. A player may not bounce the ball and then hit the serve.

6. The server's foot may not touch the line or any part of the court inside the line until after contact is made with the ball.

7. The server is allowed two attempts of serve for each point. If the server misses the first serve, it is called a "fault" and the server can make another attempt at the serve. If the server misses the second serve, it is called a "double fault" and the point is lost.

8. If the serve hits the net and then lands inside the correct service box, it is called a "let" and that serve may be attempted again. If the serve hits the net and does not land inside the service box, it is called a "fault."

The rules for doubles are as follows:

- Only one player may make contact with the ball on each side of the net.

- At the beginning of the set, the receiving team must decide which partner will receive the serve on the right side of the court (deuce court) and which partner will receive the serve on the left side (ad court). Once this has been established, the receiving positions stay the same for the remainder of the set.

- Once the serving order has been established, it remains for the entire set.

- No member of the receiving team may stand inside the service box during the serve.

This list is not exhaustive but addresses some of the most common questions that surface during match play in a beginners' tennis class. There are numerous other rules that can be introduced to students based on their age and level of play.

Etiquette

Basic etiquette is an important part of a beginner tennis program. The students may not use much of this knowledge in class or when playing with each other, but if they are exposed to tennis outside of class, either as a player or as a spectator, they should understand and be able to follow the basic rules of etiquette. The following is a short summary of some of the rules of tennis etiquette.

A high level of concentration is required to play tennis, and it is easy for players to lose this concentration during a point. For this reason it is important that there be no noise or other distractions during a point. Spectators should not talk, yell, or clap and should not move from their seats during a point. If spectators need to move from their seats or across a court, they should do so in between points. If something happens accidentally during a point to distract the players, as when a ball crosses from another court, a "let" should be called immediately and the point should be replayed. By the same token, players should not try to distract their opponents by making extraneous movements or noises.

The server has several responsibilities. The server should announce the score before every point in order to help avoid disagreements about the score later in the match. The server should always begin each point with two balls in his or her possession to keep the game moving. The server should not begin the service motion until the opponent is ready.

Only in rare cases will an umpire be present at matches. Therefore it is the players' responsibility to make all line calls. Players should make all calls on their own side of the net. They should make calls quickly and clearly so that their opponent hears or sees the call immediately. A player who has any doubt as to the call should give the benefit of the doubt to the opponent.

Because tennis is rarely officiated by a third party and players must make their own calls, it is a sport that provides great opportunity to teach the value of fair play and sportsmanship. If players do not make fair calls and do not respect their opponents, the game loses its enjoyment value, and unfair players may have difficulty finding future opponents and doubles partners.

Sample Lesson Plans

The following lesson plans illustrate a typical tennis class session at West Point. The normal sequence of events includes (1) student accountability; (2) warm-up, utilizing ball-handling games; (3) introduction and demonstration of new skills; (4) practice; (5) rule of the day; (6) cleanup of area; and (7) class dismissal. Using these lesson plans as a guide will allow you to adapt your teaching to your own setting.

LESSON 1

Ball Handling and Volleying

SCOPE

Introduction, ball handling, introduction to the volley

SEQUENCE (45-MINUTE CLASS)

1. Class administration (10 minutes)
2. Ball-handling games designed to get the students accustomed to the racket, the ball, and the surface (10 minutes)
3. Introduction to the continental grip (5 minutes)
4. Introduction to the volley (15 minutes)
5. Rule of the day and court cleanup (5 minutes)

MAJOR SKILL THEME

Ball handling

TEACHING CUES

No cues are given—guided discovery. Students are instructed to do the following:

- Bounce ball up in the air, forehand and backhand.
- Bounce ball on ground, big bounce and small bounce.

- Bounce it on a line, alternate back and forth over line, small bounce and big bounce.
- Walk in a straight line, rotate in a circle while bouncing the ball.
- Bounce ball on ground and in the air with frame of racket.
- Throw the ball in the air and "catch" it with the racket.

BALL-HANDLING GAMES

- Keep-away game, introduction to an area of the court, singles or doubles, alley
- Relay races:
  - Run the width of the court and back with the ball on the racket.
  - Run the width of the court while bouncing the ball on the ground.
  - Bounce the ball in the air.
  - Run with a partner while "passing" the ball back and forth.
  - Run with a partner using a "bounce pass."

MAJOR SKILL THEME

Introduction to the volley

TEACHING CUES

- Use the continental grip.
  - Butt of racket in navel.
  - Slide hand down top of racket to grip.
  - "V" of the hand is pointed toward the top bevel—12 o'clock.
- Keep the racket head above the wrist—"head higher than the hand."

ASSESSMENT

This is an introductory class; all of the skills that are introduced will be further developed in other lessons and will be assessed at a later date.

LESSON 2

Ground Strokes

SCOPE

Forehand and backhand ground strokes, areas of the court

SEQUENCE (45-MINUTE CLASS)

1. Warm-up drills (5 minutes)
2. Introduction to spin and grips (5 minutes)
3. Eastern forehand grip (2 minutes)
4. Forehand ground stroke drills (13 minutes)
5. Eastern backhand grip (2 minutes)
6. Backhand ground stroke drills (13 minutes)
7. Rules of the day—areas of the court and court cleanup (5 minutes)

MAJOR SKILL THEME

Forehand ground stroke

TEACHING CUES

Eastern Forehand Grip

- Butt of the racket in the navel.
- Slide hand down from the strings to the handle.
- "V" of the hand is pointed toward first bevel to the right—2 o'clock.

Ready Position

- Feet are hip-width apart.
- Weight on the balls of the feet.
- Knees are slightly bent.
- Body slightly bent at the waist.
- Racket held out in front.
- Nondominant hand supports the throat of the racket.

Forehand Ground Stroke

- Ready position.
- Eastern forehand grip.
- Pivot—racket back.
- Step out in front with nondominant foot.
- Shift weight to the front foot.
- Swing low to high.
- Make contact with the ball out in front of the body.
- Return to the ready position.

MAJOR SKILL THEME

Backhand ground stroke

TEACHING CUES

Eastern Backhand Grip

- Butt of racket in navel with strings parallel to ground.
- Slide hand down edge of racket.
- "V" pointed toward first bevel to the left—10 o'clock.

Backhand Ground Stroke

- Ready position.
- Eastern backhand grip.
- Pivot—racket back.
- Step—weight to front foot.
- Swing low to high.
- Meet the ball out in front.
- Return to the ready position.

MAJOR SKILL THEME

Areas of the court

TEACHING CUES

Teach the students the location of the following areas of the court (see figure 12.4):

- Baseline
- Service line
- Singles sideline
- Doubles sideline
- Doubles alley
- Centerline
- Center mark
- Service box
- Deuce court
- Ad court
- No-man's-land

ASSESSMENT

The forehand and backhand ground strokes will not be assessed during this lesson. Students will be given several more lessons to practice before they are assessed on this skill.

Tennis balls are fed to students standing at the baseline using the ball machines. Students must use the appropriate stroke while attempting to put topspin on the ball. Students are given a brief warm-up to adjust to the ball delivery. Each student will receive 10 balls. Ten points are awarded for each ball landing in the singles court behind the service line, and 5 points are awarded for each ball landing in the singles court in front of the service line.

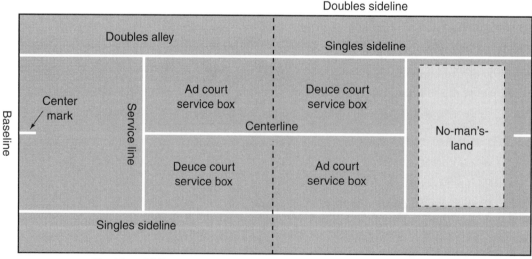

FIGURE 12.4 Areas of the court.

There are several "money balls" in the ball machine, which are balls that are a different color. These balls are worth twice as many points as a regular ball. For example, a money ball that lands in the singles court in front of the service line is worth 10 points. The idea of the money ball is to more closely mimic a real match situation. When the student sees that the machine has served the money ball, there is more pressure on the student to hit the ball well.

The maximum number of points that can be earned for each test is 100. Students may test up to three times, with the best score counting. All scores must be administered and verified by an instructor or tennis classmate.

LESSON 3

Volley

SCOPE

Volley

SEQUENCE (45-MINUTE CLASS)

1. Warm-up drills (5 minutes)
2. Discussion and demonstration of the volley (5 minutes)
3. Volley drills (20 minutes)
4. Discussion of tennis scoring (10 minutes)
5. Rule of the day and court cleanup (5 minutes)

MAJOR SKILL THEME

Volley

TEACHING CUES

Volley Footwork

- Split step
- Crossover step

Volley

- Ready position—split step.
- Continental grip.
- Crossover step.
- Very little backswing.
- Stiff wrist.
- Meet the ball out in front.
- Punch the ball—pivot from the shoulder.
- Return to ready position.

MAJOR SKILL THEME

Scoring

TEACHING CUES

Instruct the students how to keep score.

- Game scoring: love, 15, 30, 40, game—by 2 points
- Set scoring—first to six by two
- Tiebreaker at six all
- Match scoring—two out of three sets

ASSESSMENT

The volley will not be assessed during this lesson. Students will be given several more lessons to practice before they are assessed on this skill.

Tennis balls are fed to students standing halfway between the net and the service line. Students are given a brief warm-up to adjust to ball delivery. Each attempt will consist of volleying the ball at the net and then retreating to the service line and touching it. After touching the service line, students must move forward, split step, crossover step, and volley. Each student will receive five balls to the forehand and five balls to the backhand. Ten points are scored for each ball landing in the singles court behind the service line.

As in lesson 2, there are several "money balls" in the ball machine, which puts pressure on the student to focus and hit the ball well. The maximum number of points that can be earned is 100. Students may retest up to three times, with the best score counting. All scores must be administered and verified by an instructor or classmate.

LESSON 4

Slice Serve

SCOPE

Slice serve

SEQUENCE (45-MINUTE CLASS)

1. Warm-up drills (5 minutes)
2. Discussion and demonstration of the serve (10 minutes)
3. Serve drills (15 minutes)
4. Singles play (10 minutes)
5. Rule of the day and court cleanup (5 minutes)

MAJOR SKILL THEME

Slice serve

TEACHING CUES

The Serve in the Game of Tennis

- The serve begins each point.
- Two serves per point.

- Always start from the deuce court (right side).
- Must serve to the opposite court.
- With every point, alternate between the deuce (right) and ad court (left).
- One player serves the entire game.

Ball Toss

- Straight arm.
- No spin.
- At least as high as the reach of the racket.
- Nondominant hand stays pointing toward the ball.

Service Motion

- Continental grip.
- Left foot 45 degrees to the baseline.
- Right foot parallel with baseline.
- Backswing.
- Back scratch.
- Contact the ball high.
- Snap the wrist.
- Brush the back of the ball.
- Hit down into the court.

MAJOR SKILL THEME

Singles play

TEACHING CUES

- Spin the racket for the serve—winner chooses either serving order or side, loser chooses the other option.
- Start serving from the deuce court (right).
- Start positions for server and receiver.
- Switch sides—after odd-numbered games, including all games in the match.

ASSESSMENT

The serve assessment is not administered during this lesson. Students are allowed several lessons to practice the serve before they are tested.

The serve test is a two-part exam, with each part worth 50 points. On the first serve test, each student attempts five serves each from the deuce court and the ad court. Points are awarded for each serve landing inside the service box based on the location of the second bounce (see figure 12.5). On the second serve test, each student attempts five serves each from the deuce court and the ad court. Five points are awarded for each serve that lands inside the service box. Students may retest up to three times, with the best score counting. All tests must be administered and verified by an instructor or classmate.

PE 444 Tennis Server Test

First serve – 5 attempts from each court

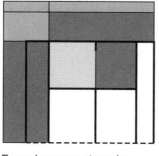
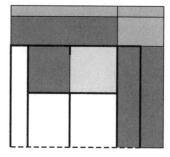

From deuce court scoring:

▢ ____ x 2 pts. = ____ pts.

▢ ____ x 4 pts. = ____ pts.

▢ ____ x 8 pts. = ____ pts.

From ad court scoring:

▢ ____ x 2 pts. = ____ pts.

▢ ____ x 4 pts. = ____ pts.

▢ ____ x 8 pts. = ____ pts.

First serve total = ____ pts.

- -

Second serve – 5 attempts from each court

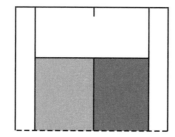

Deuce court scoring:

▢ ____ x 5 pts. = ____ pts.

Ad court scoring:

▢ ____ x 5 pts. = ____ pts.

Second serve total = ____ pts.

- -

First serve total ____ + Second serve total ____ = ____ points
(total may not exceed 100 points)

FIGURE 12.5   Serve test.

Adapting This Course for Your School

High school physical education teachers often have large classes and a limited number of courts available for instruction purposes. Classes must be modified to ensure that all students are actively engaged in a fun and safe manner. An instructor can design fun drills and games in which a number of students are playing on one court. For example, one teacher can run a series of drills by feeding balls to 12 to 16 students on one court. The instructor can begin with a warm-up drill by feeding forehand and backhand ground strokes to two lines of students. As soon as one student has hit the ball, he or she will run to the outside of the court, touch the net post, and then return to the end of the opposite line. By giving students something to do between strokes, the instructor is ensuring that they are engaged and active. This drill can also be done with volleys, lobs, and overheads. While these drills are occurring on one court, the other courts can be used for doubles or round robin play. After a designated period of time, have the students rotate. This allows one teacher to run a class on three courts with 24 to 28 students.

Another game that engages many students on one court is "Around the World." Six to eight students line up in one line on each end of the court. Each player hits a ground stroke and then runs to the opposite line. When a player has made three mistakes, he or she is automatically "out." The game continues until one or two players remain. This drill involves a lot of players on one court and keeps the students moving for a better workout. This drill can be used for ground strokes, volleys, or lobs.

If an instructor doesn't have any courts available, there are many games that can be modified so that students receive some experience with a tennis racket and ball even if they are not actually playing the game of tennis. Relay races on a hard surface emphasize racket and ball control. Players can bounce the ball on their racket, on the ground, off the side of the racket, to their partners, and so on while they are running relay races. This doesn't require a court, is a good conditioning drill, and can involve many students at one time.

An instructor's imagination is the only limit when he or she is designing exercises to teach the game of tennis. Other games that can be modified to accommodate tennis equipment include tennis volleyball, tennis lacrosse, and tennis softball.

In a game of tennis volleyball, students are divided into two teams on opposite sides of the net. This net can be a tennis net, a volleyball net, a fence, or a simple piece of rope. Students must catch the ball with their hands and then hit the ball with their rackets. It may be too dangerous to eliminate the catch as students may get hit with their teammates' rackets! If the team fails to catch the ball with their hands before the ball hits the ground, they lose the point. Advanced players may be required to catch the ball with their rackets. Players must serve from out of bounds, and teams are allowed three hits on each side. All other rules of volleyball apply.

In tennis lacrosse, the rules of women's lacrosse are used. Lacrosse sticks and balls are replaced by tennis rackets and balls. Players learn ball-handling skills when they "travel" with the ball and pass the ball. The act of "picking up the ball" from the ground with the racket and flicking it to a teammate teaches them the low-to-high stroke, which they will also use in the forehand and backhand ground stroke. This is a great game to use to introduce students to the equipment of tennis and to teach them some introductory ball-handling skills.

As with the two previous exercises, tennis softball is an exercise that is performed using rules modified from another game, in this case softball. Tennis balls are substituted for softballs, and rackets are substituted for bats and gloves. A pitcher throws the tennis ball to the "batter," who must hit the ball with the tennis racket. All players in the field can use their hands to catch the ball but must "throw" the ball by hitting it with their racket. All other rules of softball apply.

Students can and should learn other aspects of sport in addition to acquiring the necessary physical skills. Once students become familiar with the sport, the instructor can give them other roles. Students can be referees, umpires, ball boys or girls, or tournament directors. This will give them an entirely different view of the sport and will lead them to a greater appreciation for it.

Every comprehensive physical education program should include racket sports. There are a variety of racket sports, and most of them are considered lifetime sports, so it is important for young students to be exposed to them at an early age. Do not be limited by facilities or equipment. For beginning students, it is enough just to introduce them to racket sports, even if not within the strict rules of tennis, racquetball, or any of the other sports. It is possible to introduce students to tennis and to give them knowledge of the game, the rules, and a profound sense of enjoyment without having the proper equipment and courts. If students show an interest in pursuing the sport, they can take the basics that they have learned and pursue the sport of tennis on their own.

Key Terms

ad court—The service box located on the left side of the court on the same side of the net as the server, and on the right side of the court on the opposite side of the net as the server.

approach shot—The shot immediately preceding a player's movement from the baseline to the net.

Australian doubles—A strategy of doubles play in which players attempt to disguise the location of the net player.

backhand—A stroke used when the ball is hit on the left side of the body for a right-handed person and on the right side of the body for a left-handed person.

backspin—See *slice.*

baseline—The line that marks the boundary of the court farthest from the net.

Canadian doubles—Game that can be played with three players, one player against two players.

centerline—The line that divides the deuce court from the ad court.

center mark—A 4-inch (10-centimeter) line that divides the boundaries for serving into the deuce court and the ad court.

closed racket face—Position of the racket in which the hitting surface of the strings is angled toward the ground.

continental grip—Grip used for the beginner volley and slice serve; this grip is unique in that it is the same for the forehand and backhand.

deuce court—The service box located on the right side of the court on the same side of the net as the server, and on the left side of the court on the opposite side of the net from the server.

double fault—Fault that occurs when a player is not able to put the first or second serve into play and therefore loses the point.

doubles alley—An area of the court between the singles sideline and doubles sideline; the area of the court that is used only in doubles play.

doubles sideline—Outside boundary of the court for doubles play.

Eastern backhand grip—A grip used for the backhand ground stroke; this grip closes the face of the racket on the backhand side and allows the player to put topspin on the ball.

Eastern forehand grip—A grip used for the forehand ground stroke; this grip closes the face of the racket on the forehand side and allows the player to put topspin on the ball.

fault—Failure of a player to hit the serve into play.

flat serve—A serve delivered with little or no spin.

foot fault—A violation committed by a player with the foot during the serve.

forehand—A stroke used when the ball is hit on the right side of the body for a right-handed person and the left side of the body for a left-handed person.

ground stroke—The stroke used when the ball has already bounced on the same side of the court as the player; generally the player is standing near the baseline.

lob—A ball that is hit high over the net and lands deep into the opponent's court.

no-man's-land—An area of the court between the service line and approximately 2 feet (.6 meters) inside the baseline. Most balls bounce in this area of the court, so it is not recommended that players stand here. It is difficult to return a ball that bounces near the feet in this area.

open racket face—Position of the racket in which the hitting surface of the strings is angled upward toward the sky.

overhead—A shot during which contact is made high over the head, generally when the player is standing at the net, with a motion similar to that of the serve.

service line—Line that marks the back boundary of the service boxes.

singles sideline—Line that marks the outside boundary for the singles court.

slice—Spin placed on the ball that causes the ball to float during flight and to decelerate and stay low after the bounce.

slice serve—Basic serve that causes the ball to drop down into the court.

tiebreaker—A series of points played to determine the winner of the set when the score is 6-6.

topspin—Spin placed on the ball that causes the ball to drop during flight and accelerate and bounce higher after the bounce.

topspin serve—A serve delivered with topspin that travels high over the net, drops down into the court, and then accelerates toward the returner.

volley—Stroke used to hit a ball before it bounces, generally when the player is standing at the net.

Reference

Brown, J. (1976). *Tennis: Teaching, coaching, and directing programs*. Englewood Cliffs, NJ: Prentice-Hall.

Suggested Readings

American Sport Education Program. (2002). *Coaching youth series*. Champaign, IL: Human Kinetics.

Gallwey, T. (1997). *The inner game of tennis*. New York: Random House.

Gould, D. (1999). *Tennis anyone?* Mountain View, CA: Mayfield.

Hoskins, T. (1997). *1001 incredible tennis games, drills & tips: A super abundance of information for every teaching professional & tennis enthusiast*. Nantucket, MA: Hoskins and Grant.

Perlstein, S. (1993). *Essential tennis: A player's guide*. Guilford, CT: Lyons Press.

Perlstein, S. (1997). *Winning doubles: Strategies, key concepts, and shot-by-shot playbook for players at all levels*. Guilford, CT: Lyons Press.

Perlstein, S. (1999). *Winning tennis*. Guilford, CT: Lyons Press.

Pierce, K., Beebe, V.N., & Evert, J. (2002). *Introducing children to the game of tennis*. Salt Lake City, UT: Alliance House.

Professional Tennis Registry. (1998). *International book of tennis drills: Over 100 skill-specific drills*. Chicago: Triumph Books.

Professional Tennis Registry. (1998). *Munchkin tennis: A parent's guide to teaching tennis fundamentals*. Chicago: Triumph Books.

United States Tennis Association. (1998). *USTA's teaching group tennis: A practical approach to instructing large groups.* Champaign, IL: Human Kinetics.

United States Tennis Association. (2002). *Official rules of tennis.* Chicago: Triumph Books.

Vasquez, Reggie Jr. (2001). *Tennis for kids: Over 150 games to teach children the sport of a lifetime.* Charleston, SC: Citadel.

Sport-Specific Organizations

Professional Tennis Registry (PTR)
P.O. Box 4739
Hilton Head Island, SC 29938
800-421-6289
843-785-7244
Fax: 843-686-2033
www.ptrtennis.org

United States Professional Tennis Association (USPTA)
USPTA World Headquarters
3535 Briarpark Drive, Suite One
Houston, TX 77042
713-978-7782
800-USPTA-4U
Fax: 713-978-7780
www.uspta.com

United States Tennis Association (USTA)
70 West Red Oak Lane
White Plains, NY 10604
914-696-7000
www.usta.com

13

Golf

Thomas Horne

The exact origin of golf is unknown. Some historians believe that the earliest form of golf may have emerged in Greece, where ancient shepherds made a game out of hitting stones with their staffs. The Romans played a game called *paganica,* the object of which was to use a bent stick to strike a ball stuffed with feathers. However, the game we know as golf today has its true origins in St. Andrews, Scotland (Owens & Bunker, 1995). In the modern game of golf, developed around 1744, a player hits a ball from a teeing area into a hole on an area of short-cut grass called a green. The ball is struck with a variety of clubs that include metal woods used for long shots; irons for midrange and short shots; and a putter, which is used only once the ball is on the green. The goal of the game is to get the golf ball from the tee area into the hole using the minimum number of strokes. Most golf courses have 18 holes, which is the standard number for a round of golf, although there are exceptions. Some small courses may only have nine holes, while some large golf complexes have more than one course.

The popularity of golf has increased tremendously since its early days in Scotland, and the sport has a large international following and a popular appeal. Golf came to American shores in 1888, when John Reid founded the first American golf course. The United States Golf Association (USGA), formed in 1894, established game rules and guidelines for golf sportsmanship and etiquette and sponsored golf championships and tournaments for its members. Today there are several thousand golf courses and millions of golfers in the United States. Hundreds of golf tournaments for professional, amateur, and recreational players are conducted annually throughout the world. Due to the continuing popularity of golf as a lifetime physical activity and its applicability to social and business environments, golfing and golf-related activities are more relevant than ever in today's physical education curriculums.

Purpose of the Course

Most golf classes are designed as arenas for teaching this lifetime physical activity to beginner and novice golfers. These classes generally serve to develop the foundation skills and knowledge needed for playing golf successfully and to motivate students to continue practicing and playing. The basic skills taught usually include the full swing, pitch shot, chipping, and putting. In addition to these golf skills, beginning golf classes often cover information on golf equipment, terminology, rules, etiquette, and playing strategies. By the end of the course the students should be able to consistently hit the ball, play according to the rules, and demonstrate the proper golf etiquette.

Golf is a growing sport that provides opportunities for fitness, recreation, and socialization. Unlike many other popular sports, golf is truly a lifetime sport. It has broad appeal, and with time, patience, and practice, anyone can learn to become a successful player. A game of golf can be a very serious game that is played professionally, or can serve as a workplace game that is an opportunity for coworkers and clients to mix business and recreation. But most often it is simply an enjoyable game that offers a level of friendly competition to its players.

Instructional Areas

Golf can be taught in an indoor area such as a gymnasium or a multipurpose room, on an outdoor field or playground, at a driving range, or on a regular golf course. Most schools do not have easy access to a golf course or a driving range; therefore, most scholastic and collegiate instructional golf classes are taught in multipurpose indoor or outdoor facilities. The skills required to play golf do not have to be taught at a golf course, although schools that utilize block scheduling procedures for their students may be more apt to teach their golf classes at a local course.

The first golf lessons are often introductory lessons that focus on golf basics, such as mastering the correct terminology, the proper grip, stance, and club swing. Actually hitting the ball during the first lesson is not necessary, and concentration on doing so may distract the student from adequately learning the proper form, grip, stance, and swing mechanics. Beginning students tend to focus too much on where the ball goes rather than on developing the necessary technique. An instructor should challenge students' development by introducing a variety of ball striking activities, but should also concentrate on the development of basic golf skills.

Indoor Facilities

Whether indoors or outdoors, the primary consideration for golf instruction lies in providing enough space for each student to participate safely in the planned golf activities. Golf instruction, especially in a school setting, is often taught in an indoor facility. The average public school gymnasium is usually of sufficient size to teach golf classes, although all indoor facilities should be evaluated for their appropriateness in terms of the class size and the golf program's scope. Indoor golf facilities tend to have restricted space, but they are usually readily available and make for good teaching arenas when outdoor golfing facilities are affected by adverse weather conditions.

When people swing a golf club, the initial contact of the club with the floor may damage the floor, the club, or both. Golf mats are often used to protect the floor and the club and are available through a variety of commercial and Web-based sources. Restricting the flight of the golf ball is essential when the sport is being taught indoors. Using a modified golf ball is one way to restrict ball flight (see section "Golf Balls"), while carpeting or some type of synthetic turf should be placed on the floor to help control the ball bounce. Another approach to controlling ball flight is to use some type of restrictive netting. Most golf netting sets have netting on three sides and a top net. The netting restricts ball flight and absorbs the impact of the ball. Some netting used for other athletic activities, such as baseball, may also be used for golf activities if suitable golf netting cannot be found.

Putting is an essential skill for golfers—one that is simple to master and among the easiest golfing skills to teach in an indoor setting. The area needed to practice putting is smaller than that needed to practice the full swing. Almost any carpeted area can be used to practice putting. If the floor is not carpeted, carpet strips or commercial putting surfaces can be laid on the floor to protect it. A variety of commercial putting cups are available to use as putting targets. Some of the practice putting cups on the market today are electric and will send the ball back to the person putting. However, students do not need a putting cup in order to practice this essential golf skill. Putting targets can be as simple as the leg of a chair or a strategically placed cup or coin. An introductory golf unit that includes only putting materials and some basic golf rules is a good way for a novice golfer to begin to develop strong golfing skills.

Multipurpose Fields

A large athletic field or other large open space can be used to teach golf classes. If the space is exceptionally large, it can be used as a driving range. Teaching golf on an outdoor multipurpose area usually requires some safety modifications that will restrict ball flight and prevent injury. Ways to do this are to use restricted-flight golf balls; use golf nets; limit the golf skills taught; and emphasize basic swings such as putting, chipping, and pitch shots, which are done with a short iron. Precautions must also be taken to keep nonstudents from entering the golf hitting area. Beginning golfers tend to hit the ball far from the intended target area, so be sure to allow for a generous buffer zone when planning a space to teach golf classes. Target areas can be distinguished with a flag, cones, or other easily visible markers. Providing distance markings will assist new students in assessing their accuracy in hitting the ball toward the intended target.

Hitting a golf ball from natural turf can be difficult for beginning players, and an incorrect hit can cause damage to the turf. The use of a synthetic golf mat is generally a good way for beginning golfers to learn proper hitting techniques. A synthetic mat protects the turf and allows students to see progress in their study of the game. Using a synthetic golf mat that includes a rubber tee makes it even easier for beginning students to strike the ball cleanly, especially when hitting with a wood.

Driving Ranges and Golf Courses

While indoor facilities and multipurpose outdoor spaces can be used to teach golf, the ideal spot for teaching a golf class is a course or a driving range. Driving ranges are designed to support practicing golf shots using a full range of clubs and standard golf balls. Both mats with rubber tees and natural turf hitting areas are normally available for practice. Driving ranges usually have restrictive fences or nets to keep even the wildest golf shots within the hitting area. Most ranges have distance markers and a target green area to help the golfer assess the effectiveness of his or her shots. Some practice range areas also include practice putting greens and sand traps so that a full range of golf shots can be practiced.

Having access to a golf course to apply the shots practiced on the driving range, multipurpose golf area, or indoor facility is ideal. It is the instructor's responsibility to make sure that students are sufficiently prepared and well versed in golfing skills before attempting to play on a "real golf course." Beginning players must know enough about golf rules and etiquette to be able to play safely and not disturb or delay other golfers on the course.

Equipment

The type and quality of the equipment used in class are essential to success. A well-equipped golfer may carry the 14 allotted clubs in a fancy golf bag with head covers for each club, as well as dozens of golf balls, tees, ball markers, a spike wrench, a distance finder, a ball mark repair tool, extra scorecards, a ball retriever, and a host of other golf-related items. While expensive golf equipment is certainly not necessary for the beginning golfer, each instructor must determine what equipment is most necessary to teaching the game. Most instructional programs provide golf clubs, golf balls, and training materials for students and instructors.

Golf Clubs

Golf clubs have developed over time from simple bent sticks to intricately designed tools crafted with high-technology materials and computer-aided design features. Club design has been and will continue to be an evolutionary process, one that is continually developing to meet the needs of golfers (see figure 13.1). One of the first major changes in the construction of golf clubs was to manufacture the club head separately from the wooden shaft. Varying the loft (or "backward slant") of the club head and the later addition of clubs with metal heads ("irons") dramatically increased the golfer's ability to adjust the length of shots and to hit the ball high and far. A tubular steel shaft introduced in the 1920s replaced the earlier hickory shaft.

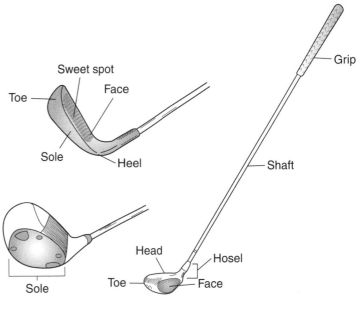

FIGURE 13.1 Parts of a golf club.

Today's clubs still use tubular steel shafts, although shafts made of graphite and other composite materials are becoming increasingly popular, especially for the woods. In the search for clubs that will hit the ball farther and have a larger hitting area (or "sweet spot"), new materials and designs have been developed, and now most woods actually have a metal club head. The USGA sets standards for golf clubs, and any golf clubs used in sanctioned tournaments must meet these standards.

Selecting the best golf clubs to be used in an instructional setting depends on a number of factors. The first factor to consider is the age, size, and skill level of the students. Young children can be provided with developmental and beginner clubs that are shorter and lighter and will make hitting the ball easier for them. Clubs to be used by young adults and adults should be full-sized clubs that are very durable and are of reasonable quality. Generally, tubular steel-shafted clubs are a good selection for instructional clubs because they are strong, relatively inexpensive, and of sufficient quality for students to learn the game of golf.

Golf Balls

The earliest golf balls were made of solid boxwood, but by the early 17th century these were replaced by feather-stuffed balls made of rawhide (Gowland, 2001). Modern golf balls originally consisted of a durable outer cover of wound rubber over a solid core. Today's golf balls rarely have the wound center; most have a solid or a multipiece center. The outside covers of today's golf balls are made of either a softer balata material or the firmer Surlyn. A one-piece or multipiece ball with a Surlyn cover is best for distance shots and is durable, while a balata cover is better for experienced golfers who want to put a lot of spin on the ball. The best choice for beginning and novice golfers is a solid-core ball with a Surlyn cover, because these are more durable and will fly farther. Many manufacturers make a "range ball," which is used primarily at driving ranges or during practice sessions. Range balls are usually of two types: One type has a very durable cover, while the other is a solid ball without an outer cover. Range balls do not fly as far as standard golf balls, but they are more durable and are much less expensive. Most scholastic, collegiate, and

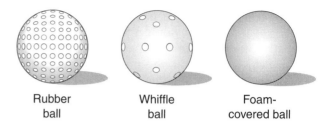

Rubber ball · Whiffle ball · Foam-covered ball

FIGURE 13.2 Commercial restricted-flight golf balls.

commercial programs give out either range balls or used golf balls, which also are considerably less expensive than new standard golf balls.

Whiffle, restricted-flight, homemade, and other nonstandard golf balls can also be used to practice golf skills and are often used for instructional programs and in personal practice. Whiffle golf balls are especially useful for teaching in small facilities such as gymnasiums, multipurpose rooms, or small outdoor areas. A variety of commercial restricted-flight golf balls are available for student purchase (see figure 13.2).

Risk Management

Golf is a relatively safe sport, but being hit with a club or golf ball does present some risks, especially with multiple students. As with any physical activity, a golfer or golf student participating in a golf activity should warm up and stretch before golfing and cool down afterward. The keys to maintaining a safe golfing teaching environment are to establish and enforce sound safety rules, reinforce staying alert, and maintain safe distances between students. Table 13.1 is a sample risk management tool for a golf class.

Skills and Techniques

The putt, chip, pitch shot, full swing, top of the backswing, and follow-through are the skills discussed in this section. Each skill is explained, as are the techniques that may be demonstrated to the students. This section also includes several useful teaching cues for each of the skills.

Table 13.1 Possible Risks in Golf

Risk identification	Reduction strategies
Muscle pulls, strains, ligament sprains	Adequate warm-up, stretch, and cool-down.
Injuries due to impact of golf ball	Post warning signs around landing area. Place restrictive barriers along hitting areas, especially close to the tee area. Teach students to call "Fore" if a shot is hit outside the landing area or near someone.
Improper positioning when a golfer yells "fore"	*Do not* look up to see the approaching golf ball. The proper position is looking down, huddling, and putting forearms overhead.
Blisters from improper grip	Blisters result if a club is gripped too tightly. A student should hold the club carefully, as if it were a tube of toothpaste with the lid removed. During a swing, the golfer does not want to place any unwanted pressure on the club. Golf gloves may also be used to prevent blisters.
Walking too close to a golfer who is swinging a club	Students not hitting golf balls must be vigilant in watching other students who are practicing. For safety, all students should remain at least 3 yards behind the golfer swinging the club. Students should swing a club only when instructed to do so. All course participants should act as "safety monitors" and must be prepared to warn fellow classmates when the potential for injury arises.
Inclement weather and lightning	If teaching outdoors, discontinue class once lightning is seen. Shelter should be sought within a lightning-protected building. High places, isolated trees, and small shelters in exposed locations are not safe and should be avoided.
Golf cart accidents	Golf carts are less stable than automobiles and are more likely to overturn. Caution should be exercised during driving, and a slow speed is recommended on slopes and side-hill locations. Be sure to set the brake on the cart when it is not in use.

Putting

A putt is a stroke made on the green with use of a putter in order to roll the ball into the hole. Most golf experts consider putting the most important skill in golf. In an 18-hole round of golf, 50 percent of the strokes allotted toward par are for putts. The putting stroke is by far the most individualized stroke in golf. Golfers at all levels use a variety of grips, stances, putter types, and putting strokes. The only true measure of a good putting stroke is whether the golfer can consistently putt the ball the desired length and direction.

Despite the wide variety of putting styles, equipment, and techniques, there are some sound teaching cues appropriate for all beginning putters. The recommended grip for putting is the reverse overlap grip. This grip is demonstrated as follows:

- Index finger of the left hand overlaps the little finger of the right hand (for a right-handed player).
- Thumbs are placed straight down the shaft.
- Palms oppose each other.
- Putter is gripped softly to enhance touch.

A square stance with the feet about shoulder-width apart is recommended for executing this grip properly. The ball should be played between the center of the stance and the toe of the front foot. The eyes should be directly over the ball to aid in accurately aligning the putt. The shoulders, arms, and hands are brought directly back from the ball as a unit without cocking of the wrists. Maintain a firm-wrist swing directly along the intended target line with the shoulders, hands, and arms again moving as a unit. The head and the body should remain as still as possible. The more moving parts in the putt, the greater the chance for error.

TEACHING CUES

- Arms, hands, shoulders, and putter swung as a unit (wrists remain firm).
- Putter reverses overlap grip.
- Head remains still and aligned over the ball.
- Square stance held, with the ball toward the front of the stance.
- Deliberate unrushed swing; straight back and straight follow-through required.

Confidence and a positive approach to putting are more important in becoming a good putter than any of the technical aspects of putting itself. Good putters are able to visualize the path the putt will travel and are confident in their ability to stroke the ball along that path. Since putting greens are not perfectly flat, a putted ball will tend to curve based on the slant of the green and the speed of the putt. Visualizing the path a putt will follow is called "reading the green" and is a skill that will develop with practice. Being a good putter is not a matter of strength, so anyone can become a good putter if he or she follows the basic mechanics of putting and is consistent and dedicated in practice.

There is no firmly established method for teaching putting, but the following are some sound strategies for practicing and improving putting skills. Students should begin their practice putting with very short putts of between 12 and 18 inches (30 and 45 centimeters). They should stroke the putts to the hole while concentrating on a smooth and relaxed stroke. As they begin to achieve success, the instructor should allow them to gradually increase the length of the putts. Another putting drill that can be practiced is the "putting ladder," which involves four to eight golf balls placed in a straight line away from the cup or target, with about 18 inches between each ball. Beginning with the closest ball, each ball is putted toward the cup until all balls have been putted. This drill exercise is especially useful in helping people to determine how hard to putt the golf ball from various distances. This skill is sometimes called a "putting touch." Another effective way to develop putting skills is to replicate putting during an actual round of golf. To do this, the instructor sets up a series of different putts and has the students putt the course for score. Students may compete with other students in the class or may simply try to achieve the lowest score possible. This format is used to assess students' skills in the West Point Golf class.

Chipping

Professional golfers consistently hit their approach shots onto the green, but most golfers are happy to get their approach shots close to the green. When taking greenside shots, golfers have three options: putting, chipping, or pitching the ball. Billy Bomar, a respected teaching professional, suggests that golfers visualize the easiest of the three shots to make and trust that it will work for them (Bomar, 2003). He recommends putting first, then chipping the ball. Pitching should be used only as a last resort. Since it is easier to judge ball roll than flight, golfers should get the ball onto the ground as quickly as possible and allow it to track toward the cup. The chip shot is the recommended shot to take when one is hitting onto the green from a distance of 1 to 15 yards (.9-14 meters).

Chip shots are short shots that use little or no wrist action. The arms, hands, and shoulders of the player are moved as a unit. The hands start out ahead of the club head and remain ahead of the club head throughout the chip swing. The club is taken back along the target line and then swung forward along the target line. An open stance, the front foot farther from the target line than the back foot, is recommended for the chip shot. The chip shot can be hit with any club, but the 7-iron and the 9-iron are recommended for most golfers. The 7-iron is used when the ball has a relatively long distance to roll to the hole. A 9-iron is the club of choice if there is less green between the ball and the hole. The novice player should develop confidence in using one or two clubs before trying to chip with multiple clubs.

TEACHING CUES

- Arms, hands, shoulders, and club swung as a unit, and wrists remain firm.
- Narrow and open stance should be maintained.
- Weight should remain on the target-side foot.
- Ball should remain back in the stance.
- Stroke is similar to a putting stroke.
- Player should chip to an intermediate target.
- Always remember: "It's easier to judge roll than flight."

The chip shot is an easy shot to include in a beginning golf class because the chip shot requires a relatively small area, uses a simple stroke pattern, and keeps body motion to a minimum. The chip shot can be practiced at an indoor or an outdoor facility. As with all other golf shots, repetition is needed to develop an effective chipping touch or feel. The mechanics of the chip shot are relatively simple, so the key elements for success involve hitting the ball in the right direction and the right distance.

Having students hit to an intermediate target is a good way for them to learn to hit the chip shot in the right direction. Instructors should have the students chip the ball in the air to intermediate targets and have them observe how far the ball rolls after it lands. Learning how far the ball rolls after hitting an intermediate target is important in calibrating how hard to hit the chip shot. Chipping the ball in the proper direction depends primarily on how closely the club swing pattern traces the target line. An effective drill for practicing chipping in the right direction is to have the students place two clubs parallel to the target line, about 8 inches (20 centimeters) apart, and then practice. The club head should remain between the clubs on the backswing, at the point of contact, and on the follow-through. Having students hit to an intermediate target will help develop the ability to hit the ball to the desired distance. Using the parallel club drill will aid students in hitting the ball in the proper direction.

Pitch Shot

The purpose of the pitch shot is to hit the ball high enough into the air that it lands softly on the green with the least possible roll. The pitch shot is a relatively short shot, hit with less than a full swing. Hitting the pitch shot accurately is more important than hitting for maximum distance. Since a pitch shot can be hit anywhere from 15 to 90 yards (14-82 meters), the challenge for students is to calibrate their swing length and speed to hit the ball the desired distance. Pitch shots are usually hit with a 9-iron, a pitching wedge, or the sand wedge. The stance for the pitch shot is slightly narrower than shoulder-width and is slightly open. Unlike the chip shot, the pitch shot is hit with considerable wrist action. Wrist action helps propel the ball high into the air. The distance the ball will travel depends on length of the swing and the wrist action and also depends, to a lesser extent, on the involvement of the hips, shoulders, and legs. The swing mechanics are the same as those used for the full swing, except that the swing length is shortened on both the backswing and the follow-through.

TEACHING CUES

- Control pitch distance with swing-length wrist action.
- Use wrist action to get the ball in the air.
- Stance should always be narrower than shoulder-width.
- Keep the head down through contact.
- Maintain a relatively high follow-through.

An effective way of practicing the pitch shot is to begin hitting whiffle golf balls. Students should maintain focus on shortening the swing, incorporating the wrist action, and contacting the whiffle ball solidly. After practice with whiffle golf balls, they can practice the pitch shot using practice golf balls. A logical progression begins with hitting very short pitch shots to a specific target. Instructors should then encourage students to gradually begin hitting to targets that are progressively farther away. After hitting groups of pitch shots to targets at a variety of distances, the students can hit a series of shots, starting with a short shot and following up with successively longer shots. Practicing pitching balls to a variety of distances will help develop the muscle memory to pitch the ball the desired distance and direction.

Full Swing

The full golf swing is a difficult skill that requires the coordination of numerous body parts. The golf swing must be built on a strong foundation that includes mastery of the proper golf grip, alignment, and stance. These fundamental techniques are taught early in the course (see Lessons 1 and 2 for review).

The backswing of a golf stroke begins with slowly taking the club head back from the ball and keeping the club on the same plane. The arms, shoulders, and hands should move as a unit. The club should remain on the same plane as the hands, arms, and club continue to rise. The head rotates, but moves very little.

TEACHING CUES

Top of the Backswing

- Left arm remains straight and tucked under the chin.
- Right forearm is perpendicular to the ground.
- Thumbs and wrists sit directly under the grip.
- Club is approximately parallel to the ground.
- Club head points toward the target.
- Club head swings back toward the target.
- Wrists remain firm.

The checkpoints at the top of the swing afford the best opportunity to provide feedback to novice golfers on the quality of their swing. The checkpoints are very specific and occur when the club is not moving very fast, so a physical educator who isn't an experienced golfer can still provide constructive feedback.

The swing begins as the target-side hip turns toward the target and the hands drop; then the wrists release as the body uncoils and the weight shifts to the target side. The hands, arms, and club are extended at impact, and the club head returns to the square position. On the follow-through, the body turns to face the target, the hands finish high, the weight is on the target-side foot, and the golfer is in balance. Swinging the club in a smooth, coordinated motion is more important than trying to swing according to prescribed checkpoints. Novice students should avoid overanalyzing the swing, since this may lead to what is called "paralysis by analysis." Good tempo, timing, and rhythm in the swing are the ultimate objectives.

Similar to the top of the backswing, the finish of the follow-through provides a good opportunity to evaluate the specific checkpoints of a good swing.

Follow-Through

- Weight is shifted to the target-side foot.
- Hips and shoulders face the target.
- Toe of the rear foot is pointing straight down to the ground.
- Hands finish high.
- Finish is balanced, with a pause at the end of the swing.

Hitting the ball both the desired distance and in the right direction are the ultimate objectives of the golf swing. One of the best forms of feedback when people hit a golf ball involves watching where the ball goes. Instructors should be careful not to make corrections after every shot. Instead, they should look for a pattern of faulty ball contact and for distance or direction problems before recommending changes in swing mechanics.

West Point Golf Instruction Model

This section describes the West Point model of golf instruction and ways to adapt the model for other school-based situations. Most of the technical information needed by golf students is covered in the first two lessons and is reinforced in subsequent lessons. The basics of the grip, the stance, and the swing are covered in detail, and students are given an opportunity to work on their technique and to provide constructive feedback to a student partner. The following two lesson plans cover the basic mechanics of the golf swing and can be used as models when one is planning a course of instruction for a beginning golf class.

Sample Lesson Plans

The typical golf lesson at West Point includes (1) student accountability, (2) review of previous skills, (3) practice and feedback, (4) introduction of new skill, (5) practice and feedback, (6) lesson closure, (7) dismissal. The following lesson plans include several teaching cues for each skill as well as creative learning activities that will help the student better understand and learn the skills.

LESSON 1

Grip, Alignment, and Stance

SEQUENCE (45-MINUTE CLASS)

1. Student accountability and administrative details (5 minutes).
2. Class procedures: Cover equipment issue, course overview, and safety procedures (5 minutes).
3. Grip: Demonstrate grip, cover instructional cues, and give time for student practice (10 minutes).
4. Alignment: Demonstrate proper alignment, cover instructional cues, and give time for student practice (10 minutes).
5. Stance: Model stance and discuss instructional cues (10 minutes).
6. Closure and student dismissal: Review key instructional points and return all equipment (5 minutes).

TEACHING CUES

Grip

- Target-side hand
  - Balance club on index finger and heel of the hand.
  - Thumb down the right side of the grip.
  - "V" made by the thumb and index finger points to the right ear.
  - Should see two knuckles on the left hand.
  - Last three fingers are the primary gripping fingers.
- Rear-side hand
  - Center groove of the hand covers left thumb.
  - "V" made by the thumb and index finger points to the right ear.
  - Should see only one knuckle on the right hand.
  - Index finger in trigger position.
- Grip types
  - Overlapping grip: Pinkie finger of the right hand overlaps the index finger of the left hand.
  - Interlocking grip: Pinkie finger of the right hand interlocks with the index finger of the left hand.
  - "Baseball grip" or "ten-finger grip": All ten fingers are in contact with the grip (not recommended).

Alignment

- Square: The feet are equidistant from the target line.
- Open: The target-side foot is farther from the target line than the rear-side foot.
- Closed: The target-side foot is closer to the target line than the rear-side foot.
- Woods
  - Feet should be slightly wider than shoulder-width.
  - Ball is played off the front heel.

- Mid to long irons
  - Feet are shoulder-width apart.
  - Ball is slightly behind front heel.
- Short irons
  - Feet are closer than shoulder-width.
  - Ball is played slightly in front of midpoint of the stance.

Stance

- Chin up
- Back straight
- Knees slightly flexed
- Bent at the waist
- Shoulders over the front of the knees
- Straight line down left arm to the club (hands in front of the club head)

SUGGESTED LEARNING ACTIVITIES

- Grip: Balance club with left hand, keeping the club on the second bone of the index finger and under both heel pads.
- Grip, alignment, stance, and partner assessments: Have students choose a partner and let the partners take turns assessing each other's golf skills and form.
- Alignment: Take two clubs, and place one parallel to the target line and the other perpendicular to the first club. Use this to assess stance alignment and ball positioning.
- Stance: Take two clubs and assume a stance. Grip one club normally and the other club with the club head toward the shoulder. The inverted club should trace up the left arm to the shoulder if the stance is correct.

LESSON 2

Full Swing

SEQUENCE (45-MINUTE CLASS)

1. Review instructional cues for the golf grip, alignment, and stance (10 minutes).
2. Introduce and practice the golf backswing (10 minutes).
3. Instructor and peers give feedback on the golf backswing (10 minutes).
4. Demonstrate and practice the full golf swing (5 minutes).
5. Analyze and assess the proper golf follow-through (5 minutes).
6. Lesson closure: Review key instructional points and return equipment (5 minutes).

TEACHING CUES

Take-Away

- Follow along target line.
- Arms, hands, and club begin to move as a unit.

- Wrists cock at waist level.
- Target heel may come off ground (this is a by-product of a good turn).

Top of Swing

- Full hip turn is completed over center of the stance.
- Turn back toward the target.
- Target arm remains straight.
- Back forearm remains perpendicular to the ground (elbow at 90 degrees).
- Club head is pointing toward the target.
- Club remains parallel to the ground.
- Target eye is focused on the ball.
- Wrists remain under the grip.
- Hands are higher than the back shoulder.

Downswing

- Arms, hands, and club start down as a unit.
- Wrists release at impact.
- Hips return to a square alignment.
- Club head, hands, and head remain aligned at the point of impact (club face square to the target).
- Swing pattern should be along target line (an "outside-in" swing will cause a slice and an "inside-out" swing will cause a hook).

Follow-Through and Finish

- Hips and chest turn toward target area.
- Rear shoulder is closer to target than target shoulder.
- Hands finish high.
- Ending is always balanced.

SUGGESTED LEARNING ACTIVITIES

- Drag drill: Have the student drag the club head back along the target line 4 to 6 inches (10-15 centimeters), prior to having the club come off the ground. (This type of exercise is used to promote a square take-away and helps to avoid lifting the club too soon.)
- Partner analysis:
  - Top of the backswing (look for instructional cues)
  - Follow-through and finish (look for instructional cues)
- Wrist motion drill: Place a tee in the end of the grip. As the wrists cock at waist level, the tee should be pointing straight toward the ground.
- Rotation drill: Place the club across the shoulders in front of the body. Rotate the body so that the club end points perpendicular to the target line. Repeat with students in the proper stance position. The club end should point about to where the ball is located.

Administrative Details

The golf classes at West Point are designed for beginning and novice golfers, so the course description states that the course is for students who shoot more than 110 strokes for 18 holes. The course is taught on an athletic field, on a practice golf green adjacent to the athletic field, or at the West Point Driving Range, which is located about 3 miles from the central campus. The course consists of 18 lessons of 50 minutes each. The beginning golf class is very popular at the Academy; therefore, relatively large classes of 30 students with two instructors per class are offered.

Each class of 30 students is divided into two sections (Section A and Section B). The first two lessons, introduction to the grip stance and swing, are usually taught together on the athletic field. Beginning with Lessons 3 and 4, Section A and Section B alternate classes on the athletic field and on the practice putting green. One section works on the pitch shot while the other section works on chipping and putting at the practice putting green. For the next class, the sections switch facilities and lessons. The remaining lessons, with the exception of the test review class (Lesson 9) and the final exam (Lesson 10), are taught using this alternating format.

Assessment

The class is a graded course, with skills tests embedded throughout. The testing protocol is designed to meet West Point's needs, but suggested modifications are provided here for adapting the testing procedures to a variety of school-based settings. Multiple trials of the skills tests are permitted, programmed, and encouraged because the instructors and students view them as focused practice sessions in addition to valuable evaluation tools.

60-Yard Pitch Test

The 60-yard (55-meter) pitch test consists of hitting six pitch shots at a target 60 yards from the hitting area. The target is located in the center of three circles (see figure 13.3).

PROTOCOL

The 60-yard pitch test requires pitching six golf balls from the same location toward a flag with three concentric circles around it. The innermost circle has a radius extending 5 yards (4.5 meters) from the flag. The next circle has a 10-yard (9-meter) radius, and the outermost circle has a 15-yard (14-meter) radius. Scoring is determined through observation of where the ball lands. If the ball lands in the innermost

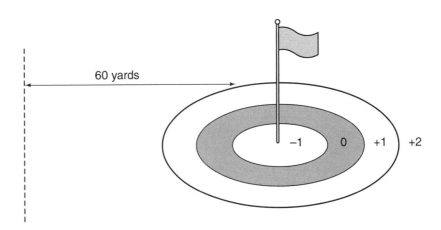

FIGURE 13.3 **60-yard pitch test.**

circle, the score is –1; in the middle circle, 0; in the outermost circle, +1; and outside all circles, +2. The total score, based on par, for the six shots is then converted to a scale score according to the Golf Skills Test Conversion Scale (see table 13.2). The 60-yard pitch test is worth 200 points out of a possible 1,000 points for the course.

The 60-yard pitch test format provides a flexible template for testing other golf skills of students of all ages and abilities. The distance of the shot, the type of ball used,

Table 13.2 Golf Skills Test Conversion Scale

CHIP AND PUTT		PITCH (60 YARDS)		FULL SWING	
Points	Score	Points	Score	In play	Score
−6	200	−6	200	10	200
−5	192	−5	190	9	180
−4	184	−4	182	8	160
−3	178	−3	176	7	140
−2	174	−2	172	6	120
−1	168	−1	168	5	100
0	164	0	164	4	80
+1	160	+1	160	3	60
+2	156	+2	156	2	40
+3	152	+3	152	1	20
+4	146	+4	146	0	0
+5	142	+5	142		
+6	140	+6	140		
+7	132	+7	132		
+8	130	+8	130		
+9 >	120	>9	120		

the size of the target area, the raw points awarded, and the conversion scales can easily be modified to accommodate the age and skill level of the students and the evaluation requirements of the course.

Chipping and Putting Test

Another skills test used in the class is the chipping and putting skills test. Students chip the ball from six different locations around the putting green to six different holes on the green itself (see figure 13.4). Once the ball is on the green, the student takes as many putts as needed to putt the ball into the hole. An effort is made to vary the distance of the chip shots, the slope of the green, and the amount of green between the hitting area and the hole. The test is designed to replicate real chipping and putting on a golf course, thus providing an "authentic assessment."

PROTOCOL

The chipping and putting skills test requires chipping from six different locations around the green. Once the ball is chipped onto the green, the ball is then putted into the designated hole. The test is scored similarly to a real golf game, with each hole being a par 3; however, the maximum score for any single hole is +2 (also known as "a double bogey"). The total score, based on par, for the six holes is then converted to a scale score according to the Golf Skills Test Conversion Scale (see table 13.2).

All six holes are played, and the raw score is determined according to the chipping and putting test protocol. As with the 60-yard pitch test, the Golf Skills Test Conversion Scale is used to convert the raw score into a scaled score (see table 13.2). Putting and chipping can easily be separated and tested independently if separate tests better suit the students' needs.

1 stroke = –2
2 strokes = –1
3 strokes = 0
4 strokes = +1
5 strokes = +2

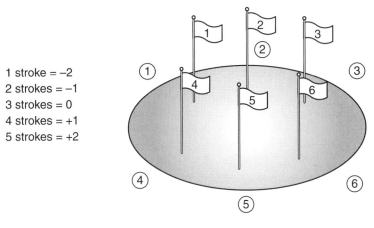

FIGURE 13.4 Chipping and putting test.

Full Swing Test

Since the West Point golf class is designed for beginning golfers, the general objectives are to have the students consistently make solid contact with the ball, hit the ball into the air, and hit the ball in the desired direction. Hitting the ball for distance is important in golf, but is not the focus of the beginning golf class. With this in mind, the full swing test was developed.

The full swing test consists of hitting five full swing shots with a 5-iron, followed by five full swing shots with a 3-wood. The objective is to fly the ball over a small creek in front of the tee area and have the ball stop in the designated range area without hitting the retaining screening on either side of the range area (see figure 13.5).

PROTOCOL

Each shot meeting the criteria just outlined is awarded 20 points. The maximum score for the test is 200 points. The conversion scale for the full swing test is also shown in the Golf Skills Test Conversion Scale (see table 13.2).

A full swing can also be assessed using a test protocol similar to that for the 60-yard pitch test. The distance and accuracy required for the full swing shots can easily be adjusted to fit the skill level of the students in the class.

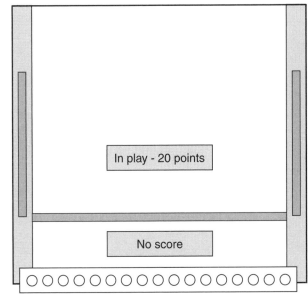

FIGURE 13.5 Full swing test.

Guidelines for Teaching Golf

There are hundreds of golf schools that enable serious golfers to fine-tune their game. Interested golfers should look into programs that provide very skilled and knowledgeable instructors, high-quality equipment and facilities, and technical training aids. However, most physical education teachers and recreation specialists with modest golf training, limited facilities and equipment, and some motivation can teach basic golf classes as part of their instructional programs, so there is not necessarily a need for students to seek expensive private lessons. A physical education teacher can provide an equally challenging and fulfilling golf lesson. The following are some general guidelines for teaching a basic golf class:

• Safety first: Swinging clubs and flying balls pose safety risks to the golf instructor and the students. As in any other physical activity class, the instructor needs to establish a safe, controlled, and disciplined environment. Sound policies, procedures, and rules need to be established that set safety guidelines. While every situation is different, all instructors need to ensure adequate space to swing a golf club, must provide a secure landing area for golf balls, and must maintain control over the class and ensure that the students conduct themselves under the guidelines of proper sportsmanship. Also, the utilization of safety equipment such as restricted-flight balls, golf netting, and warning signage will assist in maintaining a safe teaching environment.

• Keep it simple: The golf swing is built on the basics of golf: the grip, the proper alignment, and the stance. The instructor should provide adequate time for students to develop these basic skills, and should begin the lessons with the shorter shots such as putting, chipping, and pitching before having students attempt the more complex full swing, sand shots, and other specialized shots.

• Active learning and peer feedback: Schools and recreation programs usually teach golf in relatively large groups with a limited number of instructors. An effective way to teach and reinforce golf skills is to have the students work together. Instructors can pair students up or put them into small groups and provide them with specific checkpoints and teaching cues on the lesson of the day. The students will be able to give each other feedback in addition to that provided by the teacher, and this is often helpful to novice golfers as they begin to apply the various techniques they have learned.

• Avoid "paralysis by analysis": The golf swing requires the coordination of numerous body parts. Many technical articles and resources are available that analyze every aspect of the golf swing. Teachers need to avoid getting too technical when introducing the golf swing. Students who think too much about technical details tend to lack the coordination and fluid movements needed to correctly execute a golf swing, and often aim the club in the wrong direction. Emphasis should be placed on swinging the club in a smooth and fluid motion that simply allows the ball to get the full impact of the swing. Avoid trying to make corrections based on the results of a single swing. Students should hit between 5 and 10 golf shots before analyzing the swing and making changes to their swing pattern. The following quote should help instructors keep this in mind when teaching a beginning golf class: "Information overload is a common mistake when teaching golf to beginners. In a good faith attempt to correct swing errors, many instructors cloud students' minds and bring about paralysis by analysis" (Goehl, 2002).

• Appropriate assessment: If golf is taught as a graded activity, some type of evaluation is necessary. Even in a nongraded situation, students need some feedback on how effective they are in executing the desired skills. The best assessment of golf skills can be obtained through playing golf for score; however, this isn't practical for most educational situations. Putting, chipping, pitching, and the full swing are all components of golf that can be tested individually. When one is analyzing novice golfers, an objective test is better than a subjective test. Subjective tests should only be used if the evaluator is a highly skilled observer. Test protocol and grading standards must be kept simple, attainable, and reasonable.

• Use available resource material and teaching aids: There are numerous books, magazines, videotapes, DVDs, Web sites, and other materials on golf instruction. Some of the material is student focused, while other resources center on instructors and teaching techniques. These materials include information appropriate for any basic golf class and provide a variety of ideas and approaches to the teaching of golf. Teaching aids are available to assist in productive practice. Some of the teaching aids are great for individual practice but have limited use when introduced into a group setting. Be sure that the teaching aids you purchase focus on a particular instructional objective and that they are useful in a classroom setting.

• Keep golfing fun: Golf is a difficult game, and beginning golfers may become frustrated and lose interest if they do not feel as though they are making progress. Keep the students active and structure the class so as to give them many opportunities to hit the ball. Including interesting drills, golf-type games, and friendly competition will make the class informative and fun.

• Program for success: Students enjoy success and tend to continue participating in activities in which they have achieved success. Include activities in golf classes that are applicable to all members of the class, so that students will feel successful in their golfing endeavors and will want to continue with the game.

Golf is a popular sport that will no doubt continue to experience a growth in popularity in the future. There are currently more golfers and golf courses in the United States and around the world than ever before. Golf is a relatively safe and immensely enjoyable sport, and instructors should always plan a safe and informative instructional program whenever teaching it to new students.

It is recommended that potential instructors prepare a modest lesson plan and golf program that includes a general introduction to the sport and its rules. Even if funding is limited, physical education teachers can start a golf program at their school by soliciting borrowed or donated equipment from veteran golfers and established courses. Often a local golf course, sporting goods store, or parents' group will be happy to help sponsor a golf program, so it is recommended that teachers research all possible avenues when looking to form golf classes. An abundance of golf instructional material is available to students and teachers and is especially valuable when a program is just getting started. These sorts of teaching aids are often useful to students and can serve as enhancements to any golf program.

Whether the students are elementary, secondary school, or college level students, the introduction of golf to the physical education curriculum will enhance the students' physical education and provide them with a new athletic avenue to explore. All teachers are encouraged to begin golf programs at schools that are currently without one. If golf is already offered as part of a school's physical education curriculum, instructors should regularly update the quality, safety, and scope of the program so that students may continue to learn and benefit from it.

Key Terms

apron—The closely cut area surrounding the green.

away—The ball farthest from the hole.

caddie—A person who carries the clubs of a player.

casual water—An unplanned accumulation of water on the golf course, not considered a water hazard.

cup—The hole in the green into which the ball is played.

divot—The piece of turf removed by the club head during a stroke.

dogleg—A bend or curve in the fairway either to the right or to the left.

draw—A ball in flight that moves slightly from right to left for a right-handed player and from left to right for a left-handed player.

fade—A ball in flight that moves slightly from left to right for a right-handed player and from right to left for a left-handed player.

fairway—The well-mowed area of the course between the tee and the green.

flagstick—A pole inserted in the cup to indicate the number of the hole and location of the cup.

flights—The divisions into which players are grouped for a tournament.

foursome—A group of four persons playing together who are competing against par or against one another.

frog hair, fringe, collar, apron—The higher area of trimmed grass surrounding the green.

green—The area of closely mowed turf surrounding the hole.

halved—A tied score for a hole or a game.

handicap—The difference between the average game of a player and par for the course; also refers to a method of equalizing the playing ability of opponents by awarding strokes to the weaker players.

hazard—A bunker or water trap strategically arranged to increase the difficulty of the course.

hole out—A long and final stroke of a hole.

honor—The right of a side or player to drive first from the teeing ground on a hole, usually earned by having scored lower on the previous hole.

hook—A flight of the ball that curves dramatically to the left for a right-handed player and to the right for a left-handed player.

LPGA—Ladies Professional Golf Association.

match play—A type of competition based on the number of holes won or lost.

medalist(s)—The person (or persons) with the lowest score in a qualifying round.

medal play—A type of competition based on the total strokes for the round.

out of bounds—An illegal area, marked by a line or white stakes, that surrounds the golf course.

PGA—Professional Golf Association (men).

playing through—Playing in front of a slower group; the slower group extends the courtesy of standing aside and permitting the faster group to play first.

press—A shot in which a player attempts to apply more than his or her normal power.

pull—A ball hit to the left of the intended line of flight.

push—A ball hit to the right of the intended line of flight.

qualifying round—A designated number of holes played prior to a tournament in order to ascertain eligibility and classification of participants.

rough—The unkempt area of grass that parallels the fairway.

sand trap—A hazard on the fairway or around the green formed by substitution of sand for topsoil.

scratch player—A player who has a handicap of zero.

shank—A shot in which the ball is contacted with the heel and the shaft of a club and projected at a right angle to the intended line of flight.

slice—A stroke in which the ball curves dramatically to the right for a right-handed player and to the left for a left-handed player.

smothered ball or duck hook—A ball hit with a closed club face; ball immediately goes into the ground, traveling as little as 100 yards. If the ball lifts off the ground, it hooks.

stymie—A ball that has another ball or object directly in the intended line of play.

tee—An object (usually wooden or plastic) used to elevate the ball for a drive.

teeing ground—The starting area of each hole, usually designated by markers.

threesome—A group of three persons playing together who are competing against par or against one another.

topped ball—A shot in which the club head contacts the ball above the centerline, causing the ball to have a low flight or to roll along the ground.

up—The number of holes in match play or strokes in medal play by which a person is ahead of an opponent.

USGA—United States Golf Association.

water hole—A hazard of water strategically constructed and located between the tee and the green.

winter rules—The application of seasonal, local rules permitting a player to improve the lie of the ball on the fairway.

References

Bomar, B. (2003). Tips from the 50 states. *Golf Digest, 54,* 80.

Goehl, C. (2002). A simplified approach for teaching golf to beginners. *Journal of Physical Education, Recreation and Dance, 73,* 12.

Gowland, R.G. (2001). Early golf clubs and balls. *The Magazine Antiques, 160,* 184.

Owens, D., & Bunker, L.K. (1995). *Golf: Steps to success.* (2nd ed.). Champaign, IL: Human Kinetics.

Suggested Readings

Books

Adams, M. (2000). *Play golf for juniors.* Westport, CT: Firefly Books.

Anselmo, J. (2001). *A-game golf.* New York: Doubleday.

Detty Moore, B. (2001). *Teaching kids golf: The baffled parent's guide.* Camden, ME: Ragged Mountain Press.

Emerick, D. (2000). *Tiger tips: Beginners golf for kids.* Coal Valley, IL: Quality Sports.

Gordon, J. (2001). *The kids book of golf.* Toronto, ON: Kids Can Press.

Green, S. (2000). Consider it golf: Golf etiquette and safety tips for children. Troy, MI: Excel.

Hogan, B. (1985). *Five lessons: The modern fundamentals of golf.* New York: Simon & Schuster.

Ledbetter, D. (2000). *The fundamentals of Hogan.* New York: Doubleday.

Peltz, D. (1999). *Dave Peltz's short game bible.* New York: Broadway Books.

Peltz, D. (2000). *Dave Peltz's putting bible.* New York: Doubleday.

Web Sites

www.golfdigest.com

www.usga.org

www.uskidsgolf.com

Videos and Compact Discs

Akers, M. (2001). *Build your dream swing* (CD).

Barge, M. (1991). *Super golf for juniors* (VHS).

Blenz, H. (1990). *Junior golf* (VHS).

Sport-Specific Organizations

Royal and Ancient Golf Club
Fife
Scotland
KY 16 9JD
+44 (0) 134 460000

United States Golf Association
Liberty Corner
P.O. Box 708
Far Hills, NJ 07931
908-234-2300
www.usga.org

Ice Skating

Susan Tendy and Ivan Evans

Ice skating, long popular for its numerous physical benefits and for its graceful beauty, can be either a recreational or a competitive sport. There are numerous ways for athletes and recreational skaters to channel their aspirations in ice skating. Once an adequate level of skill in the basics of ice skating is obtained, the possible avenues in skating are limited only by the individual's personal desire and ambition.

Types of Ice Skating

As a competitive sport, skating can be divided into five major categories: figure skating (individuals or pairs), ice dance, speed skating, hockey, and synchronized skating. All of these except synchronized skating have competition available at the local, state, regional, national, international, and Olympic levels. Formerly known as precision skating, synchronized skating was recognized as recently as 1994 by the International Figure Skating Union. Thus, a variety of challenges for the novice as well as for the top professional are available in competitive skating. Each of the five competitive areas of skating requires specialized training techniques and equipment.

Figure skating is physically demanding and artistic. Skaters must polish the basics of skating as well as maintain proficiency in combinations of figures, jumps, spins, and turns. The use of costumes and music enables the skater to portray an artistic theme much as in ballet. There are three categories in figure skating: individual men's event, individual women's event, and pairs (one man, one woman).

Ice dance is artistically based on the concept of ballroom dancing. A male–female dance pair learns the steps of many dances, from the waltz to the tango. Ice dancing demands balance and control and involves myriad dance steps. Unlike figure skating, the purpose is not speed, spins, and the height of jumps; instead, dance pairs demonstrate artistic dynamics while complementing each other.

Speed skating is a timed event that covers a predetermined distance. Superior conditioning and training on specific competitive race techniques are key factors in developing excellence in speed skating. Speed skaters work hard to develop strong legs to maximize the power needed for each skating stroke. Nevertheless, learning the skating fundamentals is still essential to good performance.

Ice hockey, a team sport of six players per team, involves pushing a puck across the ice with a hockey stick in an attempt to score into the opponent's goal. It requires speed, balance, agility, and control. Good hockey players must possess expertise in the basics of ice skating and power skating. They must also be able to handle a stick and have the ability to work as a team member. The development of good peripheral vision is very important, as it aids in tracking other players during skating.

Synchronized (precision) skating uses formations incorporating both marching and choreography. Synchronized skating requires the mastery of skills commonly taught in basic figure and dance skating classes. It involves the performance of footwork and skating maneuvers utilizing various group formations set to musical themes. Recognized as the fifth and newest category of skating, synchronized skating entails teams who are judged on factors such as unity, accuracy, and the difficulty of the formation. Skaters display a variety of intersecting lines, blocks, wheels, and circles.

Recreational skating gives novice skaters the opportunity to get out on the ice and move! Indoor and outdoor skating rinks and frozen ponds and lakes are all areas that afford a wonderful outing for the whole family. Basic skating skills involving forward movement and the ability to stop may be the only two skills a recreational skater learns, but they are essential skills for both safety and enjoyment. Times are set aside at various local skating rinks and outdoor facilities for recreational skating. Additionally, local communities often supervise frozen ponds to ensure safety.

Skating as a spectator sport, performed by professional as well as amateur skaters, has provided entertainment for millions worldwide. Spectators flock to arenas to observe figure skating exhibitions, hockey games, and speed skating meets. Regional and national television coverage of many events has made it possible to keep up with the latest developments in the sport.

Purpose of the Course

The general purpose of the West Point skating course is to enhance and broaden the recreational interests of our students. Our goal is to create an interest in ice skating and develop a basic skill level that allows students to take advantage of ice skating as a lifetime recreational activity.

This activity can be an essential part of a lifetime of fitness, involving little to no repetitive impact and enabling a cardiorespiratory, leg, and upper body workout. Our specific course objectives are as follows:

- Develop proficiency in the basic skills of ice skating: balance, sculling, forward stroke, backward stroke, crossovers, and starts and stops
- Enable students to appreciate the need for leg strength and total-body endurance for ice skating
- Have students experience the relationship of neuromuscular control and kinesthetic awareness in moving on an ice surface
- Develop student knowledge about the care and maintenance of a variety of ice skating equipment
- Increase student understanding of the variety of ice skating specialties: figure, hockey, and speed
- Enable students to value ice skating as a lifetime activity that will enhance physical fitness

Instructional Area

Probably the most popular location at which a skate class can take place is the public indoor ice rink. The benefits of this type of facility are many. Rental skates are available for those who cannot afford, do not have, or have outgrown their own skates. Group rates can be arranged for class instruction and equipment rental. Inclement weather is not a factor for indoor skaters. Colleges may have an indoor rink that offers group lesson time or school day-trip opportunities. Municipal outdoor ice rinks are also very popular, but they close down during the warmer months. Group rates and rental equipment are also advantages of these areas. Supervised town ponds can be monitored by town authorities for ice thickness, which allows for skating under certain controlled conditions. An ice thickness test is performed to ensure that no unfortunate incidents occur. Students should always take care to exercise caution when skating on a pond or a lake and must remember to always observe the "No Skating" signs when posted. The most dangerous and often the most inviting sites are unsupervised frozen lakes. In extremely cold temperatures, the ice can be up to 12 inches (30 centimeters) thick—thick enough to support a vehicle if necessary (Graham, 1998). Again, the local authorities can survey the situation, and a group can certainly enjoy the great outdoors safely when safety issues have been addressed. The downside to outdoor facilities, aside from those already mentioned, is that students have to supply their own equipment.

Equipment

Proper equipment in all skating activities is a critical element in terms of cost, safety, and performance. Important considerations in the purchase of equipment for any entry-level skater should include issues such as how fast a young skater will grow, mandatory equipment for safety, and proper fit. Purchasing slightly used equipment is a good option if you know that the skater is growing quickly. However, the importance of proper fit and safety should never be compromised when you are faced with a financial choice. Local skate shops may help determine the life left in equipment when you are considering an individual purchase. If skating is a part of the physical education instructional curriculum, a school might consider utilizing the resources of an already established public skating program that rents skate equipment in order to allay the cost of replacement and repair.

Clothing

Clothing is an important part of a skater's equipment package. What to wear on the ice is as much a factor of safety as it is a warmth issue. Gloves protect the hands from the cold, as well as protecting the fingers of a fallen skater from the blades of other skaters. A hat keeps the head and the body warm and also provides a slight cushion in the event of a fall. Many ice rinks require beginning skaters of all ages to wear helmets during their lessons. This is a good idea, and should be enforced for adult classes as well as for younger students. It's also beneficial to wear layers of upper body clothing that can be removed as the skater warms up. Additionally, various types of leg wear will help keep the skater warm. The important point about leg wear is that pant legs should not flare at the bottom. They can easily catch on a skate blade during crossover maneuvers.

Skates

The various styles of skates have the same basic structure. Each style of skate provides advantages that suit a skater's particular needs. Once people decide on an area of interest, they can decide on what style of skate is best.

The figure skate is the recommended skate for the beginner. With a higher boot, it immediately offers more support than the dance, hockey, or speed skate; and the sole and heel make for additional support in jumps and spins. Additionally, figure skates have a wider blade and different sharpening from the other skates, allowing for additional stability on the ice. The blade is sharpened by machine, which creates two distinct edges (inside and outside). There is a slight "rock" from toe to heel on the blade, with toe picks on the front of the blade.

Hockey skates have a tendon guard on the boot and a hard toe for protection. Blades are also sharpened by machine, but are much narrower than the blades of figure skates. The blade is higher than the figure skate blade and has a quarter-curve from toe to heel.

Speed skates have a boot that is low cut and very light. The long, thin blade is sharpened by hand, which creates square edges and leads to less "rock" from front to back. The skate is designed for speed and has limited turning agility.

Risk Management

Given the proper instruction, equipment, and safety considerations, skating can be an enjoyable lifetime activity. Beginning skaters may have to be reminded of situations that can cause injury or discomfort. Horseplay and out-of-control skating contribute to most recreational skating accidents. Falling on the ice is part of every skater's initiation into the sport. Even the best skaters fall; the important thing is to learn how to avoid injury during a fall and how to recover from a fall.

It is a good policy to look for basic safety rules posted within the skating area. For example, a standard practice at most rinks is to establish an area in the center of the ice for working on advanced skills. This may not be feasible at all times, especially if the ice is crowded or many beginners are in the area. Be on the lookout for these rules and cautions when visiting your rink. The information in table 14.1 may help you identify and reduce risk of injury (Cokeley & Tendy, 2001).

Table 14.1 Possible Risks in Ice Skating

Risk identification	Reduction strategies
Falling or collisions with other skaters	• Learn to fall; learn to stand up from a fall. • Skate under control; no horseplay. • Modify activities: two feet on the ice at all times for speed-type games. • Divide class into two or more smaller groups by skill level.
Muscle strains, ligament sprains, and contusions from falling	• Warm up before class. • Cool down after class. • Review falling and recovery techniques. • Enforce clothing safety: pants, gloves, hat or helmet. • Reinforce stopping techniques taught in class. • Never grab another student when falling. • Skate at a controllable speed at all times.
Aggravation of a prior injury	• Never skate if hurt. • Report any prior injuries to instructor.
Injury due to cold temperature	• Emphasize proper clothing: sweatshirt, skull cap, gloves.
Head injuries or concussions	• Emphasize proper falling technique. • Never skate at speeds that will compromise skill level. • Wear caps for minor protection, helmets for all beginners.
Ankle injuries	• Fit skates properly. • Lace skates tightly. • Avoid advanced activities until thoroughly warmed up.
Injuries from skate blades during class	• Avoid kicking or leg-swinging activities in close quarters that increase the chance of a toe-pick incident. • Wear gloves to protect the fingers from other skaters' skates in case of a fall.
Injuries from skate blades outside of class	• Keep skate guards on blades when skates are not in use.
Injuries from objects in pockets	• Remove pens, pencils, keys, and so on from pockets during class.
Choking incidents as a result of falling	• Do not chew gum while skating.

Skills and Techniques

In this section we define the skills that are the target topics for each individual lesson. These are foundational skills that will stand all beginning skaters in good stead as they progress through a beginning skate program.

Forward Stroke

With the forward stroke, the skater skates forward by alternating the transfer of his or her weight to the outside edge of the glide foot with the toes turned out while pushing off of the inside edge of the opposite foot.

Snowplow Stop

This stop is recommended as the first stop to teach the beginner. To accomplish the snowplow stop, the skater turns the toes inward so as to gradually press down on the inside edge of both skates while flexing at the hips and knees.

Backward Stroke

With the backward stroke, the skater skates backward by alternating the transfer of his or her body weight to the inside edge of the glide foot, with the toes turned inward, while pushing off of the inside edge of the opposite foot.

Two-Foot Turn

The two-foot turn allows a change of direction from forward to backward skating or vice versa while both skates are kept on the ice.

T-Stop

In a more advanced technique, the T-stop, the skater glides on one foot in a straight line while placing the arch of the opposite foot behind and at a right angle to the skating foot. Gradually the rear foot is lowered to the ice on an outside edge. Transferring more weight to the rear foot allows the stop to become more pronounced.

Hockey Stop

The hockey stop is an advanced stop in which the skater moves from a forward two-foot glide and pivots the skates 90 degrees. The skate blades are kept parallel, and the body flexes at the hips and knees. The front skate is on an inside edge, and the back skate is on an outside edge. The upper body (arms, shoulders, head) faces the direction of travel while the lower body (from the waist down) turns at a right angle from the line of travel.

Crossovers

The crossover is a skating technique used to navigate a curve, in either a forward or a backward direction. The foot on the outer edge of the curve crosses over the foot closest to the inside of the curve. There are four crossover directions: forward right, forward left, backward right, and backward left.

Serpentine

The serpentine uses crossover and forward stroke techniques to navigate in a semicircular manner around cones or marked areas.

In addition to the skills just described, the following Web page includes video clips of many other skating skills (Tendy, 2003). The link for each major skill theme is also provided within each lesson in this chapter. Visit the site at www.usma.edu/dpe/courses/IceSkating/FlashSite/01index.htm.

Course Overview

Many skills can be taught to the beginning skater. It is important to remember that a beginning skater can be a beginner at any age; however, the primary skill instruction is the same. An instructor may adjust the lessons in terms of types of practice activities or use of games depending on the maturity of the group. Keep in mind that younger children have a shorter attention span. You may need to incorporate frequent breaks and have a larger array of practice activities for a given basic skill in order to maintain their interest. Older children may respond to more competitive types of activities. Some students may require constant feedback while others just prefer time to practice what they have learned. These issues always make teaching ice skating fun and interesting.

Table 14.2 summarizes an 18-lesson figure skating course, showing the progression of skills and the learning activities associated with each skill.

Sample Lesson Plans

The sample lessons that follow include many lead-ups to help the skater develop basic techniques needed to master the targeted skill for each lesson. These lead-ups in themselves are engaging activities that will keep the interest of the class as a whole.

Table 14.2 Overview of Skating Lessons

Lesson	Topic	Activities
1	Safety Proper fit and care of skates Falling and recovering from a fall	Lecture Lace and unlace skates Sit and recover
2	Forward stroke	T-start position Barrier drill Scooter pushes Light switch drill
3	Snowplow stop	Pigeon-toe, knock-knees Line drill, target practice
4	Backward stroke	March in place, toes in Chair sit drill
5	Review: forward and backward stroke, snowplow stop	Activities from lessons 2, 3, and 4

6	Two-foot turn	Two-foot glide
		Two-foot edge drills
		Circus elephants nose-to-tail holding hands:
		    180-degree turn: in place as a group
		    180-degree turn: together around curve

7	T-stop	One-foot glide Arms perpendicular to line of travel Land that plane! Line drill
8	Hockey stop	Line drill Two-skater relay
9	Review: stops, forward and backward stroke, two-foot turn	Activities from lessons 2-4, 6-8
10	Forward right crossovers	Scooter pushes Sculling or pumping with outside foot Keep the circle in the "V" drill Olympic medal drill
11	Forward left crossovers	Scooter pushes Sculling or pumping with outside foot Keep the circle in the "V" drill Olympic medal drill
12	Review: forward crossovers	Activities from lessons 10 and 11
13	Backward left crossovers	Backward scooter pushes Sculling or pumping with the outside foot Sports car entry, driver's side Ankle-heel steering drill Olympic medal drill

Lesson	Topic	Activities
14	Backward right crossovers	Backward scooter pushes Sculling or pumping with the outside foot Sports car entry, passenger's side Ankle-heel steering drill Olympic medal drill
15	Review: backward crossovers	Activities from lessons 13 and 14
16	Serpentine	Review of two-foot edge drills Review of scooter pushes on half-circle One-foot edge drill
17	Compulsory routine	Combine all skills taught
18	Optional routine	Student's choice of five figures

Forward Stroke

View the video: www.usma.edu/dpe/courses/IceSkating/FlashSite/elem_03.htm.

SEQUENCE (45-MINUTE CLASS)

1. Conduct warm-up exercises (5 minutes).
   - Marching in place
   - Marching and glide
   - T-start position
   - Arm carriage
2. Introduce the forward stroke (1 minute).
3. Demonstrate the forward stroke: Teacher models proper technique (see figure 14.1) (2 minutes).
4. Review key instructional cues while demonstrating (2 minutes).
5. Reinforce instructional cues during group-directed learning activity (11 minutes).
6. Student learning activities:
   - Group practice, instruction, and feedback (11 minutes). Have students line up at the end of the ice surface. Have them skate from one end of the ice to the other. You may have them change activity at the half-ice point in order to reduce fatigue and boredom.
     - Barrier drill
     - Scooter pushes
     - Skateboard pushes
   - Individual practice, instruction, and peer feedback (11 minutes). Have students pair up on one side of the rink. Have the practicing student go from one side to the other while the observing student provides feedback.
     - Light-switch drill
     - Push, extend, and hold the glide

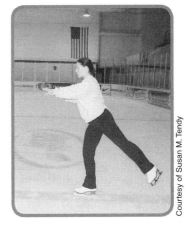

Courtesy of Susan M. Tendy

FIGURE 14.1 **Forward stroke.**

7. Closure: review of proper techniques, instructional cues, questions (2 minutes).

TEACHING CUES

- Start position: feet in T-start position, arms wide, knees flexed, weight centered over the glide foot
- Weight shift onto the glide foot
- Slight push with the inside edge of the rear skate (blade flat, no toe picks)
- Keep the rear skate at a 45-degree angle, free leg fully extended
- Recovery: bring feet close together, two-foot glide
- Stroke length: equal to or greater than the height of the skater
- Head and eyes: up and forward in the direction of travel

SUGGESTED LEARNING ACTIVITIES

Barrier Drill

Position the students so that they are facing the wall surrounding the perimeter of the ice rink (the barrier). Have them place their hands on top of the wall, palms down, about as wide apart as if they were riding a wide-handled bicycle. If there is a glass partition, have them look at themselves in the window. This approximate skating posture—head up and proper arm-carriage position—is very important for skaters. Students should hold on to the wall for support and keep the toe and knee of one leg against the wall while in a stationary lunge position. They should keep the other leg fully extended back and out to the side about 45 degrees, the flat of the blade resting on the ice. If the instructor has the students lift the rear leg, this will mimic the one-foot glide position needed for a good forward stroke. Students should then straighten the lunge leg and bring their skate blades together underneath them. Having both skates on the ice at this point will simulate the two-foot glide during the forward stroke. Instructors should next have the students repeat the lunge position with the other leg, then recover with both skates underneath them. This exercise gives students a feeling of balance during the often-difficult one-foot glide phase of the forward stroke and emphasizes the lunge position, the arm carriage, and the head position.

Scooter Pushes

Students can simulate riding a scooter by bending their knees and laterally pushing one foot back at about a 45-degree angle while keeping the other skate blade in contact with the ice. The pushing foot then recovers back next to the gliding foot into a two-foot glide.

Light-Switch Drill

Students can imagine that there is a light switch, in the "off" position, on the ice beside and just behind the midline of the stroking-leg side of their body. The object of this exercise is to extend the stroking leg completely in order to flip the switch to the "on" position with the skate blade. As the students become more successful at turning "on" the light switch they will realize the optimal power of the leg stroke (Kunzle-Watson & DeArmond, 1996).

Snowplow Stop

View the video: www.usma.edu/dpe/courses/IceSkating/FlashSite/Stop_01.htm.

SEQUENCE (45-MINUTE CLASS)

1. Warm-up exercises, practice prior skills taught (5 minutes).
   - T-start position
   - Scooter pushes
   - Push, extend, and hold the glide
2. Introduce the snowplow stop (1 minute).
3. Demonstrate the snowplow stop: Teacher models proper technique (2 minutes) (see figure 14.2).
4. Review key instructional cues while demonstrating (2 minutes).
5. Reinforce instructional cues during group-directed learning activity (11 minutes).
6. Student learning activities:
   - Group practice, instruction, and feedback (11 minutes). Have students line up on the blue line or goal line.
     - Pigeon-toe, knock-knees—stationary
     - Two-foot glide to pigeon-toe and knock-knees position for stopping
   - Individual practice, instruction, and feedback (11 minutes). Have students form pairs and line up on the blue line. Have them go from blue line to red line to blue line.
     - Line drill
     - Target practice
7. Closure: review of proper techniques, instructional cues, questions (2 minutes).

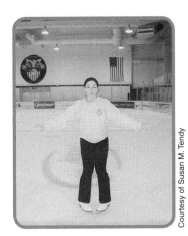

FIGURE 14.2 **Snowplow stop.**

Courtesy of Susan M. Tendy

TEACHING CUES

- Pressure even on inside edges
- Control: full 3-second stop and hold at designated spot
- Body position: toes in, hips and knees flexed

SUGGESTED LEARNING ACTIVITIES

- Pigeon-toe, knock-knees: Students can try this body position while standing still and then from a two-foot glide position.
- Line drill: Have the students push off with a T-start and one forward stroke, to a controlled two-foot glide, and then to a snowplow stop.
- Target practice: Have the students push off of one line or a designated area on the ice, sustain a two-foot glide, and then try to stop on another line or at a designated spot on the ice.

Backward Stroke

View the video: www.usma.edu/dpe/courses/IceSkating/FlashSite/elem_04.htm.

SEQUENCE (45-MINUTE CLASS)

1. Warm-up exercises, practice prior skills taught (5 minutes).
   - T-start
   - Forward stroke
   - Two-foot glide
   - Snowplow stop
2. Introduce the backward stroke (1 minute).
3. Demonstrate the backward stroke: Teacher models proper technique (2 minutes) (see figure 14.3).
4. Review key instructional cues while demonstrating (2 minutes).
5. Reinforce instructional cues during group-directed learning activity (11 minutes).
6. Student learning activities:
   - Group practice, instruction, and feedback (11 minutes). Arrange students on the side of the ice surface. Have them go from one side of the ice to the other.
     - March in place (Oppelt, 1974)
     - Toes in—stationary
     - Toes in—marching
   - Individual practice, instruction, and feedback (11 minutes). Have one student skate backward while a partner assists by holding the exerciser's hands lightly, thus assisting with balance and providing stability.
     - Shift and lift
     - Chair sit drill
     - Light-switch drill
7. Closure: review of proper techniques, instructional cues, questions (2 minutes).

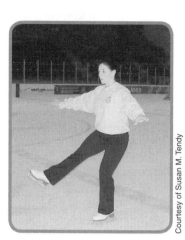

FIGURE 14.3   Backward stroke.

TEACHING CUES

- Weight shift and opposite skate lift, extending the leg forward
- Body position: knees flexed with head and eyes up, arms out
- Recovery: bring feet together—two-foot glide
- Stroke length: approximately the height of the skater

SUGGESTED LEARNING ACTIVITIES

Shift and Lift

Students have toes in and march in place (Oppelt, 1974). Gradually they shift more weight to the glide foot, lifting the opposite skate off of the ice. They recover the free leg to the "toes-in" position.

Chair Sit Drill

Students can pretend to begin to sit in a chair, but must act as though it has suddenly been pulled out from underneath them and they are trying not to fall. They should flex their legs accordingly and maintain a slight backward lean.

Light-Switch Drill

Have the students imagine that there is a light switch, in the "off" position, on the ice beside and just forward of the midline of the stroking-leg side of their body. The object is to extend the stroking leg completely in order to flip the switch to the "on" position with their skate blade. As the students become more successful at turning "on" the light switch, they will realize the optimal power of the leg stroke (Kunzle-Watson & DeArmond, 1996).

Two-Foot Turn

View the video: www.usma.edu/dpe/courses/IceSkating/FlashSite/inter_03.htm.

SEQUENCE (45-MINUTE CLASS)

1. Warm-up exercises, practice prior skills taught (5 minutes).
   - Chair drill
   - Light-switch drill
   - Snowplow stop
2. Introduce the two-foot turn (1 minute).
3. Demonstrate the two-foot turn: Teacher models proper technique (2 minutes).
4. Review key instructional cues while demonstrating (2 minutes).
5. Reinforce instructional cues during group-directed learning activity (11 minutes).
6. Student learning activities:
   - Group practice, instruction, and feedback (11 minutes). Have the students split into two groups. Position the groups in opposing corners of the ice. Have each group forward stroke to a two-foot glide through the center of the ice rink to the opposing corner.
     - Two-foot glide drill
     - "Circus elephants" nose-to-tail drill: Arrange the students in a circle, holding hands. They can then turn 180 degrees and practice pivoting in place.
   - Individual practice, instruction and peer feedback: Use student checklist (11 minutes).
     - Two-foot edge drill
     - 180-degree turns while moving
7. Closure: review of proper techniques, instructional cues, questions (2 minutes).

TEACHING CUES

- Body position: knees flexed, head and eyes up
- Edges: arms holding the circle, skater looking toward the center of the circle to get on the correct edges for direction of turn
- Smooth transition into backward stroke, crossover

SUGGESTED LEARNING ACTIVITIES

Two-Foot Glide

Students perform forward stroke and glide with proper arm carriage, knees slightly bent and shoulders over heels with most of the weight on balls of feet. Once in a good forward glide, students should lower the upper body by bending the knees further and keeping the shoulders over the heels—they should not lean forward. They may glide in this position for 2 seconds and then slowly rise up to the starting position.

"Circus Elephants" Nose-to-Tail Drill

Group members hold hands in a circle and weight and unweight the skates while performing a 180-degree turn. Holding hands in a circular formation approximates the proper arm-carriage position. An instructor can tell the students to pretend they are "holding the circle" with their arms.

Two-Foot Edge Drills

The two-foot edge exercise helps students recognize the inside and outside edges of their skate blades. Students can find a circle, skate, and then glide along the curve, looking toward the center and gliding on both skates while "holding the circle." They can try it in both directions—clockwise and counterclockwise—and, when ready, may add the 180-degree pivot turn as in the circus elephants drill.

180-Degree Turn Drill (Stationary and Moving)

While stationary, students should flex their knees. They may unweight the skates by raising the center of gravity of the body via straightening the legs, balancing on the center of both blades on the ice as they turn 180 degrees. When the students are moving, an instructor may suggest that they maintain a stationary upper body while the body rotates from the armpits down. In general, once the turn is completed, the students will be able to maintain momentum in the direction of travel by turning the toes inward, thus producing a backward glide.

T-Stop

View the video: www.usma.edu/dpe/courses/IceSkating/FlashSite/Stop_02.htm.

SEQUENCE (45-MINUTE CLASS)

1. Warm-up exercises, practice prior skills taught (5 minutes).
   - Two-foot glide
   - Two-foot turn
2. Introduce the T-stop (1 minute).
3. Demonstrate the T-stop: Teacher models proper technique (2 minutes) (see figure 14.4).

4. Review key instructional cues while demonstrating (2 minutes).

5. Reinforce instructional cues during group-directed learning activity (11 minutes).

6. Student learning activities:

   – Group practice, instruction, and feedback (11 minutes). Position students on one end of the ice. Have the students skate from one end to the other in waves. Provide group feedback at the opposite end.

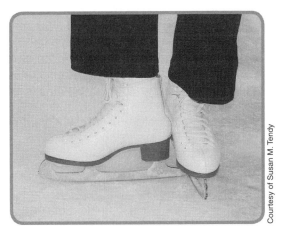

FIGURE 14.4   Foot position for T-stop.

   – One-foot glide: Students perform two forward strokes and then glide on one foot with slightly bent knee for 3 seconds, then alternate the glide foot; have them identify their most comfortable forward glide foot.

   – Arm carriage and upper body angle: Ensure that students have the arms extended but relaxed at the proper arm-carriage level. They should maintain a forward line of travel by holding their arms at an imaginary line perpendicular to the direction of travel.

   – Individual practice, instruction, and feedback: Use student checklist (11 minutes). The instructor can position students on one end of the ice and should have the students skate from one end to the other. Then the students should try to "land the plane" after taking a few forward strokes to attain some momentum. The students should be encouraged to feel and should trust that speed is their friend during the T-stop approach and execution. After they have the basic action down, students can take a few forward strokes and then attempt to stop on the blue lines on their way to the other end of the ice. Observers can provide encouragement and feedback.

     – Land that plane!

     – Line drill: target practice—stop on demand

7. Closure: review of proper techniques, instructional cues, questions (2 minutes).

TEACHING CUES

- Edges: glide foot flat, back foot on outside edge
- Control: stop and hold at designated spot
- Body position: flexed knees, gradual backward shift of body weight to rear skate

SUGGESTED LEARNING ACTIVITIES

- Land that plane!: Think of the rear skate as the landing gear on a plane, and the need to land on the runway very gradually.
- Line drill: Target practice—stop on a line as in the snowplow stop. Stop on target while maintaining a rearward lean but staying in balance.

Hockey Stop

View the video: www.usma.edu/dpe/courses/IceSkating/FlashSite/stop_03.htm.

SEQUENCE (45-MINUTE CLASS)

1. Warm-up exercises, practice prior skills taught (5 minutes).
   - Glide on one foot and rotate the upper body 90 degrees.
   - Land that plane!
   - Stop on demand—blue lines
   - Two-foot glide
2. Introduce the hockey stop (1 minute).
3. Demonstrate the hockey stop: Teacher models proper technique (2 minutes) (see figure 14.5).
4. Review key instructional cues while demonstrating (2 minutes).
5. Reinforce instructional cues during group-directed learning activity (11 minutes).
6. Student learning activities:
   - Group practice, instruction, and feedback (11 minutes). The instructor should have students line up on one end of the rink. Students should start with a T-stop and several forward strokes on their way to the other end. The instructor can send them in small groups in order to adequately observe their progress and provide feedback.
       - Two-foot glide—weighted and unweighted
       - Small lift perpendicular to line of travel, then a glide
   - Individual practice, instruction, and feedback: Use student checklist (11 minutes). Position students on one end of the rink. Have the students skate from one end to the other in waves. Peers provide feedback while observing each other and at the opposite end (line drill). Position students on lines on the ice (two-skater relay).
       - Line drill
       - Two-skater relay
7. Closure: review of proper techniques, instructional cues, questions (2 minutes).

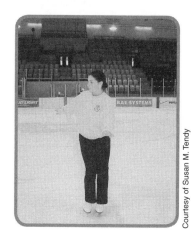

FIGURE 14.5 Hockey stop.

TEACHING CUES

- Weight on balls of feet, dip and pivot, sliding to a stop
- Control: stop and hold at designated spot
- Body position: knees flexed with arms out for balance

SUGGESTED LEARNING ACTIVITIES

Line Drill

The line drill is for target practice: stopping on a line. Students should concentrate on not turning or gliding out of the stop by sliding or by "shaving the ice" to come to a complete stop. Students must face forward, maintaining a straight forward line of travel by holding their arms over an imaginary line perpendicular to the direction of travel.

Two-Skater Relay

Two skaters stand on a line; one skates to the next line, executes a hockey stop, and returns to the partner, using a hockey stop on the partner's line. The second skater repeats the same exercise. Skaters must be careful that they do not bump into their partner upon their return.

Forward Right Crossover

View the video: www.usma.edu/dpe/courses/IceSkating/FlashSite/cross_01.htm.

SEQUENCE (45-MINUTE CLASS)

1. Warm-up exercises, practice prior skills taught (5 minutes).
   - Forward stroke
   - Two-foot turn
   - Backward stroke
   - Hockey stop
2. Introduce the forward right crossover (1 minute).
3. Demonstrate the forward right crossover: Teacher models proper technique (2 minutes).
4. Review key instructional cues while demonstrating (2 minutes).
5. Reinforce instructional cues during group-directed learning activity (11 minutes).
6. Student learning activities:
   - Group practice, instruction, and feedback (11 minutes). Position the students on one side of the rink. Have the students skate from one side to the other.
     - Scooter pushes
     - Sculling or pumping with the outside foot
   - Individual practice, instruction, and feedback (11 minutes). Position the students in one of the circles facing inward. Have the students skate one way around the circle and then the other way.
   - Keep the circle in the "V" drill
   - Olympic medal drill
7. Closure: review of proper techniques, instructional cues, questions (2 minutes).

TEACHING CUES

- Step into the circle with the left skate, push on the inside edge of the right skate as in the forward stroke.
- Step in front of and over the left foot with the right skate while gliding onto the right foot, on an inside edge.
- Push with the outside edge of the left skate while tightly crossing the thighs.
- Body position: Hold the circle, shoulders turned in.
- Recover by uncrossing the left leg, stepping into the circle, and returning to the forward stroke position.

SUGGESTED LEARNING ACTIVITIES

- Ride a scooter: Perform scooter pushes with the outside foot.
- Sculling or pumping with the outside foot.
- Keep the circle in the "V" drill: Using any of the face-off circles on a hockey ice surface, the instructor can have the students extend their arms to shoulder height, with their right arm out front. This is much the same as "holding the circle." This will ensure the proper rotation of the hips and shoulders and thus maintain the proper edges. The instructor should tell the students to make a fist and extend only their thumbs and index fingers, making a "V" shape with their hands. The object of the drill is to keep the painted circle lines passing through the "V" shape of their hands. This drill will naturally keep the students' shoulders at the optimal rotation (preventing the shoulders from becoming square and facing outward) inward toward the circle (turning radius). In addition, the students will be using the correct lean of the upper body in order to optimize the turning radius.
- Olympic medal drill: Using any of the face-off circles on a hockey ice surface, have the students extend their arms shoulder height, right arm out front, much the same as in "holding the circle." This will ensure the proper rotation of the hips and shoulders, enabling the skater to turn in toward the center of the circle. While the students are doing this they can imagine that they have an Olympic medal hanging around their necks. The object is to keep the medal hanging free of their body and out over the sternum. In this drill the students will naturally lean inward toward the center of the circle or turning radius. In addition, they will be on the inside edge of the inside skate, which will optimize their weight distribution prior to executing the crossover.

Forward Left Crossover

SEQUENCE (45-MINUTE CLASS)

1. Warm-up exercises, practice prior skills taught (5 minutes).
   - Two-foot glide
   - Hockey stop
   - Sculling with the outside foot around a circle
   - Olympic medal drill
2. Introduce the forward left crossover (1 minute).
3. Demonstrate the forward left crossover: Teacher models proper technique (2 minutes).
4. Review key instructional cues while demonstrating (2 minutes).
5. Reinforce instructional cues during group-directed learning activity (11 minutes).
6. Student learning activities:
   - Group practice, instruction, and feedback (11 minutes). Position the students on one side of the rink. Have the students skate from one side to the other.
     - Scooter pushes
     - Sculling or pumping with the outside foot

- Individual practice, instruction, and feedback (11 minutes). Position the students in one of the circles facing inward. Have the students skate one way around the circle and then the other way.
    - Keep the circle in the "V" drill
    - Olympic medal drill
7. Closure: review of proper techniques, instructional cues, questions (2 minutes).

TEACHING CUES

- Step into circle with the right skate, and push on the inside edge of the left skate.
- Step in front of and over the right foot with the left skate.
- Push with the outside edge of the right skate and tightly cross thighs.
- Body position: hold the circle, shoulders turned inward.
- Recover by uncrossing the right leg, stepping into the circle, and returning to the forward stroke position.

SUGGESTED LEARNING ACTIVITIES

- Ride a scooter: Scooter pushes with the outside foot.
- Sculling or pumping with the outside foot.
- Keeping the circle in the "V" drill: Using any of the face-off circles on a hockey ice surface, the instructor can have the students extend their arms shoulder height, with their left arm out front, much the same as in "holding the circle." This will ensure the proper rotation of the hips and shoulders, thus maintaining the proper edges to stay on the curve. The instructor should then tell the students to make a fist and extend only their thumbs and index fingers, making a "V" shape with their hands. The object of the drill is to keep the painted circle lines passing through the "V" shape of their hands. This drill will naturally keep the students' shoulders at the optimal rotation (preventing the shoulders from becoming square and facing outward) inward toward the circle (turning radius). In addition, the students will be using the correct lean of the upper body in order to optimize the turning radius.
- Olympic medal drill: Refer to page 328 for an explanation of the drill.

Backward Left Crossover

View the video: www.usma.edu/dpe/courses/IceSkating/FlashSite/cross_03.htm.

SEQUENCE (45-MINUTE CLASS)

1. Warm-up exercises, practice prior skills taught (5 minutes).
   - Two-foot turn
   - Backward stroke
2. Introduce the backward left crossover (1 minute).
3. Demonstrate the backward left crossover: teacher modeling (2 minutes).
4. Review key instructional cues while demonstrating (2 minutes).
5. Reinforce instructional cues during group-directed learning activity (11 minutes).

6. Student learning activities:
   - Group practice, instruction, and feedback (11 minutes). Position the students on a painted circle.
     - Backward scooter pushes
     - Sculling or pushing with the outside foot
   - Individual practice, instruction, and feedback (11 minutes). Students continue to work around the existing painted circles.
     - Sports car entry—driver's side
     - Ankle-heel steering drill
     - Olympic medal drill

7. Closure: review of proper techniques, instructional cues, questions (2 minutes).

TEACHING CUES

* Step into the circle with the right foot, turning the toe slightly away from the circle.
* Lead with the heel.
* Step or scull over with the left foot, balancing on the left blade.
* Extend the crossover portion by pushing away with the right outside edge as the thighs are tightly crossed.
* Body position: knees flexed, arms holding the circle.

SUGGESTED LEARNING ACTIVITIES

* Sculling (pumping) with the outside foot.
* Scooter pushes with the outside foot.
* Sports car entry—driver's side: Students should sit into the circle as if they were entering a low sports car on the driver's side.
* Ankle-heel steering drill: The instructor can have the students glide backward around a face-off circle. As they work their left foot crossover, they should concentrate on lifting their back-inside right ankle-heel and should steer it to their right before placing it on the ice on the painted circle. This is a crucial step in getting skaters to lead with the right hip, which allows them to lean in toward the circle or turning radius. This skill will teach them to counter the centrifugal forces that are forcing them outside the circle or turning radius.
* Olympic medal drill: Refer to page 328 for an explanation of the drill.

Backward Right Crossover

View the video: www.usma.edu/dpe/courses/IceSkating/FlashSite/cross_04.htm.

SEQUENCE (45-MINUTE CLASS)

1. Warm-up exercises, practice prior skills taught (5 minutes).
   - Two-foot turn
   - Backward stroke

2. Introduce the backward right crossover (1 minute).

3. Demonstrate the backward right crossover: Teacher models proper technique (2 minutes).

4. Review key instructional cues while demonstrating (2 minutes).

5. Reinforce instructional cues during group-directed learning activity (11 minutes).

6. Student learning activities:
   - Group practice, instruction, and feedback (11 minutes). Position the students on a painted circle.
     - Backward scooter pushes
     - Sculling or pushing with the outside foot
   - Individual practice, instruction, and feedback (11 minutes). Students continue to work around the existing painted circles.
     - Sports car entry—driver's side
     - Ankle-heel steering drill
     - Olympic medal drill

7. Closure: review of proper techniques, instructional cues, questions (2 minutes).

TEACHING CUES

- Step into the circle with left foot, turning the left toe slightly away from the circle.
- Lead with the heel.
- Step or scull over with the right foot.
- Exaggerate the crossover position by pushing away with a left outside edge as the thighs are tightly crossed.
- Body position: knees flexed, arms holding the circle.

SUGGESTED LEARNING ACTIVITIES

- Sculling (pumping) with the outside foot.
- Scooter pushes with the outside foot.
- Sports car entry—passenger's side: Sit into the circle as if you were entering a low sports car on the passenger's side.
- Ankle-heel steering drill: The instructor can have the students glide backward around a face-off circle. As they work their right foot crossover, they should concentrate on lifting their back-inside left ankle-heel and steer it to their left prior to placing it on the ice on the painted circle. This is a crucial step in getting them to rotate the left hip, which allows them to lean inward toward the circle or turning radius. This skill will teach them to counter the centrifugal forces that are forcing them outside the circle or turning radius.
- Olympic medal drill: Refer to page 328 for an explanation of the drill.

Serpentine

View the video: www.usma.edu/dpe/courses/IceSkating/FlashSite/cross_05.htm.

SEQUENCE (45-MINUTE CLASS)

1. Warm-up exercises, practice prior skills taught (5 minutes).
   - Backward crossovers
   - Front crossovers
   - Front spiral—one-foot glides
2. Introduce the serpentine (1 minute).
3. Demonstrate the serpentine: Teacher models proper technique (2 minutes).
4. Review key instructional cues while demonstrating (2 minutes).
5. Reinforce instructional cues during group-directed learning activity (11 minutes).
6. Student learning activities:
   - Group practice, instruction, and feedback (11 minutes). Have students position themselves in the circles.
     - Two-foot edge drill
     - Scooter pushes
   - Individual practice, instruction, and feedback: Use student checklist (11 minutes).
     - One-foot edge drill
7. Closure: review of proper techniques, instructional cues, questions (2 minutes).

TEACHING CUES

- Take T-start position facing the circle, leading with the outside arm and the inside foot.
- Push off to front crossover step pattern at the apex (height) of the circle.
- Use forward stroke patterns between the cones.
- Foot-change step-in stroke preparation for front crossover pattern.

SUGGESTED LEARNING ACTIVITIES

- Review two-foot edge drills.
- Review scooter pushes on a half-circle.
- One-foot edge drill—one-foot glide on a circle, facing into the circle. Alternate feet at the halfway mark and snake the circle in the other direction.

Teaching the basics of beginning skating should be essentially the same regardless of the age of the students. The wonderful thing about skating is that it does not require the development of tremendous upper or lower body strength before one sees results from a series of well-taught lessons. The individual student's attention span and motivation are probably the two key ingredients that determine the rate of success. Incorporating safe and creative games can add an important element of fun to any skating class. People are never too old to perform routines with costumes or themes, which can be a fun way to celebrate the culmination of a course and to demonstrate to others what has been achieved.

Key Terms

backward stroke—Skating backward by alternating the transfer of one's weight to the inside edge of the glide foot with toes turned in, while pushing off of the inside edge of the opposite foot.

crossover—A skating technique used to navigate a curve, in either a forward or a backward direction, in which the foot on the outer edge of the curve crosses over the foot closest to the inside of the curve. There are four crossover directions: forward right, forward left, backward right, and backward left.

forward stroke—Skating forward by alternating the transfer of one's weight to the outside edge of the glide foot with the toes turned out, while pushing off of the inside edge of the opposite foot.

hockey stop—An advanced stop in which the skater moves from a forward two-foot glide and turns sideways 90 degrees. The skate blades are kept parallel, and the body flexes at the hips and knees. The front skate is on an inside edge, and the back skate is on an outside edge. The upper body (arms, shoulders, head) faces the direction of travel while the lower body (from the waist down) turns 90 degrees from the line of travel.

serpentine—The use of crossover and forward stroke techniques to navigate in a semicircular manner around cones or marked areas.

snowplow stop—A stop that is recommended as the first stop to teach the beginner. The skater accomplishes the snowplow stop by turning the toes in so as to gradually press down on the inside edge of both skates while flexing at the hips and knees.

T-stop—A more advanced technique than the snowplow stop; skaters perform the T-stop by gliding on one foot in a straight line while placing the arch of the opposite foot behind and at a right angle to the skating foot. Gradually the rear foot is lowered to the ice on an outside edge. Transferring more weight to the rear foot allows the stop to become more pronounced.

two-foot turn—A change of direction from forward to backward skating or vice versa, with both skates kept on the ice.

References

Cokeley, K., & Tendy, S. (2001). Ice skating safety techniques—from risky business to fun and games. *Strategies, 14,* 10-11.

Graham, G. (1998, Winter). Ice safety. *The Ohio State University Extension Environment Task Force Newsletter, 1(4).* Retrieved 5 June, 2006, from http://ohioline.osu.edu/enviro/wi98/enviro_7.html.

Kunzle-Watson, K., & DeArmond, S. (1996). *Ice skating: Steps to success.* Champaign, IL: Human Kinetics.

Oppelt, K. (1974). *Oppelt standard method of therapeutic and recreational ice skating.* State College, PA: Private Printing.

Tendy, S. (2003). Ice skating video Web page. Retrieved 5 June, 2006, from www.usma.edu/dpe/courses/Ice Skating/FlashSite/01index.htm.

Suggested Readings

Bezic, S., & Hayes, D. (1996). *The passion to skate.* Atlanta: Turner.

Hagen, P., Clark, S., Cashen, J., Kollen, P., Lamb, S., Morris, K., & Wright, B. (1995). *Figure skating: Sharpen your skills.* Indianapolis: Masters Press.

National Safety Council. (2001). Skating safely on ice. Retrieved 5 June, 2006, from www.nsc.org/library/facts/iceskate.htm.

Petkevich, J.M. (1989). *Figure skating: Championship techniques.* Lanham, MD: Sports Illustrated Books.

Shulman, C. (2002). *The complete book of figure skating.* Champaign, IL: Human Kinetics.

Yamaguchi, K. (1997). *Figure skating for dummies.* Foster City, CA: IDG Books Worldwide.

Sport-Specific Organizations

International Skating Union (ISU)
Chemin de Primerose 2
CH 1007
Lausanne, Switzerland
Phone: (+41) 21 612 66 66
Fax: (+41) 21 612 66 77
E-mail: info@isu.ch

Skate Canada (previously Canadian Figure Skating
Association, CFSA)
865 Shefford Road
Gloucester, Ontario K1J 1H9
613-747-1007
888-747-2372
Fax: 613-748-5718
Toll-free fax: 877-211-2372
www.skatecanada.ca/
E-mail: skatecanada@skatecanada.ca

United States Figure Skating Association (USFSA)
20 First Street
Colorado Springs, CO 80906-3697
719-635-5200
Fax: 719-635-9548
www.usfsa.org

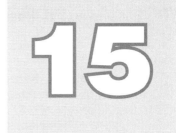

Rock Climbing

Edmund Crossley and Scott Bovee

We are all faced with rock climbing-like activities on a daily basis. Like a rock climber, when you get out of your chair, you position your feet and hands, redistribute your weight, and then stand up. Each of these movements—repositioning hands, foot placement, and weight redistribution—is applicable to rock climbing. In climbing in our adult lives, we use the natural skills developed from childhood. These skills start when we learn to climb out of the crib, progress as we climb and descend stairs, and develop further when we climb trees as young children. As adults, we use the climbing skills developed during childhood to accomplish everyday tasks such as ascending a ladder to change a lightbulb, to hang objects, to retrieve items off a high shelf, to clean windows, and even to paint. Thus, a person's innate balance, hand–eye and foot–eye coordination, and the fear of and respect for a vertical environment serve as developmental learning experiences for rock climbing.

Today, the sport of rock climbing takes place on cliffs outside and on walls, both indoors and outdoors. Regardless of the type of rock climbing activity, people of both genders across the full spectrum of ages and abilities are participating. Rock climbing has played a significant part in the "adventure sport" phenomenon over the last 15 years. The increased popularity of rock climbing activities is indicated by the rise in the number of both indoor and outdoor climbing facilities, climbing Web sites, videos, challenge rope courses, adventure sporting equipment stores, and advertising and media exposure such as the ESPN X-Games.

Hundreds of climbing walls, from homemade versions to expensive industrial-quality commercial and public climbing walls, have been constructed over the past 15 years. Rock climbing activities have mainstreamed into schools, fitness centers, YMCAs, campgrounds, and even the neighborhood backyard.

Constructing a climbing wall for your school or community center may be as simple as attaching handholds to an existing wall. Look around: You may be able to use the block wall on the backside of a gymnasium. All that is needed is a basic wall with handholds and footholds for beginners of all ages.

The editors wish to thank Dawes Strickler for his contributions to this chapter.

Climbing activities range from bouldering to roped "free" climbing, mountaineering, ice climbing, and rappelling. All climbing adventures are offered by commercial guide services or can be done "on your own."

Bouldering entails ropeless climbing between 4 and 12 feet (1.2 and 3.7 meters) above the ground and takes place on low walls either indoors or outdoors. This type of climbing has become popular because of its freedom from ropes and because it requires little economic investment or much training and also is relatively safe. Bouldering can be done alone, in pairs, or in large groups, with no belayers or rope work needed. In addition, bouldering can offer a strenuous workout or a convenient way to learn or improve on technique.

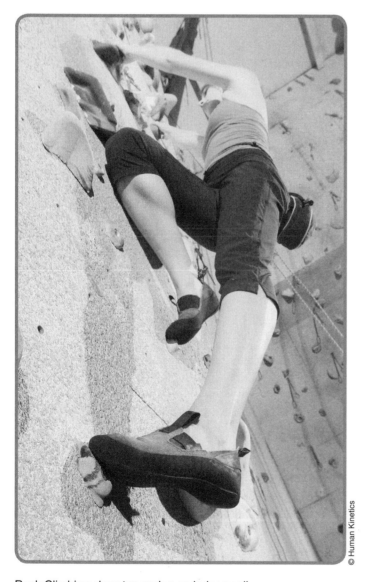

Rock Climbing class top roping on indoor wall.

© Human Kinetics

Roped "free climbing" utilizes harnesses, ropes, belayers, and other equipment for safety. However, this equipment is not used to assist in climbing but as a backup should a fall occur. Free climbing, especially top-rope climbing, has grown in popularity in part because of the advances in and availability of climbing equipment that makes climbing safer. The rope, anchors, and belayer provide safety to the climber in the event of a fall.

Mountain climbing is ascending and descending various sizes of hilly terrain requiring advanced hiking and climbing skills, as well as the use of technical equipment and systems. Snow, ice, rock, glaciers, altitude, and weather present objective dangers to the climber in the form of avalanches; ice and rock falls; effects of altitude, cold, and heat; and dehydration. Technical mountaineering involves all the basics of rock climbing. Ice climbing involves the use of pointed crampons attached to the feet and the use of handheld ice tools with picks. Using the ice tool picks and kicking in the front points of the crampons allow the climber to ascend sheer ice faces. Vertical and overhanging ice is now commonly climbed. Roped technical ice climbing is becoming common in alpine settings worldwide.

Rock climbing on cliffs and indoor walls, either roped or via bouldering, can challenge everyone from the novice to the most experienced climber. Utilize the information in this chapter and the wide variety of available resources to join the thousands of people enjoying rock climbing activities. Challenge yourself and your students to explore the vertical world!

Purpose of the Course

West Point offers six rock climbing programs for students. Climbing opportunities include a physical education Basic Rock Climbing advanced sport course, a three-week lead climbing camp offered during the summer, a one-day Basic Training Rappel Site class during students' first summer, two indoor wall bouldering classes for all freshmen, open climbing sessions on the indoor wall, and membership in a 50-cadet mountaineering team that climbs year-round.

Six climbing facilities are utilized as a part of the climbing program: four prepared bolted outdoor rock cliffs; the USMA Class of 1979 Indoor Wall (48 feet tall, 8,000 square feet [14.6 meters tall,

745 square meters]); and the world-famous Sha-wangunks climbing area located just 45 minutes to the north of West Point.

The remainder of this chapter outlines the Basic Rock Climbing course offered at the U.S. Military Academy on its new indoor climbing wall. This is one of the most popular advanced sport courses offered to students. The primary purpose of the course is to teach the novice climber the skills and techniques of basic rock climbing in eighteen 45-minute lessons. Students learn physical rock climbing skills and the basic rope systems. They learn how to boulder, top rope, belay, rappel, mock lead climb, and lead climb on the indoor rock wall using various techniques.

Students build confidence through their abilities to overcome fear and take calculated risks. Finally, students are exposed to real rock climbing situations that demand sound judgment, emotional control, physical application, and teamwork, all of which contribute to their growth as leaders.

Upon completion of this course, students will demonstrate the following and show by action:

- The basic concepts of climbing safety as demonstrated by their actions near, on, off, and on top of the 48-foot (14.6-meter) indoor cliff with full ledge system

- The basic skills of climbing footwork and handholds, in combination with the positioning and repositioning of the center of mass of the body

- The ability to climb or the attempt to climb color-coded climbing routes that will test their physical fitness and coordination

- Understanding usage and features of various types of climbing equipment

- Recognition of proper climbing and falling techniques

- Proper verbal signals and buddy checks

- Adherence to proper safety practices and behaviors necessary for participation in basic rock climbing

- Management of fear, overcoming fear, and dealing with fear, and using experience and knowledge, as well as trust in others and the gear systems

- Appreciation of rock climbing as a participant and knowledgeable observer

Instructional Area

The West Point primary facility is the 8,000-square-foot (745-square-meter) USMA Class of 1979 Indoor Climbing Wall. It is 48 feet (14.6 meters) tall by 110 feet (34 meters) long, complete with a full-length ledge system on top with anchors. A 12-foot (3.7-meter) indoor bouldering wall is 110 feet long. The outdoor cliffs are used for the climbing team. These outdoor cliffs consist of 1 million square feet on four outdoor crags of natural rock. The crags have countless stainless steel bolts and bolt hangers as anchor points that support multiple roped routes for large-group and class climbing. Students hike to all locations with their backpacks and their issued rock climbing equipment. The rock climbing staff and students of the mountaineering team maintain both the indoor wall and the cliffs, setting them up for individual and group climbing and practice.

Devising an instructional area for any rock climbing course or experience can be as simple as using a masonry wall on an existing building or constructing small or large walls either indoors or outdoors (see figure 15.1). It is important to assess what is currently available, visit existing climbing programs, or use the Internet to get ideas.

Identify the vertical space or natural terrain to develop your program and then consult the section "Adapting This Course for Your School" in this chapter to get started.

Equipment

Although it is possible to climb rock without equipment, it is safer and more productive to climb on prepared indoor and outdoor walls with proper gear and footwear. For the lowest-cost climbing experience, bouldering is a good choice. A program can be effective when climbers use only sneakers but will be most effective when participants have rock climbing shoes and a chalk bag. To ensure safety when people jump or fall off a boulder climb, a spotter can be employed along with a gymnastics-type mat. For free rock climbing higher than 8 to 12 feet (2.4-3.7 meters), ropes should be used.

For a climbing course with top roping or rappelling (or both) that uses indoor walls or cliff heights of more than 12 to 100 feet (3.7-30 meters), the following equipment is recommended.

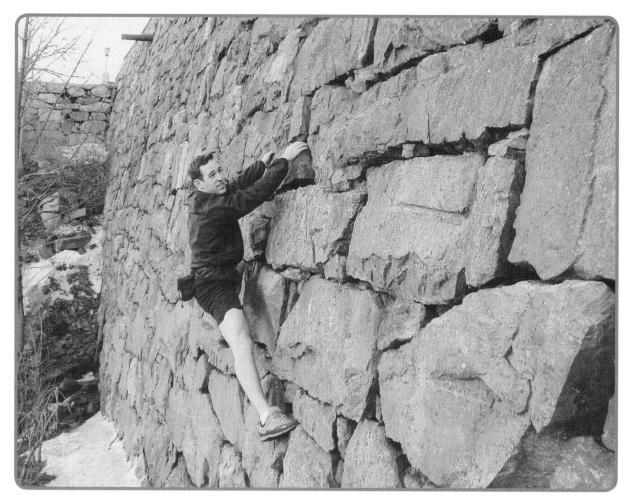

FIGURE 15.1   Masonry wall with inserts for climbing holds.

Climbing Shoes

A close-fitting pair of real rock climbing shoes with high-friction rubber and with no welt allows the participant to learn proper foot placement techniques. Rock climbing shoes are much better than sneakers and are safer because they have higher foot-to-wall friction rubber. Climbing shoes are not necessary for beginning programs, but they enhance skills and confidence because they lead to less handhold dependence and more footwork balance and friction.

Climbing Rope

A climbing rope is usually 10.5 millimeters in diameter and 60 meters (198 feet) in length. The rope has dynamic qualities, so when holding the force of a falling climber it stretches to absorb the load. Climbing ropes are usually tested out well above a 4,000-pound (~1,800-kilogram) working load.

Climbing Harness

A climbing harness is made of nylon sewn into a seat that surrounds the waist, pelvis, and upper legs. The climbing rope is attached to the harness via a knot, usually a figure-eight trace-through knot. The harness attaches the rope to the body.

Belay Device

A belay device is made of metal and is designed to create a loop of friction that can hold a falling climber; the device connects to the harness via a large pear-shaped carabiner. The climbing rope is inserted into the belay device slot and the pear-shaped carabiner in the proper manner: The rope usually forms an "S" through the belay device and carabiner. The belay device allows the belayer to lock off the rope in the event of a fall. Via friction and tension applied by the belayer, the rope through the belay device can hold a falling climber.

Or, the belayer can feed the rope through the belay device in two directions in a controlled manner to provide for slackening or tightening of the rope. The belayer can also take in rope slack, give rope slack, hold a climber, or lower a climber. To rappel, climbers simply belay themselves down the rope using the belay device.

Carabiner

A carabiner is a chainlike link of aluminum alloy, usually shaped like a "D," with a side that opens via a spring-loaded gate. Carabiner links are used to connect and link together climbing gear like ropes, slings, and harnesses. Carabiners come in different sizes, strengths, and styles for specific uses.

Slings or Runners

A loop of nylon or Spectra-nylon webbing material is used to make bigger links in connecting together carabiners, ropes, and other gear.

Helmet

A helmet is worn to protect the head if a climber falls or if a rock or gear falls down while he or she is climbing or belaying. A helmet should be worn whether one is belaying or climbing, although many climbers, boulderers, and indoor wall climbers choose not to wear them in many situations.

Chalk Bag and Belt

The chalk bag contains magnesium carbonate or gymnastic chalk. Climbers reach into the bag to coat their hands with the chalk, which absorbs sweat and oils from the hands so that the holds feel more positive to hold on to. The chalk bag is secured to the body with an adjustable waist belt.

Leash

A leash is a sling that is girth hitched to the harness and has a locking carabiner on its end. The leash is used to anchor the climber to a bolt in lieu of a rope, somewhat like a tether. The leash can be extended or lengthened with another sling or shortened by halving of the sling.

Risk Management

Getting everyone involved in the safety program of any rock climbing activity is crucial for accident and injury prevention. A written safety warning document informs students of potential risks and requires them to actively comply with the safety procedures. Safety in any sport depends on sound risk management procedures. To create a safe yet challenging teaching–learning environment, one needs to answer the following questions:

1. What are the abilities, sizes, ages, and levels of experience of the participants?
2. What is the planned activity?
3. What equipment is available?
4. What is the instructor's knowledge and experience?
5. How much time is available?

The process of answering these questions facilitates sound decision-making procedures. Once risk management strategies have been established, *always provide written and verbal warnings to students.*

The risk scenarios outlined in table 15.1 are merely a starting point for new climbers. All rock climbing programs need to address the questions just listed, taking into account their facilities, program contents, staffing, and climbing wall users.

Table 15.1   Possible Risks in Rock Climbing

Risk identification	Reduction strategies
Falling off climbing surface	• An alert belayer. • Appropriate route selection. • Demonstrate proper climbing techniques for all skills. • Enforce three points of contact. • Supervise all climbing and belaying activities and intervene when necessary.

(continued)

Table 15.1 *(continued)*

Risk identification	Reduction strategies
Falling rocks, equipment, or other climbers	• Alert climber and belayer. • Enforce helmet usage. • Proper route selection. • Verbal alerts. • Supervise all climbing activities and intervene when necessary.
Equipment systems errors	• Always double-check the final product. • Use buddy and partner checks. • Demonstrate proper equipment systems setup and operations. • Supervise all climbing activities and intervene when necessary. • Conduct periodic inspections of equipment. • Conduct regular maintenance of equipment.
Engaging in skills beyond ability	• Instruct students to do only the skills demonstrated in class. • Appropriate route selection. • Demonstrate proper technique for all climbing skills. • Provide proper progressions for all climbing skills. • Provide a variety of skills that are appropriate for all students. • Supervise all activities and intervene when necessary.
Horseplay	• Instruct students about rules prior to activity. • Maintain a safe environment through a specific discipline plan. • Warn students that they will be asked to cease activities if horseplay occurs. • Supervise all climbing activities and intervene when necessary.
Student attire	• Ensure that students wear proper attire for climbing. • Ensure that students use rock climbing shoes. • Instruct and enforce that students not wear jewelry. • Request students with long hair to tie it back.
Environmental factors	• Have standardized procedures for any inclement weather condition. • Supervise all climbing activities and cease climbing when appropriate.

Participant involvement in risk management from the start is important. A comprehensive risk management document ensures that all participants are actively informed and engaged in their own safety program.

Skills and Techniques

Instruction in a rock climbing class must focus on the five actual skills or zones of learning.

- Skill 1: rock climbing movement skills
- Skill 2: belaying and basic gear systems
- Skill 3: rappelling
- Skill 4: climbing difficulty and rated climbs
- Skill 5: judgment and safety systems

Students learn climbing experientially through a step-by-step and system-by-system approach. Each student is issued his or her own set of gear. Climbing pairs are designated a top rope at the base of the indoor wall or a station at the top of the indoor climbing wall. Climbing rules and climbing judgment are taught through a progressive, integrated series of lessons. Instructors provide precise demonstrations of skills and tasks in a progressive sequence. Students learn experientially through trial and error with formative feedback from instructors. The student climbers are constantly using judgment and foundation skills in successive lessons to learn new skills and remain safe. The following is the basic sequence of the indoor wall lessons:

- Arrival and gearing up
- Getting the lesson task and lesson
- Executing the lesson task
- Reviewing and repeating the previous lesson

Rock Climbing Movement Skills

The climber uses handholds and footholds to move up, down, left, right, under, and over the rock. Climbers must exhibit good balancing skills on the footholds with one or both feet. Precise footwork and the proper use of footholds require significant practice. Likewise, proper use of one's hands, arms, and the handholds is critical, as the harder climbs tend to place an increased demand on the upper body. Most climbs require a moderate level of upper body strength; however, footwork and technique allow a climber to be successful on a wider variety of climbs. Several footholds, handholds, and movement combinations are described next. Additional descriptions are presented in the list of key terms at the end of the chapter. Complete descriptions of all foothold, handhold, and movement combinations may be found in popular how-to climbing books and videos.

To move over rock, a climber uses five body reference points to climb in all directions. The five reference points of a climber's body are the center of mass, the two hands, and the two feet. Other body parts are utilized; however, the center of mass in combination with the hands and feet is the most important. The most effective climbers use the five reference points of the body efficiently in various rock climbing movement combinations.

Climbers redistribute their weight by flexing, extending, rotating, pulling, pushing, leaning, and bracing, in combination with handholds and footholds. A climber has three arms and three legs: A leg can be used like an arm, and an arm can be used like a leg. Balanced motion and use of the five reference points in both static and dynamic ways are the keys to successful, effortless climbing.

Many climbing combinations are dependent on counterpressure. Counterpressure, or one force in opposition to another, dominates good climbing. For example, counterpressure is used as the hands and feet are pulled and pushed in opposite directions. Pinching a handhold, when the thumb is pressed one way and the fingers the other way in a pinching fashion, is counterpressure. Balancing the center of mass over a tiny foothold with a smearing action and leaning out is counterpressure; that is, the weight of the body presses down and in, and the friction of the rubber and foot pushing down and in gives a smear the purchase on the wall.

Good footwork requires precise weight redistribution of one's center of mass in loading the foot placement. What separates good climbers from great climbers is often "artistic" footwork. Smearing, inside edging, outside edging, toe edging, foot jamming, heel hooking, toe hooking, rest stepping, back stepping, crossover stepping, dropping the knee, and flagging the leg are the primary foot maneuvers required for good footwork for climbers.

Handholds and uses of the arms have hundreds of names and movement variations. The five basic handgrips, according to climbing expert John Long, are the "open grip, the cling grip or 'crimp,' the vertical grip, the pocket grip, and the pinch grip" (Long, 1998). Other common types of handholds include the mantle, the undercling, the side pull, finger jamming, hand jamming, finger stacking, fist jamming, hand stacking, and forearm jamming.

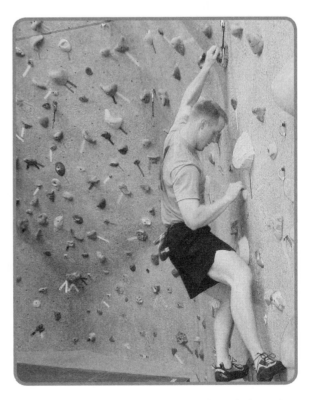

The infinite combinations on the chessboard of climbing possibilities.

When learning to rock climb, one of the fastest ways to improve is to practice downclimbing. In doing so, climbers are forced to look down at their feet, place them precisely, and shift weight onto the foot. Climbing is not always straight up; many climbs require side-to-side movements as well as vertical movements.

Some common movement patterns using the body, footholds, and handholds are known as chimmeying, lie-backing, and stemming. Climbers move in and out of these patterns constantly.

These movement patterns require a combination of the five climbing reference points.

Using climbing movement skills, a successful climber is able to effectively assess the rock and mold the climbing movements into a sequential series of handholds, footholds, body shifts, and weight redistributions. When a climber can move well in all directions using a variety of movement skills, problem solving on the rock using climbing combinations leads to a successful climbing experience.

THE 14 FUNDAMENTAL COMMON CLIMBING SKILLS

The following lists the 14 basic common climbing skills to be taught. These skills are a part of millions of combined rock climbing maneuvers and movements. Learn these 14 basic skills and you will know how to do and analyze most climbing movements.

1. **Balance:** Balance your center ("nugget") over a precisely placed foot (or feet). The climber must be balanced in all dimensions: fore–aft, left–right, up–down.

2. **Look, precisely place the foot, and shift the nugget (your center of mass) over the foot:** Precise placement of feet and hands followed by a shift of the nugget is what happens in lots of climbing maneuvers.

3. **Rest or positions of less strain:** Climbers must find positions of rest or less strain such as standing on a straightened leg as opposed to standing in a 3/4 squat on one leg. Another example is hanging with a straight arm as opposed to bent arm.

4. **Downclimbing:** Downclimbing creates a good climber really fast. Practice downclimbing; it also adds to safety.

5. **Counterpressure:** One force opposing another force. Hundreds of climbing movements require counterpressure; a pinch, a layback, a stem, leaning back out from the wall and smearing with the feet, pulling in opposition, jamming, dropping knees, and underclinging are examples.

6. **Hip turn:** The pelvis turns 180 degrees in both directions. In this respect the climber differs from X-Man. X-Man keeps his hips square to the climbing surface at all times. X-Man is good at climbing a straight ladder but is limited as a rock climber.

7. **Footwork:** Learn to smear, front point, inside edge, outside edge, toe hook, heel hook, and foot jam. Basic footwork rules in climbing.

8. **Handholds:** Learn the crimp, open grip, and palm climbing holds. Finger jamming and hand jamming are also needed, as well as combined handholds with pinch and side pulls.

9. **A climber has three to four arms and three to four legs:** When hanging by your arm or arms, you can use either or both legs as a third hand, as in a heel hook. You can push down with an arm and hand and bring up a foot to replace them—hence, the third leg.

10. **Your eyes should look between your hands and your feet 60 percent of the time:** Climbers who look up only above their hands tend to struggle.

11. **Climb the compass:** Move in all directions as if you were the center of a compass on the climbing surface. A climber should think that all directions are usable as opposed to relying on straight-up thinking.

12. **Feel the rock:** Kinesthetic climbers feel what holds can give them.

13. **Use your flexibility:** Flexibility is important for making climbing moves like a high step, wide stemming, arching, hanging straight armed, dropping the knee, heel hooking, and toe hooking.

14. **Breathing:** "Blow air out and stay calm." Holding one's breath and climbing is very ineffective and draining.

Belaying and Basic Gear Systems

The first three lessons on the indoor wall address bouldering; students learn the 14 fundamental climbing skills and do color-coded bouldering routes up to 12 feet (3.7 meters). In Lesson 4, students learn to top rope and belay a climber. Gearing up is a basic system for climbing tasks like top roping and rappelling. Students arrive and gear up by putting on the harness, buckling it correctly, and putting on their personal equipment, which includes rock shoes, shoulder sling with carabiners and quickdraws, chalk bag, and leash.

Then the buddy check system is used; each student is "checked out" by his or her climbing partner to ensure that the harness, leash, tie-in knot, and belay device are correctly linked and assembled. The buddy check system is crucial to safe climbing and teaches students to examine assembled, linked gear systems.

The students are paired up, and each pair selects one of 24 top ropes at the bottom of the indoor wall. Tying the end of the rope into the climbing harness via the figure-eight follow-through knot is taught next through demonstrations and practice.

Next, the belayer and climber duties relating to the top-rope safety system are taught. *Belaying* is the act of handling the rope with two hands in both directions as it flows through the belay device in an "S." Belaying a climber is an important part of climber safety. Proper belayer handwork and focused responsibility are paramount. A belayer performs the following handiwork with the belay device:

- Takes in the slack rope as the climber climbs up the top rope
- Locks off the belay when a climber falls, thereby arresting or catching the fall

- Gives slack to the climber who might be downclimbing
- Lowers the climber who wants to be lowered down on the weighted rope

A *horizontal* demonstration of climber and belayer is given: The climber walks away from the wall as if downclimbing, and the belayer feeds out rope through the belay device. Then the climber slowly approaches the wall as the belayer takes in the slack with proper handiwork. The belayers are taught a specific hand sequence so that they can belay the rope correctly in all directions. This horizontal, on-the-floor belaying drill is known as the horizontal belay drill. All students do this repeatedly before going vertical on the climbing wall.

The correct stance and anchoring of the belayer are very important, and the belayer is leashed to a ground anchor in the floor. The belayer should stand with a wide base of support, one foot in front of the other. The belayer should keep most of his or her body weight on the back foot and knees flexed.

After the horizontal belay drill, the 15-foot (4.6-meter) drill is taught to the top-roped, belayed climber who climbs *vertically* up to 15 feet on the wall. In step 1, the climber, while being belayed on the top rope, climbs up, left and right a bit, and then downclimbs to the floor. In step 2, the climber climbs up again to 15 feet and then requests to be lowered and weights the rope, and the belayer lowers the climber to the floor. In step 3, the climber again climbs up to 15 feet and takes a calculated short fall with no slack in the rope, and the belayer catches the tiny fall.

Then the belayer and climber switch roles and practice the correct sequences for steps 1 through

3. The instructors are constantly monitoring the belayers' handiwork, as it must be precise and correct in order for the top-rope system to operate correctly. Then, once the belayers have been trained and are trusted, the students go high, downclimb, get lowered, and fall.

Rappelling

After the eight lessons in bouldering and top roping color-coded routes, rappelling is taught. The entire class is walked up to the top ledge of the indoor wall, and the students rappel to the bottom. Rappelling is the act of descending a rope by running the rope or both ropes through the belay device in an "S." Performing a rappel is simply belaying oneself down a fixed rope or a retrievable halved twin rope. Many times, the rappel rope is not fixed but rather is looped through the anchors so that one can retrieve it by pulling down on the end. All rappels are done with an autoblock friction knot attached to the harness leg loop, which serves as a "third-hand" backup. Rappels are used in many situations:

- Getting down a top rope to start climbing after setting up the top rope.
- Avoiding a long, sometimes dangerous walk or climb down
- Getting to anchors, ledges, and other vertical places
- Exiting or escaping a climb when other choices are not possible
- Rescue

In rappelling, most of the weight is on the harness, with some on the feet. The harness is linked to the rope via the belay device and the carabiner. The rappeller lets the rope slip through the belay device while lowering him- or herself down a vertical surface or through the air. When the climber is rappelling off top ropes, he or she uses the leash backup system to get attached to the rappel point and get into the rappelling position. The student disengages the leash backup system and "raps" down. Rappelling can be very dangerous to the unprepared, although the basic rappel is not difficult. A link that fails in the rappel system will have dire consequences for the user.

Climbing Difficulty and Rated Climbs

The students attempt indoor wall color-coded rock climbs or routes of various difficulties. Some routes may be climbed many different ways; but as the difficulty increases, fewer and fewer routes exist. Experienced climbers rate rock climbs using various common scales of difficulty. Although their ratings are fairly subjective, common difficulty ratings or adjustments do exist. Rock climbing guidebooks are available that rate the difficulty of outdoor climbs. Students may actually attempt climbs that are rated above their skill level because of the safety provided by a top rope and belayer. Students who climb using sound techniques will have much more success over more difficult rock surfaces. There is no tolerance for mistakes in tying the rope into the harness, belaying, anchoring, and rappelling down in any course.

Varying levels of difficulty are important in a climbing program. Students like to be challenged to solve more difficult rock problems with strength, agility, balance, and discovery. The solutions to some climbs or climbing problems are oriented toward footwork, handwork, flexibility, technique, balance, or "raw power." Most solutions require a sequence of movements that add up to a successful gain. To assist the beginner in determining the difficulty of a climb, it is common practice to mark color-coded, taped routes indoors and then have experienced climbers rate the routes. For outdoor climbs, climbers rate routes or select routes based on difficulty ratings in guidebooks. If an artificial wall is available, regularly changing the handholds creates freshness in your routes and changes the difficulty.

Judgment and Safety Systems

Although not a specific physical skill like climbing, or a basic system like belaying, rappelling, or just gearing up to climb, *judgment and safety* clearly constitutes a zone of behavior that needs to permeate all rock climbing sessions. Students must know and demonstrate the sequential actions and steps that indicate knowledge and understanding of climbing safety and judgment. One example is conducting a buddy check on a partner's harness, tie-in knot, and leash system. Another example is checking that the belayer has threaded the rope correctly through the belay device. Verbal communications and signal double-checking are other examples of safety systems. Miscommunication and assumptions are causes of many climbing accidents.

The basic safety principle is to double-check every link, knot, anchor, and system to ensure that it is assembled correctly and looks right. We say: "Inspect the final product of all assembled and linked climbing gear." In short, *always check the final product.* Climbers must perform a self safety check every time they assemble their climbing gear. A climber must learn to visually recognize what correct looks like in setting up and using climbing gear. Just getting to the climb, selecting an appropriate climb, and setting up the top rope correctly require constant safety precautions and sound climbing judgment.

Course Overview

The following lesson overview (table 15.2) illustrates the overall purpose of the Rock Climbing course, which is to introduce the students to the sport of basic rock climbing. This is accomplished during each lesson through the introduction of basic climbing techniques and skills. Upon completion of the course, the students have be-

come familiar with, and are able to demonstrate, basic top-rope setup, rappel, belaying, and climbing skills. The students are also required to demonstrate baseline knowledge of climbing, systems, and proper judgment to ensure safety on and around the cliff.

Sample Lesson Plan

The following lesson is typical of the way a rock climbing lesson is conducted at West Point. Following student accountability and getting the appropriate gear and equipment, class begins. This includes (1) a safety reminder; (2) introduction and demonstration of new skills; (3) climbing and experimenting; (4) introduction and demonstration of additional new skills; (5) practice climbing, experimenting, and feedback; (6) lesson summary; (7) storing of gear; and (8) dismissal.

Table 15.2 Overview of Rock Climbing Lessons

Lesson	Outline of contents
1 Boulder	• Introductions and course overview. • Gear issue (shoes; harness; chalk bag, ball, belt; belay device; belay carabiner; three shoulder slings; rope, two locking carabiners; rope bag or pack; books; and optional helmet). • Administer hand receipts. • Safety awareness sheet. • Safety for indoor wall. • Climbing and movement techniques (14 basics). • Cover bouldering and spotting techniques.
2 Boulder	• Review bouldering and spotting techniques. • More climbing and movement techniques.
3 Boulder	• Marked bouldering routes. • M traverse—4 minutes.
4 Top rope	• Harness fit and double back buckle. • Add leash plus locker to harness. • Parts of the harness: belay loop, adjustable leg loops, and gear loops. • **Rule 1: Always double-check final product!** • Buddy checks. • Figure-eight follow through-knot tie-in. • **Rule 2: Never let go of the belay side of the rope even for a millionth of a second!** • Belay practice horizontally on the ground. • Belay signals. • Lowering command sequence. • Belay anchored to floor tether using harness leash. • Climber on top rope up, down, right, left, lowering, jacking, falling.

(continued)

Table 15.2 *(continued)*

Lesson	Outline of contents
5 Top rope	• Teach half leash, one and one-half leash, and double leash. • Students do all three leash systems to floor tether. • Review lesson 3 thoroughly. • Add to climbing techniques. • Belay and climb on set-up top ropes.
6 Top rope	• Review lessons 4 and 5 thoroughly. • Add to climbing techniques. • Teach marked top-rope route.
7 Top rope	• How to leash off and lower a bight of rope to get tool to tighten handhold ("spinner"). • Review lessons 4 and 5 thoroughly. • Add to climbing techniques. • Do marked route and record grade.
8 Boulder	• Video—bouldering. • Climbing exercises and climbing games like relays, follow the leader, add a move. • Belay and climb on set-up top ropes. • Do marked route and record grade.
9 Rappel	• Issue cord/prusik for third-hand device (to be returned at end of class). • Climb or walk to top of wall. • Either use top ropes by pulling up, with staff rethreading them after rappels, or have class bring up lead ropes, pull them and backpack coil them, then store them. • Students observe how to set and rappel with third-hand backup above belay device. Do three leg wraps and across chest with slack in third hand above. • Students rappel from rap lines with third-hand backup. • Top-rope belay and climb. • Do marked route and record grade.
10 Rappel	• Issue cord/prusik sling third-hand device (to be returned at end of class). • Climb or walk to top of wall. • Either use top ropes by pulling up, with staff rethreading them after rappels, or have class bring up lead ropes, pull them and backpack coil them, then store them. • Review and repeat lesson 9. • Students observe how to set and rappel with third-hand backup below rappel device with extended rap device. Use autoblock with cord sling. • Students rappel from fixed lines with third-hand backup below rap device. • Top-rope climb and belay.
11 Double rappel	• Students pull top ropes, backpack coil top ropes, and walk to top of wall. • Issue cord/prusik third-hand device (to be returned at end of class). • Show double rappel sequence with third-hand backup and set up a top rope. • Students rappel via double rappel with third hand using top rope from back anchors to set top ropes at anchors on the face of wall. • Using lead ropes, teach backpack uncoil and backpack coil. Put lead ropes away. • Top-rope climb and belay.

Lesson	Outline of contents
12 Climb	• Video—leading. • Climb marked top rope. • Climb marked boulder route.
13 Lead	• Demonstrate lead climbing on bolts—discuss clipping, belaying, rests, leg position, and falling. • Show a lead climb with mock lead (two belayers used for demonstration only, then one used for actual mock lead). • Students use gym lead rope. • Students mock lead on top rope and lower off.
14 Lead	• Redemonstrate lead climbing on bolts—discuss clipping, belaying, rests, leg position, and falling. • Show a lead climb with mock lead. • Students use gym lead rope. • Students mock lead on top rope and lower off anchor carabiner (one belayer).
15 Lead	• Review of leading techniques. • Lead climb. • Students climb at or above their level, and belayer feeds slack to leaders if or when they fall and then lowers off anchor carabiner.
16 Speed	• Video—other like trad. • Top rope for timed laps on either rainbow or taped route. • Students lead a climb below their ability.
17 Lead	• Students pair up to lead a climb below their ability and lower off anchor carabiner. • Graded lead climb on marked route or rainbow route.
18	• Do graded boulder and top-rope route. • Gear turn-in. • Course review.

Fourteen Fundamental Common Climbing Skills

This is the students' first 45-minute lesson at the indoor climbing wall. Students get shoes from shelves marked by shoe size. Students wear socks. Students also get a chalk bag with waist belt. The chalk bag contains a chalk ball as opposed to loose chalk. Once students have their shoes on and the chalk bag around the waist, class begins.

SEQUENCE (45-MINUTE CLASS)

1. The instructor covers safety policies and rules for the indoor wall, such as no climbing above the 12-foot (3.7-meter) mark, watching for spinning holds, down-climbing versus jumping off the wall, using extra pads, and not being under a climber. Also covered are the concepts that the climber is responsible for his or her landing (nobody else) and that uncontrolled falling is not the objective.

   The 14 fundamental common climbing skills listed on pages 342-343 are covered for the gathered class. Usually the first four skills are demonstrated and explained, and immediately the students actually boulder up to the 12-foot mark using the entire indoor wall and bouldering wall.

Instructors make safety corrections and ensure that climbers stay low and climb down. The class usually traverses left first, staying under 8 feet (2.4 meters), rather than going straight up to 12 feet (3.7 meters).

2. After students have climbed and experimented for a while, skills 5 and 6 are demonstrated and explained, and the students record and then copy the movements shown.

3. Students gather and get another demonstration and explanation of the other eight common climbing skills and work on them immediately. This process is repeated as climbing skills and concepts are blended into the students' performances.

4. A lesson summary is given at the end of the class. Students tie their climbing shoes together and return the shoes and chalk bag to the shelves in the storage closet built inside the indoor climbing wall.

TEACHING CUES

- Find those counterpressures.
- You want to get good . . . downclimb!
- Footwork rules. Push with legs.
- Keep the nugget balanced (body center over the foot).
- Look down 60% of the time.
- Find positions of less strain and rest.
- Feel the rock.
- Climb quietly and move across the rock in a smooth flow as opposed to "grab and crank!"
- Try not to overgrip your handholds but rather use just enough grip and stand on your feet.
- Climb in all directions.

SUGGESTED LEARNING ACTIVITIES

- Students traverse right and then left.
- Students demonstrate climbing up and immediately downclimb.
- Show climbing up in a zigzag fashion, as opposed to straight up, to emphasize that a climber moves in all directions to achieve new places on the climbing surface.

Your lesson plans will be different based on your outcome goals, student age, student experience, facilities, time, and program. Your climbing lessons should involve active learning with a great deal of time on task, as opposed to a format involving one climber and one belayer at a time and lots of waiting for a turn.

Adapting This Course for Your School

Before starting a climbing program at your school, instructors should observe and try climbing at a gym, commercial store, fitness center, camp, or another school. Once you personally experience a quality climbing program, you will be inspired to incorporate a climbing program into your curriculum. Implementing the West Point rock climbing curriculum in your school or community may not be feasible; however, there are parts of the program that may be adopted. The key point is to include climbing activities in your instructional program.

• Reverse map your classes or group to an imagined climbing facility and program. For example, you have 30 elementary school children, ages 6 to 10, and 30-minute periods. Climbing on 30 feet (9 meters) of low bouldering wall, 8 feet tall (2.4 meters), with sneakers may be the approach for you. In this instance, doing ropeless bouldering would more likely meet your outcome objectives than having a 30-foot (9-meter) climbing wall only 8 feet wide with two climbs for top-roped climbing, which would involve more safety considerations and some students getting only one chance at best to climb per period.

• Check out the readings and Web sites listed at the end of the chapter for diagrams and specifications for homemade and manufactured climbing walls, for both indoor and outdoor applications. Some Web sites have directions on how to build a framed wooden climbing wall. Some manufacturers have 4- by 8-foot (1.2- by 2.4-meter) plywood panels that are predrilled when you buy them. Just attach them to framing or hang them; then screw the artificial holds into the T-nuts and predrilled holes. Engage the shop class to help build the wall. Some climbing walls require only drilling holes directly into existing masonry walls and inserting threaded anchors for climbing holds that are simple and quick to install.

Surf the Web for commercial climbing gyms and fitness facilities. You will find incredible pictures and design ideas. Look for low ropeless caves and bouldering areas. Review the Web sites and get catalogs from the various climbing wall manufacturers and climbing hold manufacturers. Consider low ropeless climbing and bouldering that is lower than 10 to 12 feet (3-3.7 meters) in height. Create a low bouldering cave and overhanging wall, and then consider top-rope climbing with belayers and rappelling.

• Visit climbing gyms at commercial, college, school, outdoor challenge course, and camp facilities.

• Assess what you have already. Most buildings have indoor and outdoor masonry walls to which a climbing wall or holds could be attached. Use masonry inserts for climbing holds. Use retaining walls, improve a current climbing facility, or add a climbing wall to your adventure training ropes course. Take a look at local outdoor rock that can be cleared and gardened into a climbing area. Even in geographic areas with flatter terrain, a silo or barn wall can be turned into a climbing wall.

• Visualize what you have and how you might sell your vision to get a climbing or bouldering wall. A safe climbing program is a winner with parents. Team up with your industrial arts program or PTA to help construct a climbing wall.

• If the budget allows, have a climbing consultant review and assess your facilities and program goals and suggest ways to accomplish the climbing goals.

• Consider your landing zone. Do you have mats? Are the ground, terrain, and grass adequate for safety along a low outdoor wall? Check out ground-up tires for a landing surface.

• What climbing gear is needed? At minimum, you will want to have shoes, ropes, harnesses, helmets, belay devices, carabiners, slings, and anchors for top ropes.

• Build climbing wall panels; use screw-on climbing holds or glue-on climbing holds with industrial highway epoxy. From cheap to expensive, it is possible to create a vertical climbing experience that will challenge your students.

• Make your own handholds from rock and hardwoods.

• Commercial indoor and outdoor climbing walls can be bare or painted sheets of plywood, sheathing with cementitious coatings, resin-based fiberglass rocklike surfaces, cast concrete, or regular masonry walls with inserts for climbing holds.

Key Terms

aid climbing—A climbing practice in which climbers make upward progress by using the rope or equipment to help in the ascent. Aid is any man-made artificial material used to assist in climbing.

anchor—A temporary or permanent security point that does not move, used by a climber or belayer to "deadend" part of the climbing system. Anchors are usually capable of holding several thousand pounds and can come in many forms, including trees, pitons, bolts, chockstones, and camming devices.

artificial climbing hold—A manufactured or home-made handhold or foothold that is attached to some surface by a threaded hex-head bolt or is screwed in or glued on. Also, a feature built into an artificial climbing wall that is used for a climbing hold. These are either homemade, manufactured by climbing hold companies, or created by wall builders.

back stepping—A footwork technique whereby a climber steps backward to a foothold or brace to get better purchase, stem, or a rest (or a combination of these) by dropping a knee.

belaying—Holding, with reference to a system of devices and techniques that combine to protect a climber from being injured in a fall by locking the rope and holding the falling climber.

belly button shift—The redistribution of the center of one's body in alignment with one's foothold and handhold.

bolt—A metal bolt hanger (anchor to which a carabiner can be clipped) that is attached to the rock by some form of bolt, either glued or expanded into a hole drilled for that purpose. Modern bolts and bolt hangers rate at 4,000- to 6,000-pound (~1,800- to 2,700-kilogram) working load strength as anchors and are typically made from stainless steel.

chimmeying—A climbing technique used in cracks large enough to place body parts in; body parts are pressed against opposite walls in order for the climber to ascend. The most common chimmey move is with one's back and hands on one wall and the feet on the other wall in a counterpressured manner.

climbing hold—A feature on a rock cliff or indoor wall that can be used for a handhold, foothold, or body hold.

crack climbing—The use of climbing techniques in cracks in rock, including hand jamming, foot jamming, or body jamming; the practice of expanding or wedging (or expanding and wedging) one's hands, feet, or the body into cracks in the rock in order to ascend.

crimp—One of the most useful handholds, most commonly employed on tiny flat-topped holds. The fingertips are bent at the first knuckle, and the thumb is wrapped over the index finger if possible.

downclimbing—The act of climbing down below a horizontal line in any direction. Downclimbing is key to getting better at "upclimbing" and is needed to complete some routes, to escape for a rest, to prevent a fall, or to save oneself from injury or a long night out. It forces the use of the three arms and three legs in a climber's movement patterns.

dynamic—In the context of climbing, referring to any part of a system that will yield, give, or move when activated, typically reducing forces—like a dynamic climbing rope that stretches when loaded. For example, when a top-roped climber falls and the climbing rope stretches 10%, the tie-in knots tighten and the body compresses, making the fall to a stop dynamic as opposed to static. The climber's body and harness gear also have some give and flex.

free climbing—Climbing using only the hands, feet, and body without the aid of the rope or other gear to ascend a route or section of rock. The rope in this situation is used only as a safeguard against injury.

heel hook—Using the foot as a third arm and hand. Climbing shoes have friction rubber on the heel just for heel hooking.

jam—Wedging, twisting, and expanding the feet, hands, or other body parts to gain purchase in a crack.

lead climbing—A system of climbing from the ground up; a climber ascends by free climbing and trailing a rope belayed by a partner. By clipping the rope into intermediate protection anchor points along the way, the climber creates a backup system for his or her lead-free climb. In the case of a fall, the belayer holds the fall, which will be caught by the last, closest piece of protection, usually below. In general, the leader anchors the rope at the end of the pitch at a belay point and belays up the second climber. The process is then repeated until the top of a climb is reached. Lead climbing requires a great deal of skill and is much more serious and dangerous than other climbing systems with respect to a fall.

lie-backing—A climbing maneuver that entails pulling with the hands while pushing with the feet, with an offset center of the body to the side.

lowering—A method of descent; the climber weights the rope and is let down by his or her belayer, who lets the rope slide through the belay device in a controlled manner. This is the most common method of descent from a top-rope climb.

matching—Positioning in which hands or feet are placed on the same climbing hold.

move—A climbing movement; one part of a sequence of movements required in climbing progress and for motion in any direction on climbing surfaces.

pinch—A handhold; the climber uses the thumb and fingers to grip the surface. This counterpressure grip is similar to the action a lobster uses when engaging its pincers.

pocket grip—A handhold most often found on limestone or volcanic rock, which is typically pocked with small holes. Because it is rare that a pocket will accommodate all fingers, anywhere from one to as many fingers as possible may be used.

quick draw—A short sling with two carabiners clipped to each end so that it can be clipped to an anchor on one end and the rope on the other end. This is easy to place on the gear loops of the harness.

rappel—Any of various methods of descending a single rope or twin ropes using controlled friction. Using the friction of the rope running through a rappel or belay device, usually in some "S" shape, climbers lower themselves down a single or twin rope in a controlled manner.

ratings—A guidebook and communication method of rating the human climbing difficulty of established routes in comparison to other routes; the basic numeric yardstick reflecting how difficult a given climb is. There are hundreds of climbing scales: Some are for ice, some for time, some for rock difficulty, some for bouldering difficulty, and some for mountaineering.

screw-on handhold—An artificial rock climbing hold that requires two to four deck screws to be attached to plywood or other wooden surfaces.

side pull—A climbing technique used when a handhold is oriented vertically, or near vertically, with one's palm pointing either left or right. The idea is to lean away from the hold with the hands and upper body and to counterpressure that with the feet or some other body part in opposition.

smear—To stand on the front half of the foot and gain friction against the rock across the breadth of the sole in order to adhere to the rock by pushing the foot in, as well as down, to gain friction in a counterpressured manner with the upper body.

stance—A position that climbers assume in order to free up one or both hands or their arms and legs in order to rest or assemble climbing gear; also a standing rest spot, often the site of the belay.

static—Referring to a lack of give or elongation in the climbing equipment or system for all practical purposes. A static climbing rope has basically no give or stretch. This can hurt a falling climber who is coming to a sudden stop via the rope system, whereas a dynamic rope has stretch and elongation under load, and this cushions the shock load of a falling climber. Most carabiners and anchors have no give or stretch and thus are static in nature.

stem—To bridge or brace across the gap between two widely spaced holds with feet, hands, body, or any combination of parts of the body. Stemming is great for resting and making hard climbs easier.

T-nut—The T-nut acts like a fixed nut on the backside of the plywood in climbing wall panels. A very common metal insert placed on the backside of plywood in a 7/16-inch hole, whereby climbing holds are attached with a bolt threaded into the 3/8-inch T-nut permanently attached to the back of the plywood. Used on climbing walls to allow the attachment of numerous holds onto the wall; the more T-nuts per square foot, the greater the variety and the climber's ability to change the handholds. T-nuts are available in most hardware stores.

top rope—A climbing rope that goes from a belayer on the ground up through some anchored carabiners or other turning point and back down to the tied-in climber. The climber can climb, be lowered, and in case of a fall be "held" by the belayer without much danger or consequence.

traverse—Move the center of the body, feet, and hands sideways, as opposed to up or down, during climbing.

undercling—A handhold technique in which the climber grabs a hold with the palm facing up.

Reference

Long, J.,& Leubben, C. (1998). *How to climb: Advanced rock climbing.* Helena, MT: Falcon Publishing, Inc.

Suggested Readings

Burbach, M. (2004). *Gym climbing: Maximizing your indoor experience.* Seattle: The Mountaineers Books.

Horne, T.F., & Crossley, N. (1999, September). This way up. *Athletic Business.*

Huddleston, E. (2001, March). Safety at the summit. *Athletic Business.*

Leavitt, R. Home climbing walls. *Climbing Magazine.* www.climbing.com.

Long, J. (1998). *How to rock climb.* (2nd ed.). Helena, MT: Globe Pequot Press.

Rohnke, K. (2003). *The complete ropes course manual.* Dubuque, IA: Kendall/Hunt.

Rohnke, K. (2003). *Cowstails and cobras II.* Dubuque, IA: Kendall/Hunt.

Rohnke, K., Tair, C., & Wall, J. (2003). *The complete ropes course manual.* Dubuque, IA: Kendall/Hunt.

Sol, N., & Foster, C. (1992). *ACSM's health/fitness facility standards and guidelines.* Champaign, IL: Human Kinetics.

Thomas, R. (1995). *How to climb: Building your own indoor climbing wall.* Helena, MT: Falcon Press.

Webster, S.E. Project adventure safety manual. Project Adventure, www.pa.org.

Web Resources

Adventure Unlimited, Inc.: www.adventureropes.com

Alpine Towers International: www.alpinetowers.com

American Bouldering Series: www.rockcomps.com

Climbing Magazine: www.climbing.com

Eldorado Wall Company: www.eldowalls.com

Groperz Handholds: www.groperz.com

Indoor Climbing: www.indoorclimbing.com

Metolius Climbing Products: www.metoliusclimbing.com

Outdoor Network: www.outdoornetwork.com

Passe Montagne: www.passemontagne.com

Project Adventure: www.pa.org

Rock and Ice Magazine: www.rockandice.com

Rock Climbing: www.rockclimbing.com

Rock List: www.rocklist.com

Ropes Courses, Inc.: www.ropescoursesinc.com

Ropes Online: www.ropesonline.org

Solid Rock Wall Systems: www.srws.com

Traverse Wall: www.traversewall.com

Sport-Specific Organizations

Access Fund: www.accessfund.org

American Alpine Club: www.americanalpineclub.org

Association for Challenge Course Technology (ACCT): www.acctinfo.org

Outdoor Industry Association: www.outdoorindustry .org

16

Soccer

Paul Gannon

Soccer is one of the world's most popular sports. It is overwhelmingly popular in Europe and the Middle East, as well as in Central and South America, where it has millions of devoted fans. It is slowly acquiring a popular following in the United States. Soccer is a sport that is played at many ages and at every kind of competitive level. There are "pee-wee" and "snoopy" soccer programs, recreational leagues, travel and select soccer leagues, school teams, and semiprofessional and professional teams. The most common form of soccer is informal, or "pickup" soccer. The cost for this sort of game is relatively low because all that is required is a ball. Soccer can be played alone, with two- or three-person teams, or in a full-sided match with 11-person teams.

Purpose of the Course

Back in the mid-1980s, soccer was selected as the official sport of the United States Army. Those in command looked at the benefits of soccer and assessed what it could offer to soldiers and Army officers in terms of physical development and the enhancement of basic Army skills. First and foremost, soccer is an excellent aerobic activity for troops of all ages and ability levels and both genders. It gives soldiers an alternative to daily calisthenics and group runs. The game can also have a tremendous impact on a unit's morale. The game is continuous and requires commitment and teamwork. This sort of game requires soldiers to learn how to read a situation, evaluate the situation, and make a decision based on team goals and objectives. Soccer also encourages hard work and cooperation among its players. These are the primary reasons that soccer is being taught as a lifetime sport at the U.S. Military Academy.

Instructional Area

Soccer can be played on just about any type of surface. Flat grassy fields are the preferred playing surfaces. Flat dirt areas, Astroturf fields, wooden gymnasium floors, and asphalt playgrounds are also suitable playing surfaces.

The size of the field depends upon availability and condition of resources, the age and skill level of the participants, the number of participants, and type of activity being performed. For five versus five pee-wee players, a 50- by 30-yard (46- by 27-meter) field is recommended. With 6- to 11-year-olds, an 11 per side game would require about a 70- by 50-yard (64- by 46-meter) field. For 12- to 15-year-olds, a 100- by 60-yard (91- by 55-meter) field would suffice, and for players ranging in age from 16 years old to adults, a full-size field measuring 120 by 75 yards (110 by 69 meters) would be appropriate.

For programs with increased numbers of players and fewer playing spaces available, several small-sided games could be an option. For a class of 24 students, playing on a square field that measures 50 by 50 yards (46 by 46 meters), two games of six versus six could be played on separate 50- by 25-yard fields. The objective would be to maximize the number of students playing within the given playing area.

The age and skill level of the students have a direct bearing on the size of the instructional area. Obviously, the smaller and younger the student, the less space required. The bigger the field, the greater the chance that young players have to just kick and chase the ball. However, there are times when one may want to use a smaller field for the older players. This will increase pressure on the players to better control the ball. Field or grid size is dependent upon facility availability, number of participants, and the objectives of the lesson.

Equipment

Soccer does not require a great deal of equipment—just balls, shin guards, goals, and shoes. However, the age and skill level of the participants are important considerations when one is determining the quality and type of equipment to be selected.

Soccer Balls

Soccer balls vary in size, material, and price. When purchasing soccer balls, one should consider the age and skill level of the average student. Soccer balls come in three sizes. Size three is used for 5- to 7-year-olds, size four for 8- to 11-year-olds, and size five for ages 12 and over. Soccer balls are constructed primarily of leather or synthetic leather.

Balls made of leather are of a higher quality and last longer than those made of synthetic leather.

Shin Guards

Shin guards are the only protective gear required for a game of soccer. Players' skill levels and budgetary considerations will determine the type and style of shin guards used. Some shin guards are made of hard plastic and contain thin foam cushioning. The downside to these types of shin guards is that they have a tendency to crack when kicked hard. A second type of shin guard is made of a thick cloth material, with plastic or metal strips sewn inside. These guards usually have a sock stirrup on the bottom and an elastic strip at the top to keep them in place. Higher-priced shin guards usually have ankle and Achilles protection built in.

Soccer Goals

Soccer goals come in a variety of sizes and styles. Goals can be either fixed (permanently attached to the ground) or portable. The size of soccer goals will vary based on the size and age of the players. For players 5 to 7 years old, a 4-foot, 6-inch by 9-foot (1.4- by 2.7-meter) goal can be used. Eight- to 11-year-olds can use a 6-foot, 6-inch by 18-foot, 6-inch (2- by 5.6-meter) goal, and there are 8-foot by 24-foot (2.4- by 7.3-meter) goals that are appropriate for players ages 12 and over.

Soccer Shoes

Most school programs do not issue soccer shoes. The type of shoe worn on the playing field should be applicable to the student's age and ability, as well as appropriate for the playing field. Basic gym sneakers, indoor soccer shoes or flats (flat-soled soccer shoes designed specifically for indoor play), turf shoes (for use on artificial turf or hard soil with little grass), and molded or screw-in cleats are all options to consider when purchasing soccer shoes. Molded cleats work well for games that are played on normal grassy fields, while screw-in cleats work best for players in games being conducted on a wet or damp field.

Risk Management

One does not normally associate soccer with a lot of injuries. However, if you don't pay attention, injuries can occur. Table 16.1 describes areas that

Table 16.1 Possible Risks in Soccer

Risk identification	Reduction strategies
Ankle bruises	• Insist that all students wear shin guards for all activities. • Teach proper defending and tackling techniques. • Ensure that students wear proper footwear.
Sprained ankles	• Inspect field for potholes, ruts, clumps of grass, and depressions. Fill, cover, and level these as needed. • Ensure that students wear proper footwear. • Manhole covers and drainage grates should be covered with dirt or with a padded cover.
Injuries due to falling goals	• Ensure that goalposts are properly secured to the ground with pegs or stakes.
Head injuries	• Teach proper offensive and defensive heading techniques.
Miscellaneous injuries	• Teach sound and proper technical soccer (kicking, heading, trapping). • Make sure there are no obstructions (fences, trees, trash cans, cars, etc.) within 10 feet of sidelines or end lines. • Do not allow sliding tackles or tackling from behind. • Ensure that soccer balls are not overinflated.

the teacher needs to focus on to ensure that there are as few injuries as possible.

Skills and Techniques

The skills and techniques of receiving, passing, dribbling, heading, shooting, goalkeeping, and juggling are basic soccer skills. Clear explanations of each allow people to get a mental picture of the skills.

Receiving (Trapping)

Receiving or trapping the ball is a fundamental technique in soccer and involves the player's ability to collect the ball and immediately place it under control. Aside from the arms and hands, one can receive the ball with any portion of the body: the head, the chest, the top of the thigh, the inside of the thigh, the instep, or the inside or outside of the foot. To increase control, a player should choose a large, soft, fleshy portion of the body with which to receive the ball. When receiving the ball, a player should reach out to "catch" the ball and should gradually bring the ball to the centerline of the body so that it is under control. This movement is similar to catching a baseball with one's hand. This allows players to redirect

the ball in any direction, increasing the range with which they can play. One primary consideration when receiving the ball is to turn the ball away from defensive pressure and into open space. This allows the player to protect the ball and maintain better possession and allows for more time before the player makes the next play on the ball.

Passing

Passing is the act of kicking or heading the ball toward one's teammates. When passing the ball, a player must take several things into consideration. How far is the pass to be made? What kind of pace do I put on the ball? How do I get the ball around obstacles?

The three most common areas of the foot used for passing are the inside of the foot, the instep, and the outside of the foot. The inside of the foot is used for short to midrange passing and can produce a very accurate pass.

The instep is used for distance passing. When a player kicks with the instep, only a small amount of surface area strikes the ball, and accuracy is somewhat compromised.

The outside of the foot is not used as often as the inside of the foot or the instep. Because the shape of the outside of the foot naturally curves away from the ball, not a lot of surface area strikes the ball, making this way of passing somewhat inaccurate. Also, because it is difficult to lock the ankle in place when kicking with the outside of the foot, not a lot of power can be generated. The outside of the foot is ideal for bending the ball. Players usually hit a bent ball by striking or slicing the outside of the ball. The more the ball is sliced on its outside portion, the more spin will be generated, resulting in more bending of the ball.

Dribbling

Dribbling is the act of running and carrying the ball with the feet. The portion of the foot used to dribble depends upon the speed of dribble and the space available in which to dribble. A player wants to speed dribble when dribbling in open spaces and trying to get the ball downfield in a hurry, or trying to outrun an opponent while carrying the ball. When dribbling in crowded, tight spaces, a player wants to use both the inside and outside portions of the foot for better ball control and the ability to change the direction of the ball in a hurry.

Heading

Heading is the act of striking the ball with the head to pass, shoot, or clear. The progression for learning to head the ball should be slow and deliberate. The player wants to head the ball on the hairline and avoid heading it square with the face. Poor heading technique can cause players to become fearful of heading.

Shooting

Shooting is the act of "passing" the ball into the back of the net. As with passing, shots may be made with any part of the body except the arms and hands. The type of shot taken will depend on placement of the ball, angle to goal, distance from goal, defender's positioning, and the goalkeeper's position. The most common type of shots attempted are these:

- Instep drive—most powerful, least accurate (see "Passing")

- Inside of foot—least powerful, most accurate (see "Passing")
- Outside of foot—usually used to bend balls (see "Passing")
- Full volley—instep drive, striking the ball out of the air
- Half volley—instep drive, striking the ball on the short hop
- Bent ball—usually hit by slicing the side of the ball with either the inside or outside of the foot (the more the ball is sliced, the more it will swerve)
- Head shot—used for shots above the waist (see "Heading")

Goalkeeping

The goalkeeping position is unlike any other position on the field. Goalkeepers are considered the last line of defense. Goalkeepers wear special gear, wear uniforms that look different from their teammates', and have rules specific to their position. Goalkeepers are the only players on the field allowed to handle the ball with their hands.

Juggling

Juggling is the ability to keep the ball off the ground using multiple touches with multiple parts of the body. Juggling is not a major portion of the game. It is a supplemental skill used to soften one's touch and develop timing. Juggling encourages quickness and rhythm. The parts of the body most commonly used for juggling are the head, thigh, and instep.

Sample Lesson Plans

For the sake of space, only seven lesson plans are presented here. These are lessons pertaining to basic skill acquisition and development. At the middle or high school level, skill development should be the focus of the course.

LESSON 1

Receiving Balls

SEQUENCE (45-MINUTE CLASS)

1. Warm-up and stretching (5 minutes).
2. Discuss and demonstrate proper technique for receiving balls—teacher modeling (10 minutes) (see figure 16.1).
3. Partner play (10 minutes).
4. Four versus two keep-away (15 minutes).
5. Review key points of receiving balls (5 minutes).

TEACHING CUES

- Use large surface areas.
- Use soft, fleshy surface areas.
- Give way to deaden ball.
- Receive the ball away from defensive pressure.

SUGGESTED LEARNING ACTIVITIES

- Partner play: Players partner up, one ball per pair. Partners get 10 yards (9 meters) distance between them. Player 1 tosses the ball to player 2, who receives it with a specific part of the body. Player 2 then picks up the ball and serves it back.

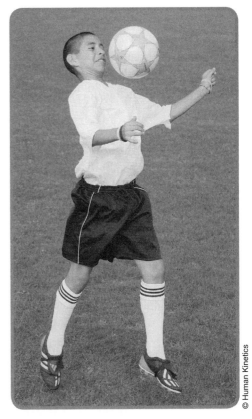

FIGURE 16.1 **Receiving on the chest.**

© Human Kinetics

- Circle drill: Players, each with a ball, form a circle with one player (without a ball) in the center. The center player runs to the outside players, who toss the ball for the central player to receive with the various parts of the body and return. The center player then runs to a different player. Play continues for a specified number of touches or a specified time period. More than one player can also be used in the center.
- SPUD: Two players per ball. Player 1 tosses or kicks the ball high into the air and runs away. Player 2 collects the ball, places his or her foot on top of the ball, and yells "SPUD." Player 1 freezes, turns, and faces player 2 and spreads legs wide. Player 2 has two passes to hit or get the ball through the legs of player 1. If this is accomplished, player 1 receives the letter "S." If player 2 misses, he or she gets the letter. Player 2 now kicks or throws the ball into the air and runs away. Play continues until one player has spelled the word "SPUD."
- Four versus two keep-away: Place four offensive players and two defenders within a confined grid. The offensive players position themselves on the outside portion of the grid, while the defenders run inside. The objective is for the offensive players to pass and receive the ball while attempting to keep the ball away from the defenders. Should an attacking player have his or her pass intercepted, or should the ball go out-of-bounds, that player switches roles with the defender who has been in the middle the longest. This activity is good for both passing and receiving.

LESSON 2

Passing

SEQUENCE (45-MINUTE CLASS)

1. Review receiving balls (5 minutes).
2. Discuss and demonstrate passing using the inside, outside, and instep of the foot—teacher modeling (10 minutes).
3. Pass and follow, and rotation passing (15 minutes).
4. Soccer golf (13 minutes).
5. Review key points of passing the ball (2 minutes).

TEACHING CUES

Inside-of-Foot or Push Pass

- Plant foot 6 to 12 inches (15-30 centimeters) to the side of the ball.
- Plant toe pointed toward target.
- Have kicking foot toes up and out to the side.
- Lock the ankle.
- Square hips toward target.
- Strike the ball slightly higher than the center of the ball.
- Follow through toward target.

Instep Pass

- Plant foot 6 to 12 inches to the side of the ball.
- Plant toe pointed toward target.
- Point kicking foot toes down.
- Lock the ankle.
- Square hips toward target.
- Strike ball slightly under center of ball.
- Short follow-through.

Outside-of-Foot Pass

- Plant foot 12 inches to the side of the ball.
- Plant toe pointed toward target.
- Point toes of kicking foot down and in.
- Lock the ankle.
- Slice through the inside of the ball with the outside portion of the foot.
- Follow-through is across the body.

SUGGESTED LEARNING ACTIVITIES

- Rotation passing: Four or more players per group, one ball. All players within the group are given a number. Player 1 passes the ball to player 2. Player 2 receives the ball and passes it to player 3, who collects it and passes to player 4. After the last player receives the ball, he or she passes it to player 1 and play continues.

- Keep-away: Divide the group into two or three equal teams. The team in possession of the ball attempts to keep the ball away from the other two teams by passing and dribbling. Once the team loses possession of the ball, they try to steal the ball back from the new offensive team. This game can also be played by having two teams combine and keep the ball away from the third team. To encourage passing, a touch restriction can be placed on the players. For example, if any player makes more than three consecutive touches on the ball before passing, that player's team automatically becomes the new defensive team.

- Soccer golf: Each player has a ball. Players are divided into groups of two or three. One player within the group selects the first hole to play. A hole may be any natural object in the area such as a trash can, a telephone pole, the side of a soccer net, or randomly dispersed playing cones. Players then take turns kicking their ball until all players have hit the target. Each kick counts as a stroke. The person with the lowest number of strokes wins the hole and gets to select the next hole, or players can rotate as to who gets to design the next hole. The game is won by the person with the lowest cumulative score at the end of the time.

LESSON 3

Dribbling

SEQUENCE (45-MINUTE CLASS)

1. Review passing (5 minutes).
2. Discuss and demonstrate controlled dribbling versus speed dribbling—teacher modeling (10 minutes).
3. Practice the various types of dribbling across the field (15 minutes).
4. Minefield (13 minutes).
5. Review key points of dribbling (2 minutes).

TEACHING CUES

Controlled Dribble

- Use inside and outside of foot.
- Take short steps.
- Touch ball quickly but softly.
- Carry the ball on the shielded side.

Speed Dribble

- First touch should be long and into open space.
- Point toes down and in.
- Hit the ball with the instep or outside of the foot.
- Touch the ball in stride.

SUGGESTED LEARNING ACTIVITIES

- Knockout: Each player dribbles his or her ball within a confined area. Should a player not maintain close enough ball control, another player within the grid can kick the loose ball out of the grid and the player who had the ball is temporarily out of the game. In order to rejoin the game, the player knocked out must first speed dribble the ball around the grid.

- Minefield: Each player dribbles his or her ball within a confined area. One player walks the grid randomly, laying mines by dropping down playing cones. Each player must dribble his or her ball throughout the minefield without hitting or touching any of the mines with the ball. Should a player hit or touch a mine with either the foot or the ball, that player leaves the playing area, performs a physical challenge (sit-ups, push-ups, or other activity), then rejoins the game. To increase the pace of the activity, one can add roving mines. Roving mines are players who run throughout the grid trying to touch any soccer ball with their feet. Should a ball be struck by a roving mine, the person dribbling the ball leaves the grid and completes whatever physical challenge in order to rejoin the game.

- Freeze tag: All players dribble the ball within a confined area. A number of players, without a ball, are designated taggers. The taggers run throughout the grid trying to touch the soccer balls with their feet or the dribblers with their hands. When a dribbler or his or her ball gets tagged, that player picks up the ball with the hands, holds it high over the head, and spreads his or her legs wide in a frozen stance. It is up to the free dribblers to dribble and push pass the ball through a frozen set of legs. This unfreezes the frozen person, who continues to dribble and look to unfreeze other people. Play continues until all dribblers are frozen or a predetermined time period has elapsed.

LESSON 4

Heading

SEQUENCE (45-MINUTE CLASS)

1. Review dribbling (5 minutes).
2. Discuss and demonstrate heading—teacher modeling (10 minutes) (see figure 16.2).
3. Head juggling (5 minutes).
4. Heading in pairs (10 minutes).
5. Head ball tag (10 minutes).
6. Review key points of heading (5 minutes).

TEACHING CUES

- Watch the ball.
- Arch the body.
- Strike the ball with the hairline.
- Rock through the ball upon impact with head.
- Turn head in the direction you want the ball to travel.

SUGGESTED LEARNING ACTIVITIES

- Head bongs: Each player holds a ball firmly in the hands at arm's length. The player then pulls the arms in and strikes the ball with the proper portion of the forehead. As the players get comfortable with this, they can increase the power with which they strike the ball.

- Head juggling: Each player tosses a ball into the air and sees how many times he or she can consecutively head the ball back into the air before it hits the ground.

- Heading in pairs: This is the same concept as head juggling, only players pair up and see how many times they can head the ball back and forth before the ball strikes the ground.

- Head ball tag: Players, identified as taggers, each pick up a ball with their hands. The remaining players, without a ball, randomly run throughout a grid. It is up to the taggers to chase the runners and hit them with the ball below the shoulders by first bouncing the ball off their own heads. When a tagger hits a runner, roles reverse.

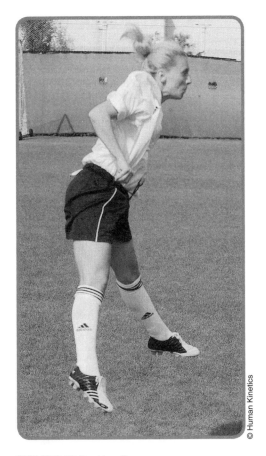

FIGURE 16.2   **Heading.**

LESSON 5

Shooting

SEQUENCE (45-MINUTE CLASS)

1. Review heading (5 minutes).
2. Discuss and demonstrate different types of shots using different portions of the foot—teacher modeling (10 minutes).
3. Line shooting (10 minutes).
4. Scramble shoot (18 minutes).
5. Review key points of shooting (2 minutes).

TEACHING CUES

- Instep drive—see "Passing"
- Inside of foot—see "Passing"
- Outside of foot—see "Passing"
- Bent ball—see "Passing"
- Head shot—see "Heading"

SUGGESTED LEARNING ACTIVITIES

- Circle shoot: Players, each with a ball and a number, randomly dribble within a grid. When a person's number is called out, that person dribbles the ball outside the grid and shoots on goal, then retrieves the ball and rejoins the group of dribblers.

- Line shooting: Players, each with a ball, form one or two lines a specified distance from goal. Players take turns dribbling toward the goal and shooting on net. They then switch lines.

- One versus one: Players begin by forming two groups. One group, the defenders, take all the balls and form a line off the end line near goal. The other group, the shooters, form a line 20 yards (18 meters) downfield away from goal. The first defender serves a ball to the first shooter. The defender then runs out onto the field to defend the shooter, who has collected the ball and is dribbling toward the goal for a shot. After the ball has been shot or the defender steals the ball, play is halted, and both players switch lines and roles.

- Scramble shoot: Two goals are placed face to face, approximately 18 yards (16 meters) apart. The distance between goals depends on the number of players participating and their age and skill level. Players are divided into teams. One person is identified as the server and stands off to the side of the field of play with all of the soccer balls. Two teams step into the playing grid while the other players or teams spread out behind the goal to retrieve missed shots, return them to the server, and wait their turn to play. The server then randomly serves a ball into the grid. The teams fight for possession of the ball and look to shoot as quickly as possible. Should a goal be scored, or if the ball goes out-of-bounds, play is dead and the server quickly sends in a new ball. Should the goalkeeper make a save, he or she can roll the ball to a teammate for a shot in the opposite direction or can throw the ball to the server on the sidelines, who will kick a new ball into play. After a specified time or a specified number of goals, new teams come onto the field and old ones leave.

LESSON 6

Goalkeeping

SEQUENCE (45-MINUTE CLASS)

1. Discuss and demonstrate the goalkeeping skills of catching, punching, and deflecting the ball, and also diving for the ball—teacher modeling (20 minutes).

2. Pair up students and work on various goalkeeping techniques (25 minutes).

TEACHING CUES

Catching

- Form a "W" around ball; fingertips face up.
- Thumbs touch, fingers spread wide.
- After catching a high ball, hold the ball above the heads of the players.

- After catching a low ball, cradle the ball between the chest and forearms.
- When catching a ball between the waist and the knees, fingertips face down.
- Pinkie fingers touch while the remaining fingers spread around the ball.
- When catching a rolling ball off to the side, one hand is positioned behind the ball while the other hand is placed on top of the ball.
- Press the ball into the ground.

Punching

- Make a fist.
- Punch the ball with the flat portion of the fingers.
- Punch the ball as far and as wide downfield as possible.
- Punch through the ball.

Deflecting

- Deflect the ball over the crossbar on high shots.
- Deflect the ball around the goalpost on low shots.
- Use the hand closest to the ball.
- The palm of the hand should face the front and be positioned behind the ball.
- Palm and fingers angle over the crossbar or to the outside of the goalpost.

Diving

- Lower center of gravity.
- Power step to the ball.
- Hands to the ball.
- After the catch, use the ball to break the fall.
- Pin the ball to the ground with the top hand on top of the ball and the bottom hand behind the ball.

SUGGESTED LEARNING ACTIVITIES

- Shooting: Goalkeepers can be placed within any shooting activity.
- Goalkeeper wars: Two goals are placed facing each other approximately 20 yards (18 meters) apart, with one goalkeeper per goal. The objective of the game is for the goalkeepers to throw, shoot, or drop kick the ball at the opposing goalkeeper or goal in an attempt to score a goal. Goalkeepers alternate turns trying to score upon one another. Each goal scored is 1 point. A game can be played until a certain score is reached or for a specified amount of time.

LESSON 7

Juggling

SEQUENCE (45-MINUTE CLASS)

1. Review goalkeeping (5 minutes).
2. Discuss and demonstrate the various techniques and body parts used in juggling—teacher modeling (10 minutes).

3. Practice individual juggling using the various parts of the body (10 minutes).
4. Juggling in pairs (5 minutes).
5. Individual and pair juggling contest (10 minutes).
6. Review key points of juggling (5 minutes).

TEACHING CUES

Head Juggling

- Keep the head up and eyes on the ball.
- Stagger legs.
- Have a slight bend at the knee.
- Put weight on the balls of the feet.
- Strike ball on hairline of forehead by gently extending legs.
- Move body to stay centered under the ball.

Thigh Juggling

- Put weight on the balls of the feet.
- Strike ball by lifting the knee so the thigh is parallel to the ground.

Instep Juggling

- Put weight on the balls of the feet.
- Lift the toes of the juggling foot slightly upward so the top of the foot is parallel to the ground.
- Gently kick the ball upward by lifting the leg.

SUGGESTED LEARNING ACTIVITIES

- Individual juggling: Each player with a ball tries to juggle the ball as many consecutive times as possible without letting the ball touch the ground. This activity can be restricted to individual body parts (e.g., thigh juggling) or a combination of body parts (e.g., left instep, right instep, right instep).
- Team juggling: Players are divided into teams of two or more. Each team is given a ball and is required to juggle the ball as many times as possible. As with individual juggling, restrictions can be added, such as these:
  - Players must head juggle only.
  - Each player must touch the ball a certain number of times before passing off to a teammate.
- HORSE: This game uses a specified number of players and one ball. One player starts the game with a single-, double-, or unlimited-touch juggle. At any point, that player passes the ball in the air to any other player, who must resume the juggling without letting the ball touch the ground. If a bad pass is made, or if a player allows the ball to hit the ground, that player receives the letter "H." The ball is then picked up and play resumes. A player is out of the game when he or she spells out the word "HORSE." As with individual and team juggling, restrictions can be placed on the type and number of touches taken.

Adapting This Course for Your School

First determine the focus of the course. Basic skill development through fun, gamelike activities is crucial. There is a saying in the soccer world, "Let the game be the teacher." Avoid lectures and stagnant drills in which players wait their turn in line to perform a skill. Describe the skill, demonstrate the proper way of performing the skill, and then organize an activity in which repetition of the skill is inherent, such as the skill of dribbling in the game known as "Knockout."

Each skill should be broken down into a two-lesson block of instruction. The first lesson includes instruction, teacher modeling, and some baseline activities to give students a basic comprehension of the skill. The second day of instruction includes a review along with higher-level activities. An example is the skill of dribbling. On day 1, have students dribble the ball across the field by themselves, using various parts of their feet. Introduce speed dribbling and dribbling for control. On day 2, play a form of keep-away in a designated grid.

When looking to play small-sided training games, keep numbers low; this will encourage maximum participation. Three versus three, or four versus four, helps keep everyone involved. Eventually introduce the 11 per side game.

Children should begin to learn the basic rules of soccer, but at a slow pace. Take one rule a day, describe it, and demonstrate it. One day talk about a throw-in, the next day a corner kick. Be careful not to overload children with too much technical jargon or too many tactical principles. They won't hear and they won't understand. Remember, "Let the game be the teacher."

Key Terms

back pass—A pass made to a supporting player who is behind the ball.

caution—A flagrant foul for which the official issues a warning (yellow card) to the offending player. Two yellow cards in the same game for the same player constitutes an automatic ejection from the game. That player cannot be substituted for.

center back—Another term for a central defender.

center circle—A circle in the middle of the field that has a 10-yard radius. This area of the field is used to start each half of a game and to restart the game after each goal is scored.

center forward—A player who plays in the middle of a three-person front line.

changing the point of the attack—After a particular portion of the field has been attacked, the ball is switched and a new part of the field is attacked.

chip pass or shot—A soft, floating pass or shot with arc and backspin.

combination—The act of connecting more than one pass together in sequence using two or more players.

contain—Keep an attacking player who has the ball from penetrating the defense with a pass or dribble.

corner kick—A free kick taken by the attacking team when the ball is knocked over the attacking team's end line and is last touched by the defensive team. The kick is taken from the corner of the field on the side of the end line where the ball went out.

counterattack—A strategy used by the defensive team; when they win the ball they immediately go on the attack before the opposition can organize defensively.

defenders—Players who line up in the backfield in front of the goalkeeper with a primarily defensive responsibility. They initiate the attack after they win the ball.

direct kick—The act of kicking the ball directly into the goal on a restart after a foul.

dribble—The act of carrying or running the ball with the feet.

eighteen-yard line—The line that is 18 yards from the end line and constitutes the top of the penalty box.

far post—The goalpost that is farthest away from the ball.

first attacker—The attacking player with the ball.

first defender—The defender who defends the attacking player with the ball.

first time—The act of shooting or passing the ball on one's first touch.

formation—A system of play; as an example, 4-4-2 is four backs, four midfielders, and two forwards.

forward—A player who plays on the front line. Primary responsibility is attacking and scoring goals.

foul—An infraction of the rules. The two types of fouls are direct and indirect (see *direct kick* and *indirect kick*).

free kick—The method according to which play resumes after a foul. Kicks can be either direct or indirect.

give and go—A two-person combination in which one player gives the ball to the other and runs into a different position to receive a return pass.

goal—The act of causing the ball to completely cross the goal line.

goal box—The 6- by 20-yard rectangular box inside the penalty area where goal kicks are taken.

goal kick—A kick performed when the attacking team is the last to have touched the ball before it goes over the end line; the defending team puts the ball back into play with a free kick from inside their own goal box.

goal line—The line that is between the two goalposts at each goal, 8 yards in length. The ball must entirely cross the goal line for a goal to be scored.

half volley—The act of kicking the ball the instant it rebounds off the ground; can be likened to a drop kick.

hand ball—Touching of the ball with any part of the arm or hand. This is a direct kick violation.

heading—The act of striking the ball with one's head.

indirect kick—A restart in which the ball needs to be touched twice before a goal can be scored.

kickoff—A way of starting or restarting the game at the beginning of each half and after each goal. A kickoff is taken from the kickoff spot in the middle of the center circle.

linesmen—Two referees who run the sidelines in a three-man officiating system. Responsibilities include calling throw-ins, corner kicks, and goal kicks and assisting the center referee with the calling of fouls and goals.

man-to-man—A style of defensive play in which defenders mark opponents all over the field. They do not mark space.

mark—Another term for the word "defend." A player can mark a player or a space depending on whether a team plays man-to-man or zone.

midfielders—Players who position themselves between the forwards and defenders. Their primary responsibility is to support the attack and help the defenders or fullbacks.

near post—The goalpost nearest to the ball.

near support—A position taken by supporting offensive players who are near the ball; used as short pass outlets.

obstruction—The use of the body to block an opponent from playing the ball; this is an indirect kick violation.

offside—An infraction in which an attacking player is in his or her offensive half of the field, is ahead of the ball, and does not have a minimum of two defensive players between him- or herself and the goal.

one-touch—Another term for "first time."

one-two—A two-man combination in which one player passes the ball to another and the receiving player touches the ball back.

pass—The act of kicking, heading, or chesting the ball to one's teammate.

penalty—A rules infraction; results in a direct or indirect kick for the opposing team.

penalty area—The large 18- by 44-yard box in front of each goal. It is only in that area of the field that a goalkeeper may handle the ball with the hands. All direct kick violations by the defending team within this area result in a penalty kick from the 12-yard line.

penalty kick—A direct free kick from the 12-yard line. Only the goalkeeper and shooter are allowed within the penalty box at the time of the kick.

penalty spot—The 12-yard spot within the penalty area from which all penalty kicks are taken.

penetration pass—A forward pass made that gets behind defenders.

referee—The official in the center of the field. There may be one or two.

restart—The act of putting the ball back into play after a dead ball situation.

save—The act of a goalkeeper who gets any part of his or her body on the ball to keep it from going into the net.

schemer—A withdrawn center forward; acts as an attacking center midfielder. Often considered the quarterback of the front line and given much flexibility as to responsibilities.

second attacker—The offensive player who provides near support to the ball; usually involved with wall passing and give-and-go plays.

second defender—The defensive player who provides cover for the first defender.

shield—The act of protecting the ball by keeping one's body between the defender and the ball until a pass, shot, or dribble can be made.

shootout—A way of determining a winner for a contest should the game be tied after regulation and overtime. Having teams alternate penalty kicks, up to five each, is the most common form of shootout.

sideline—The line on either side of the field that indicates out-of-bounds. All balls out-of-bounds over the sideline are restarted with a throw-in.

six-yard line—The line that is 6 yards away from the end line and constitutes the top of the goal box.

slide tackle—The act of a defensive player who slides feetfirst on the ground in an attempt to dispossess the attacking player of the ball.

square pass—A pass made directly to the left or right of the passer.

stopper—A central defender who plays in front of the sweeper and behind the central midfielder; his or her marking responsibility is either the center forward, the schemer, or center midfielder.

striker—Another term for "forward." Usually the team's most powerful and best-scoring forward.

sweeper—A player who plays behind the marking defenders and positions him- or herself between the ball and the center of the goal. A sweeper has no marking responsibilities but picks up and marks attackers when the attackers beat the defenders who are marking them.

tackle—The act of trying to take the ball off the foot of an attacking player. Defensive players stick their foot solidly in front of the ball, creating a barrier with which to stop the ball.

takeover—A player's taking of a ball from a teammate who has the ball and dribbles toward the player; similar to a handoff in football.

throw-in—The way in which all restarts are made on balls that go over the sideline. Both feet must be firmly planted on the ground, and the ball must be released with both hands over the head for all throw-ins.

touchline—Another term for "sideline."

tracking—Staying with and following the player that a defensive player is defending.

trap—The act of bringing a moving ball under control.

two-on-one—The situation in which two attackers go against one defender.

volley—Kicking the ball in the air before it hits the ground.

wall—A formation of defenders who line up side by side in order to block or obstruct a direct or indirect free kick on goal. All walls must be set up a minimum of 10 yards from the point of the kick.

wall pass—A pass of the ball by an attacker to a near supporting player who then touches the ball back to the original attacker behind the defender; similar to a "give and go." This is an effective way to isolate and get the ball behind the defense.

winger—A player who plays on the front line, out on the flanks. Usually used in a 4-3-3 or 3-4-3 formation.

zone defense—Defensive strategy in which the defensive team marks space, or zones, and the attackers who come into their space.

Suggested Readings

Dewazian, K. (1992). *Fundamental soccer practice.* Clovis, CA: Fun Soccer Enterprises.

Schum, T. (1992). *Coaching soccer.* Indianapolis: Masters Press.

Simon, J.M., & Reeves, J. (1982). *Soccer games book.* West Point, NY: Leisure Press.

Yannis, A. (1980). *Inside soccer.* New York: McGraw-Hill.

Sport-Specific Organizations

American Youth Soccer Organization (AYSO)
12501 South Isis Avenue
Hawthorne, CA 90250
800-872-2976
www.soccer.org

Federation Internationale de Football Association (FIFA)
P.O. Box 85
8030 Zurich, Switzerland
www.fifa.com

National Soccer Coaches Association of America (NSCAA)
6700 Squibb Road, Suite 215
Mission, KS 66202
913-362-1747
www.nscaa.com

United States Soccer Federation (USSF)
1801-1811 South Prairie Avenue
Chicago, IL 60616
312-808-1300
www.us-soccer.com

17

Volleyball

Lynn Fielitz

Volleyball is a game that can be played at any age. The game is played competitively at the junior high, high school, collegiate, and Olympic levels and is also played simply for entertainment and enjoyment at the intramural level or in the backyard. Volleyball is also played on beaches throughout the world, and beach volleyball has been recently added as an Olympic sport.

The average size of a volleyball team can vary with the level of interest, skill level, and abilities of the students. Beach volleyball is typically played with two players per side, while competitive indoor volleyball is played with six players per side. Backyard volleyball games can have as few as two players per side and as many as nine players per side, depending on the number of players available.

The object of volleyball is for each team to send the ball over the net to ground it on the opponent's court, and to prevent the ball from being grounded on their own court. The ball is put into play by the right back-row player, who serves the ball by hitting it over the net into the opponent's court. A team is allowed to hit the ball three times (in addition to the block contact) in order to return it to the opponent's court. A player is not allowed to hit the ball twice consecutively except when attempting to block. The rally continues until the ball touches the ground or the floor, or goes out-of-bounds, or if a team fails to return the ball to the opponent's court or commits a fault. The team winning the rally scores a point. When the receiving team wins a rally, it gains a point and the right to serve, and its players rotate one position clockwise. Rotation ensures that players play both the net and the back zone of the court.

A team wins a game by scoring 25 points with a 2-point advantage in nondeciding games and 15 points with a 2-point advantage in the deciding game. (The nondeciding game is the third game in a three-game match or the fifth game in a five-game match.) A team wins the match by winning the best of three or five games (Lenberg, 2006).

Volleyball has increased in popularity since the U.S. men's volleyball team won back-to-back gold medals in the 1984 and 1988 Olympics. In addition, portable systems have allowed volleyball nets to be erected on almost any flat area of ground and in any climate. Volleyball is a sport enjoyed by participants and spectators alike. Students at the U.S. Military Academy may take a Volleyball course as part of their Physical Development Program.

Purpose of the Course

The purpose of the Volleyball course is to introduce students to the sport and to develop individual skills and foster team play. Due to the nature of the sport, teamwork and communication are important concepts that are stressed in the course. The course introduces students to the basic rules of volleyball and provides them the opportunity to serve as an official.

The objectives of the course are as follows:

- Demonstrate competency in individual volleyball skills including underhand passing, overhead passing, serving, spiking, blocking, and defense
- Develop and apply knowledge of team formations and basic volleyball skills used for serving, serve reception, defense, offense, and transition play
- Develop knowledge of drills for developing individual and team volleyball skills
- Demonstrate knowledge and proper application of the rules of volleyball, as well as an understanding of the duties and responsibilities of volleyball referees

Instructional Area

The dimensions of a regulation volleyball court measure 18 meters by 9 meters (59 feet by 29 feet 6 inches). A 5-centimeter (2-inch) centerline divides the court. The space over the court should be free from obstructions to a recommended minimum height of 7 meters (23 feet) above the playing surface. All boundary lines are 5 centimeters and are a contrasting color from the floor and the surrounding lines. The boundary lines are drawn inside the dimensions of the court. An attack line is located 3 meters (9 feet 10 inches) from the axis of the centerline. This line delineates the front-row players from the back-row players so that back-row players cannot attack or spike the ball while positioned in front of the attack line (see figure 17.1).

Volleyball can be played indoors or outdoors, and the game varies slightly depending on the court surface and number of players. Outdoor volleyball can be played on grass or sand. Outdoor players have to be able to adapt to the sun, wind, and weather, while indoor players must adapt to the lighting, ceilings, and sideline space. The playing surface has an impact on team play and skills. Indoor volleyball is often preferred, as players can react quickly and jump higher on indoor courts than they can on sand or grass surfaces.

The recommended learning environment for a volleyball class consists of a minimum of two courts and two net systems. After the class is divided into teams, each team is assigned a court on which to practice. If space is limited, teams can share a court and work on team concepts and volleyball skills, with appropriate guidance provided by the teacher.

The net height should be adjusted depending on the age group. High school classes can use the regulation heights listed in table 17.1. An alternative for a coed class would be to use an intermediate height of approximately 7 feet 8 inches (2.4 meters). If the nets are too low in a coed class, a variation of the rules for spiking should be implemented. If there are exceptional students who can easily spike the volleyball on a lower net, they should be allowed to attack the volleyball only from behind the 3-meter line (10-foot line). This modification (referred to as "reverse coed" rules) provides a more competitive environment.

Equipment

Even for a sport like volleyball with few equipment requirements, just balls, shoes, and a net, certain considerations need to be kept in mind. The proper selection of equipment can improve the quality of the experience for the students.

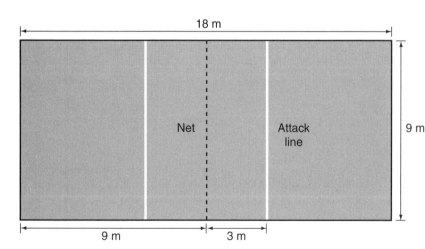

FIGURE 17.1 Volleyball court dimensions.

Table 17.1 USA Volleyball Competitive Net Heights (USA Volleyball Rules 2005-2006)

Age group	Females/Reverse coed	Male/Coed
15-18 years and under	2.24 m (7 ft 4 1/8 in.)	2.43 m (7 ft 11 5/8 in.)
13-14 years and under	2.24 m (7 ft 4 1/8 in.)	2.24 m (7 ft 4 1/8 in.)

Balls

The recommendation is that there be one volleyball per student. Additional volleyballs are useful in conducting drills. Volleyballs can be kept in portable carts, which are useful for transporting balls during class, collecting balls during drills, and storing them after class.

Footwear

Proper footwear is important for volleyball players. The three most important considerations for footwear are safety, traction, and cushioning. Since a great deal of play during a volleyball game is conducted at the net and in close proximity to other players, stepping or landing on another player's foot is a common problem. Volleyball shoes need to provide lateral support to reduce the chance of sprained ankles. Running shoes or shoes with a raised sole should not be worn. Traction is important because volleyball requires very quick, reactive movements. Players must move quickly to various locations on the court; therefore, good traction on the playing surface increases performance. In addition, good shoe cushioning is important to assist in dissipating the landing forces of the players. Spiking and blocking are two repetitive skills, and the impact of landing can injure the knees and ankles if it is not done correctly. A good pair of shoes cushions the landing and reduces the chance of injury or pain. For indoor games, look for a shoe that has the label "nonmarking sole." Many shoes can leave a mark on the playing surface that might not be removable, and this can ruin the appearance of the floor.

Clothing

Athletic clothing should be worn for volleyball. Clothing should be comfortable and allow for a full range of motion, especially around the shoulders and upper body. For beach volleyball, swimming suits are acceptable playing attire. For grass volleyball, clothing should be worn not only to keep the body cool and to provide coverage from the sun, but also to provide protection from the grass. Indoor volleyball sometimes requires the team to wear uniforms with numbers. In addition, long-sleeved shirts can be worn on any surface or at any venue. Long-sleeved shirts help to protect the forearms during passing and to absorb some of the force from hard-driven spikes. Knee pads are also used quite extensively in volleyball at all levels and arenas.

Accessories

Accessories may help to make the game more enjoyable. For an outdoor game, sunglasses can improve the vision of the players when they look upward toward the volleyball. Hats and sunscreen also provide additional comfort and increased protection from the sun and allow players to thoroughly enjoy the sport in an outdoor setting.

Additional items that are nonessential to conducting a successful class are net antennas and a referee's platform. The net antennas are flexible rods, fastened on each side of the net directly above the outside boundary lines. The ball must pass completely inside the antennas when crossing the net. A padded referee platform located in line with the net makes officiating easier.

Risk Management

The game of volleyball is unique in that opponents do not generally touch each other. Contact at or under the net with an opponent is the most common cause of injuries. The most common injury is sprained ankles, which result from landing on the opponent's foot during play at the net.

Shoulder injuries are also common when students do not properly warm up their arms prior to serving or aggressively spiking the volleyball. A gradual 5- to 10-minute warm-up of the spiking arm alleviates the majority of these types of injuries.

Performing a gradual warm-up and cool-down of 10 to 15 minutes also lowers the chance of muscle pulls or strains.

Additional safety considerations involve padding the poles and the referee stand. Most indoor net systems have pads that fit closely around the poles to protect the participants. If the net system does not have pads, these can be purchased from any sports equipment supply company. Padding thickness and ease of use are two important considerations for purchasing pole pads. Also, the referee stand should be padded on all exposed surfaces.

The final safety consideration is to keep the court free of obstacles and loose volleyballs. Equipment, chairs, bleachers, and other items should be at least 15 to 20 feet (4.6-6 meters) away from the playing surface. Students tend to chase the volleyball during play and can injure themselves if hazardous obstacles are not removed. Rolling volleyballs also pose a possible hazard. Although infrequent, injuries due to rolling volleyballs can be significant. Extra care must be taken during spiking and blocking activities to ensure that balls do not roll onto the court underneath jumping activities.

Table 17.2 identifies several common areas of concern in volleyball. Identifying these areas and removing risk factors, along with discussing them with students, lower the chance of injury.

Skills and Techniques

To achieve a high level of performance in volleyball, the mastery of a foundational set of skills is important. These skills include ball contact, communication, body positions, and movement.

Individual Skills

Players use individual skills when contacting the ball. These skills can be practiced alone, with a partner, or in a team setting. In order to achieve a high level of team play, all students must have proficiency in the individual skills. Individual skills provide the basis on which team skills are built. When a team is having trouble competing, the reason usually comes down to the deterioration of the individual skills. An instructor should always emphasize the individual skills and should include them in each class.

Communication

A key element in the game of volleyball is teammate communication. Students must constantly be communicating, both verbally and nonverbally. The most important aspect of communication on the volleyball court is "calling the ball" each time a player passes the ball. The most common words or

Table 17.2 Possible Risks in Volleyball

Risk identification	Reduction strategies
Sprained ankle	• Instruct students to stay off centerline when practicing and playing. • Enforce centerline violations in competition matches. • Enforce the wearing of court shoes for class—no running shoes. • Ensure that loose volleyballs are kept off the court.
Slipping on a wet floor	• Inspect floor prior to class. • Provide towels to wipe up wet spots during play.
Sore forearms from passing	• Have students ice forearms after class. • Have students wear long-sleeved shirts when passing.
Shoulder injuries	• Instruct students on proper warm-up prior to spiking activities. • Instruct students on proper arm swing mechanics of the spike and serve.
Muscle strains and pulls	• Have students perform proper warm-up and stretching prior to class. • Instruct students on proper skill mechanics.
Obstacle on sidelines	• Move or remove obstacles prior to class. • Pad obstacles.

phrases used in calling the ball are "mine," "I've got it," or "me." The words used are not as important as the actual call made by the player passing the ball. By calling the ball, the player making the pass lets everyone on the team know that he or she is definitely making the play on the volleyball.

Teammates can "support" the passer by telling the passer that the ball is "in" or "good." One word that should never be heard on the volleyball court is "yours." If a ball is too high to be played by a front-row player, that player should open up and turn to face the player in the back row who is making the play on the ball. Front-row students should never "duck" when not playing a ball because the back-row player cannot see the ball and is usually "faked out" of the play by thinking that the front-row player is going to play the ball. The usual result of this lack of communication is that the ball drops between two teammates and the opposing team scores a point.

Not only should students making the play on the ball communicate with one another by calling the ball; they should also make an assertive movement with their body to physically pass the ball. They should not just reach with the arms to pass the ball but should move the entire body behind the ball when making the pass. Moving the body, in addition to calling the ball, lets everyone else know that a player is going to pass the volleyball. By making a forceful move, the passer physically blocks the other players from making a play on the ball.

Communication is a skill that can be practiced, trained, and improved upon. From the very first touch on the ball, students need to get into the habit of calling the ball each time they make a pass. Through this continual reinforcement the communication becomes routine and occurs every time a player passes the volleyball.

Body Positions

The ability to move to and make contact with the ball effectively is a key component of volleyball. The students need to understand and practice high, medium, and low body positions.

High Volleyball is played in three different postural positions: high, medium, and low. The high body position is used in the skills of serving, blocking, and spiking. The body is fully upright with feet shoulder-distance apart (see figure 17.2). In spiking and blocking, the player leaves the ground and must maintain the full upright position while in the air to properly execute the skill.

Medium The medium body position is used in the underhand and in the overhead pass. The body is flexed at the knees and the waist, with the right foot slightly in front of the left. The right foot is slightly forward of the left for consistency during teaching of the set; and since most people still serve from the right back, this position allows the optimal body position for making the pass to the setter. This is true for both right- and left-handed players. Weight should be evenly distributed over the balls of the feet. A good method to get students in a medium body position is to have them put both hands on the front of their thighs and slowly drag their hands down to their knees. Once the hands are at the knees, they take the hands off the legs and put them in the proper position for either the underhand or the overhead pass. This position, with the hands in either the underhand or overhead passing position, is the correct medium position (see figure 17.3).

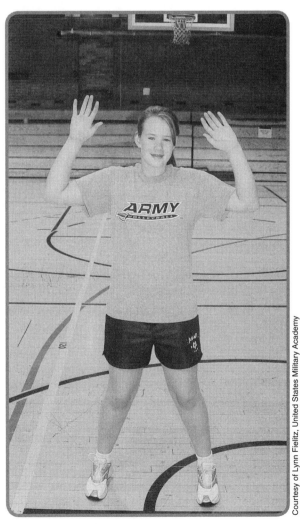

FIGURE 17.2 High body position.

Courtesy of Lynn Fielitz, United States Military Academy

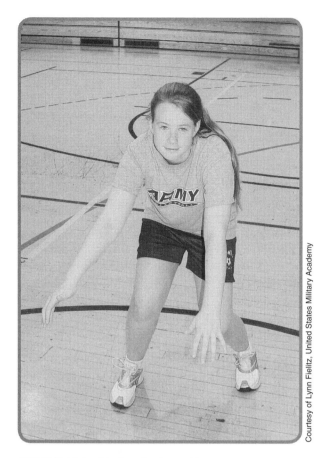

Courtesy of Lynn Fielitz, United States Military Academy

FIGURE 17.3 Medium body position.

Low The low body position is used in defense. The feet are even and very wide, at least two shoulder-widths apart. Knees and waist are bent, while the back remains straight. The weight should be slightly forward and on the balls of the feet. If the students are able to reach down and touch the ground without additional bending, they are in the proper position. It is better for students to be too low to the ground, and to have to move up to a higher position to make a defensive play on the volleyball, than for them to be too high and have to move down to play the ball. Students have to hold this defensive position for only a short time, so the instructor should encourage them to get as low as possible while still being able to move forward from this position (see figure 17.8 on page 384).

Movement

The object in the game of volleyball is to put the ball on the floor of the opposing team. Students need to be able to move to the ball as quickly and as efficiently as possible. Efficient movement means moving to the correct position as quickly as possible in the fewest steps. It also means that each movement is completed with the players in a balanced position, ready to play the ball. Many students can move quickly to the proper position but are off balance when they complete the movement, and therefore are unable to make the appropriate play on the ball. In order to execute a good play on the ball, players need to fill empty areas quickly while maintaining correct body position.

The most important aspect is to complete each movement in a balanced position. The first cue is a "hop-step to a balanced position." This is executed by a simple hop and landing with the weight evenly distributed on both feet. From this balanced position, the requisite skill can be properly executed. The key is to be balanced and to not be leaning in one particular direction. This movement can cover short distances of 1 to 2 feet (.3-.6 meters).

In order to cover longer distances up to 5 feet (1.5 meters), a movement called the "step-hop" is utilized. Usually taking a medium body position with the right foot slightly forward of the left, the player steps with the foot in the desired direction and finishes the movement with a hop-step to a balanced position. In the medium body position, a player leads with the right foot to move forward or to the right, and uses the left foot to move backward or to the left. Leading with the foot in the direction of the movement keeps the body facing the ball while facilitating efficient movement. These two movements are most frequently utilized in passing and blocking.

A third type of movement used in volleyball is the "shuffle step." A medium body position is assumed, and the feet are shuffled together but not crossed as the player moves to the proper position. This movement is used for distances up to 10 feet (3 meters) and is slow, but should still be completed with a hop-step to a balanced position.

For distances of up to 15 feet (4.6 meters), a step-crossover-hop movement is utilized. This type of movement is usually done with blocking or when a player is moving to proper defensive positions. The player takes a step with the foot in the direction of travel. The trail foot crosses over in front of the other foot while the player turns the body 90 degrees in the direction of travel. Turning the body back into the original stance and finishing with a hop-step to a balanced position completes the movement. The three steps can be lengthened or shortened to accommodate the requisite distance. When this movement is used in blocking, finishing with a hop-step to a balanced position is important so that the moving player does not collide with the other blocker, thereby knocking both players off balance and making for an incorrect execution of the blocking skill.

Course Overview

Table 17.3 illustrates the lesson sequence of the course.

Sample Lesson Plans

The following lesson plans represent a typical volleyball lesson at West Point. The lessons include (1) student accountability, (2) introduction of new skill, (3) warm-up and review of previous skill(s), (4) demonstration of new skill, (5) review of instructional cues, (6) practice and feedback, (7) closure and review, and (8) class dismissal.

Table 17.3 Overview of Volleyball Lessons

Lesson	Lecture	Activity
1	• Course introduction. • Introduce communication, movement, and underhand pass.	Individual movement Underhand pass
2	• Review underhand pass. • Introduce overhead pass.	Underhand pass Overhead pass
3	• Review underhand and overhead pass. • Introduce serve and individual serve receive.	Underhand pass Overhead pass Serve Individual serve receive
4	• Review serve and serve receive. • Introduce spiking.	Serve Individual serve receive Spiking
5	• Divide class into five teams. • Review spiking. • Introduce blocking.	 Spiking Blocking
6	• Review blocking. • Introduce six-on-six offense and team serve receive. • Discuss rules and court dimensions.	Blocking Six-six offense Team serve receive Scrimmage
7	• Review six-on-six offense. • Introduce player-up defense. • Practice games. • Review rules.	Six-six offense Player-up defense Wash drills
8	• Review player-up defense. • Introduce four-on-two offense. • Practice games.	Player-up defense Four-two offense Wash drills
9	• Review four-on-two offense. • Volleyball video.	Four-two offense
10	• Practice games. • Discuss skills tests.	Scrimmages

(continued)

Table 17.3 *(continued)*

Lesson	Lecture	Activity
11	• Tournament play.	Team 1 versus team 2 Team 3 versus team 4 Team 5 officiates
12	• Tournament play.	Team 2 versus team 3 Team 4 versus team 5 Team 1 officiates
13	• Introduce and practice skill tests.	Skill tests practice
14	• Tournament play.	Team 3 versus team 5 Team 1 versus team 4 Team 2 officiates
15	• Skill tests.	Conduct skill tests
16	• Tournament play.	Team 1 versus team 5 Team 2 versus team 4 Team 3 officiates
17	• Tournament play.	Team 1 versus team 3 Team 2 versus team 5 Team 4 officiates
18	• Written test.	Classroom

Overhead Pass-Set

SEQUENCE (45-MINUTE CLASS)

1. Student accountability.
2. Introduce the overhead pass as the second skill element, primarily used to set the ball to the spiker (5 minutes).
3. Warm-up exercises reviewing the underhand pass (5 minutes).
4. Demonstrate the overhead pass and movement: Teacher models proper technique (5 minutes).
5. Review key instructional cues for the overhead pass while demonstrating (5 minutes).
6. Allow for adequate student practice and individual instruction on the overhead pass-set (20 minutes).
7. Closure: general review of proper passing techniques, questions (5 minutes).

TEACHING CUES

- Begin in a medium body position; finish in a high body position.
- Create a "basket" over the forehead.
- Maintain contact with the ball with all fingers of each hand.

- Extend the arms toward ceiling and lift with the legs.
- Right foot moves forward.
- Hands rest on the sides of the ball.
- Absorb impact with the wrists and extend with the arms.
- Finish the set so the ball has very little spin.

SUGGESTED LEARNING ACTIVITIES

- Students pair up; one student tosses the ball to the passer, who returns the ball to the tosser via an overhand pass-set. The tosser provides feedback on the passer's performance and form. The tosser can vary the location of the toss to force the passer to move to the ball and execute a good overhand pass.
- Place students in groups of three. Within each group of three, two of the students pair up. These two students stand in a line approximately 15 feet (4.6 meters) away from the third student, whom they will face. The first student in the pair passes the ball overhead to the single player. The first student in the pair then quickly runs behind the single student in order to follow the pass. The single player then passes the ball back to the second student in the pair and follows the pass. In this way the ball goes back and forth constantly while the three players are moving into new positions each time they contact the ball. Once this has been practiced, the teacher can make a contest of the drill to see which group can keep passing the ball overhead the longest.
- In another exercise, students pair up and use the underhand and overhead passing techniques in various combinations, that is, they alternate underhand and overhead passing technique. One student passes the ball underhand while the other passes it overhand.

Underhand Pass (Forearm Pass)

The underhand pass is the most frequently used skill in volleyball. Almost every time the ball crosses the net, an underhand pass is used to play the first of the team's three contacts. While a recent rule change allows serves to be taken with the overhead pass, the underhand pass is still used quite extensively in defensive measures and by novice volleyball students.

The main concept stressed during the execution of the underhand pass is the importance of keeping the forearms even. By keeping the heels of the hands and thumbs together and level, the player keeps the forearms in the proper position. The remaining fingers of each hand should be in contact with each other; to maintain this contact the player either interlaces the fingertips, places one hand inside the other in a "cup," or makes a fist with one hand and wraps the other hand around the fist. The fingers should then be pointed toward the ground, which flattens the forearms and produces a better surface for contacting the ball. Lastly, the ball should contact the middle of the forearms and be directed toward the target.

TEACHING CUES

- Maintain a medium body position.
- Heels of both hands and thumbs are pressed together.
- Fingers are pointed toward the floor.
- Contact ball in the middle of the forearms.

For consistency with the overhead pass, the right foot should be slightly in front of the left foot during underhand passing. The arms should never swing higher than shoulder level; keeping the arms lower forces the passer to use the legs and produces less arm swing. These additional points should be included in the teaching progression:

- Pass with the right foot in front of the left foot.
- Lift with the legs during the pass—remember, "less arms and more legs."
- Transfer weight from the back foot to the front foot.

Overhead Pass (Set)

All students should be able to execute an overhead pass. The overhead pass is used to pass volleyballs that do not have a great deal of force behind them. Stronger students are able to receive serve and play defense with an overhead pass, but younger students and beginning students use the overhead pass primarily for free balls and to set. The primary use of the overhead pass is to set the ball for a spike.

In executing an overhead pass or set, the player moves to the proper position underneath the volleyball. The hands should form a "basket" the size of the volleyball over the forehead in preparation for contacting the ball. The fingers of each hand should be relaxed and spread, and the hands should be slightly cupped. As the ball contacts the fingers, the player should extend the arms while lifting with the legs to direct the ball to the desired location.

TEACHING CUES

- Start in a medium body position; finish in a high body position.
- Make a "basket" over the forehead.
- All fingers contact the ball (see figure 17.4).
- Extend arms upward toward ceiling while lifting with the legs.

When setting the ball, the player should be positioned with the right shoulder facing the net, ready to set the pass from a teammate. The right foot should be slightly in front of the left, which assists in keeping the set from drifting over the net. As the set is made, a slight transfer of weight should occur from the left foot to the right foot. Also, the setter's hands should be on the sides of the ball rather than behind the ball, providing greater control of the set.

As students feel more comfortable with the overhead pass or set, they should absorb the momentum of the ball with their hands while the arms and legs provide the force to direct the ball to the hitter. Also, the setter should try to set the ball so that it has very little spin. The way to accomplish this is to finish the set without snapping the wrists.

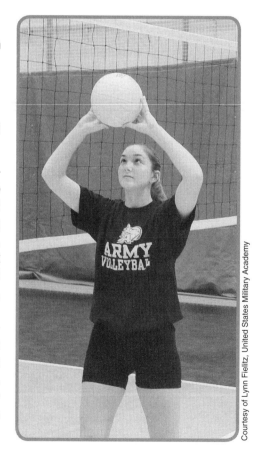

Courtesy of Lynn Fielitz, United States Military Academy

FIGURE 17.4 Overhead pass.

These additional points should be included in the teaching progression:

* Right foot remains forward.
* Hands are on the sides of the ball.
* Absorb impact with the hands and extend with the arms.

Serve

The serve should be thought of as a way to score points and to keep the opposing team off balance with serves to weak areas of the court. A serve that has a flatter trajectory is harder to pass than a serve that maintains a high arc. With the introduction of rally scoring, service errors are more costly in that the opposing team scores a point on each service error.

When introducing the serve, instructors should emphasize the toss because the majority of service errors are caused by a bad toss. Spend time working on the toss before working on actually serving the volleyball. A good toss is one that is directly in front of the serving arm and has enough height that the arm can swiftly contact the ball. The extra time spent on perfecting the toss pays dividends with good serves. Students who do not have the strength to serve overhand should use the underhand serve when first learning how to serve. Also, the service area can be moved closer to the net to facilitate success.

Underhand Serve

For beginning students, the serve should be kept simple. The footwork for the serve involves stepping with the foot opposite the serving hand (i.e., left foot for right-handed servers, right foot for left-handed servers). The ball is held in front of the serving arm and tossed only about 1 foot into the air. The arm swing should look like the swinging of a pendulum—straight backward and forward. The player contacts the ball with the heel of the hand in the center of the ball. The hand is open, with a stiff wrist. Finally, the server faces the direction of the intended serve. In this manner, the server can serve "the line" or "cross-court" by simply changing the way he or she is facing.

TEACHING CUES

* Maintain a high body position.
* Ball is in front of the serving arm.
* Toss is always low.
* Make the arm swing straight.
* Contact the ball with the heel of the hand.
* Player faces where the serve is to go.

Overhand Floater Serve

For high school students, the overhand floater serve is the easiest and most effective serve. Although some students may be able to perform a topspin or a jump serve or both, these skills are beyond the scope of this chapter. In utilizing the overhand floater serve, the server attempts to serve the ball so that it does not spin and actually floats side to side as it moves toward the receiving team. The concept is to get the volleyball to act the way a "knuckleball" does in baseball. If this serve is done correctly, the ball shows an erratic pattern as it moves toward the receiving team, thus making it much harder to pass successfully.

The footwork and body position are similar for the underhand and the overhand serve; but with the overhand serve, the serving arm is kept as high as possible so that the arm is fully extended on contact with the ball. The server begins the arm swing and toss at approximately the same time while stepping with the foot opposite to the serving arm. After the toss, the serving arm is brought forward quickly to contact the ball. The toss is 2 to 3 feet high and directly in front of the serving arm. As soon as contact is made with the ball, the serving hand is stopped so that the ball does not spin. Also, the back foot (the right foot for a right-handed server) stays in contact with the ground. By keeping the back foot in contact with the ground, the server maintains a more balanced position, which translates into more control on the serve. The back foot can be "dragged" behind the server but must remain in contact with the ground during the serve.

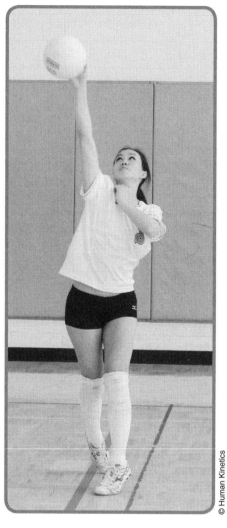

FIGURE 17.5 Overhand floater serve.

TEACHING CUES

- Maintain a high body position.
- Toss the ball 2 to 3 feet high and in front of the serving arm (see figure 17.5).
- Contact with the heel of the hand at the center of the ball.
- Stiff wrist is maintained and fingers are spread during contact with the ball.
- No follow-through.
- The back foot remains in contact with the ground.
- Player faces the direction of the serve.
- The arm is fully extended on contact with the ball.

Individual Serve Reception

Serve reception is an important aspect of volleyball because it is a method of initiating the offensive portion of the game. A good pass off of serve reception makes the entire offense work better. The rotation for the game should be set up such that the students who have the best serve reception skills are in position to receive the most serves.

Using the appropriate movement pattern, the passer should move as quickly as possible to the area where the ball is being served, completing the movement with a hop-step to a balanced position. Once in the correct position, the player should present the platform (the forearms) to the ball as soon as possible. Finally, depending on the location on the court, the passer needs to angle the platform so that the pass goes to the setter. The farther the passer is to the left side of the court, the greater the platform angle required to make a good pass to the setter.

TEACHING CUES

- Move into position as quickly as possible.
- Hop-step to a balanced position.
- Present platform early.
- Angle platform to target.

Above the Net

Volleyball is primarily played with the players' feet planted firmly on the ground. However, there are times when players leap high into the air to spike or block the ball.

Spike

The most exhilarating and challenging skill in volleyball is the spike. Many students would like to practice spiking for the entire class period. A good pass, set, and spike are things of beauty, and when done at a high level, grace in motion. In order to achieve a successful spike, players must bring many components together in a well-timed, fluid motion.

Although the spike is hard to master, the approach and the spike itself can be learned without the jump. As students progress in their ability, the jump can be added. Using the part–whole teaching progression, teach the approach without the arm swing and the arm swing without the spike approach. You can then combine the approach and the arm swing without using the volleyball. Once mastery of the individual components has been achieved, the entire approach, arm swing, and spike can be combined more effectively. While younger students often have difficulty with the jump, most high school students should be able to add the jump with the spike approach.

The spiker begins in the high body position, moves into a medium position during the takeoff phase of the approach, and becomes airborne for the contact of the spike. The spiker should start at the 3-meter line, depending on the size and age of the students. For a right-handed spiker, the approach should be from left to right. The strongest position for a right-handed player is spiking in the left front position of the court.

The simplest method of teaching the approach is to use three steps. For a right-handed spiker, begin with the left foot. The left step should be approximately 2 to 4 feet in length and should be toward the anticipated location of contact with the ball. The final two steps are a quick right-left, sometimes referred to as a "plant step," with the feet turned parallel to the net and an "arm's distance" away from the net. This plant step is important in that it transfers the horizontal momentum of the approach to the vertical lift needed for the spike. By turning the feet parallel to the net, the spiker does not "float" forward into the net but rather goes straight up in the jumping phase of the approach.

In the transition phase of the plant step, both arms should swing upward to assist in the jump. Using both arms increases the height of the jump as well as producing a better arm swing during the contact phase with the ball. Once the spiker is airborne, the nonhitting arm should point toward the volleyball while the hitting hand is simultaneously cocked near the ear. When the ball starts to descend, the nonhitting arm drops toward the ground as the hitting arm comes up and forward to contact the ball. The ball should be contacted slightly in front of the head, with the hitting arm fully extended in order to hit on top of the volleyball and direct it down into the opponent's court. The player should contact the ball with the heel of the hand while snapping the wrist on top of the ball in order to generate topspin. Once the ball is contacted, the arm swing should continue through the ball and stop by the spiker's waist. Lastly, the spiker should land evenly on both feet and absorb the landing by flexing the knees and ankles.

The timing of the approach varies with the player. Depending on the ability and speed of the player, the spiker should initiate the approach at the approximate peak of the set. This general rule varies depending on the speed of the approach, the height of the set, and the ability of the player. Timing the set is one of the most difficult aspects of the spike and takes a great deal of practice.

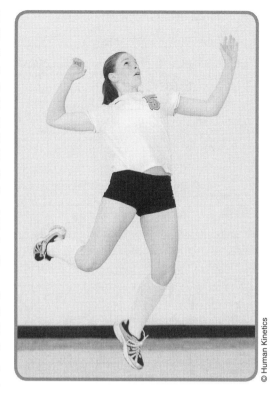

FIGURE 17.6 **Spike.**

© Human Kinetics

TEACHING CUES

- Start in the high body position.
- Start at the 3-meter line.
- Use a three-step approach.
- Begin approach when set reaches its peak.
- Take off from the medium body position.
- Swing both arms up.
- Point with the nonhitting arm and cock hitting hand by the ear (see figure 17.6).
- Contact ball at the peak of the jump, in front of the head and with hitting arm fully extended.
- Contact the ball with the heel of hand and snap the wrist.
- Follow through to the middle of the body.
- Land on both feet.

For more advanced students, sets in the middle of the court may be introduced. The height of the set can be lowered to provide a better opportunity for the spiker to be successful. The lower the set height, the less time the blockers have to adjust to the set and the greater opportunity the spiker has for a successful spike. Not only can set height be varied, but set location along the net can give an offensive advantage to the spiker.

Block

Blocking is the first line of defense for the team. If the volleyball is blocked at the net, defense is easy to play. An effective block may not always block the ball, but it does take away a particular area of the court and directs the ball toward the defenders. Blockers can reach as far as possible over the net as long as they do not contact the net or touch the opposing player.

Blockers should move into the proper position quickly and finish with a hop-step to a balanced position. If blockers are off balance when leaving the ground, either they jump into the net or their teammate, or they will not be in the correct position to block the ball. The blockers should be approximately 6 to 8 inches (15-20 centimeters) away from the net, and their shoulders and hips should be parallel with the net.

The ready position is usually one in which the hands are at shoulder level, and the preparatory arm swing for the jump should be to the side rather than forward and back. By swinging the arms to the side, blockers are able to utilize their arm swing to gain height on the block jump but avoid contacting the net. Blockers should leave the ground just after the spiker has left the ground so that they are at the peak of their jump at the same time the spiker is attacking the ball.

Once they are in the air, the blockers should extend their arms by bringing their biceps to their ears. Their hands should be about 6 inches (15 centimeters) apart so that the ball cannot fit in between the hands. The fingers should spread in order to take as much area of the court as possible away from the spiker. Utilizing two students on the block takes an additional area of the court and reduces the available shots for the spiker.

TEACHING CUES

- Maintain high body position.
- Move to position quickly.
- Finish with a hop-step to a balanced position.
- Body is parallel to the net.
- Hands begin at shoulder level, arm swing is to the side.
- Biceps to ears.
- Hands and fingers are spread (see figure 17.7).
- Blocker jumps after the spiker has jumped.

As the opposing player is spiking the ball, the blockers should reach over the net as far as possible. Also, the blockers' arms should be as close to the top of the net as possible without touching the net, so that the ball cannot fit in between the net and the blockers. The farther the blockers can reach over the net, the fewer options the hitter has for the spike. In addition, the palm of the outside hand of the blocker should be turned toward the middle back of the opponent's court. If a ball contacts the outside hand, it is directed into the court rather than out-of-bounds.

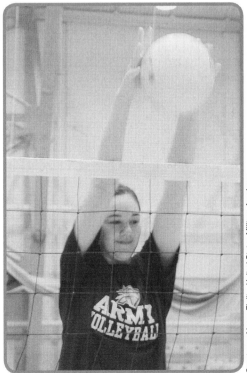

FIGURE 17.7 **Block.**

Courtesy of Lynn Fielitz, United States Military Academy

ADVANCED BLOCKING

* Blocker penetrates over the net.
* Blocker turns the outside hand toward the middle of the court.

Defense

Defense is the skill of keeping hard spikes from contacting the floor. Many students feel that once they move into defensive position, they never have to move from that spot, which is not the case. Getting into defensive position is the starting point of defense, and students will probably have to move to play the ball. The two most common mistakes are not being low enough when the ball is spiked and not being able to move from the defensive position to play a ball that is not hit directly to the defender.

Defense is one of the lowest positions used in volleyball, but students need to stay in this position for only a short period of time. The player should hop-step to a low body position with the weight on the balls of the feet. The shoulders should be slightly in front of the knees, and the knees should be slightly in front of the toes. In this position, students are able to move from the defensive position in case the ball is not hit directly at them. The platform should be ready to receive the spike and direct the ball to the setter. Since the spike comes with a great deal of force, little arm swing is needed to direct it to the setter.

Students need to get into the mind-set of going after every ball. Players should not hesitate when going for a ball. When playing defense, students need to react to the ball and must do everything possible to keep the ball from hitting the ground.

TEACHING CUES

* Maintain low body position (see figure 17.8).
* Have weight forward.
* Arms are in front of the body.
* Have the mind-set of going for every ball.

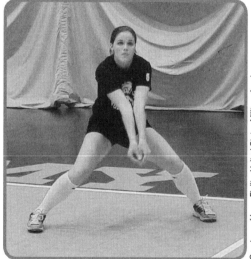

FIGURE 17.8 Defense.

Team Skills

Players depend on each other in order to be successful in the game of volleyball. On offense, the setter depends on the passers for a good pass, and the hitter depends on the setter to place the ball in the proper location for a good spike. On defense, the defenders depend on the blockers to block in the correct location and at the proper time, while the blockers depend on the defenders to be in the proper position around the block. Teamwork is the key to success in volleyball.

Team Serve Reception

The first and most important method of keeping the opposing team from scoring is through serve reception. Although one player is receiving the service, the other players have an active role in helping the passer make the best pass possible to the setter.

Students need to communicate using verbal and nonverbal cues as to which player passes the serve. The player who is actually passing the ball should call the ball "mine" while the other students are calling the ball in-bounds or out-of-bounds. In addition to the player receiving the serve, the surrounding students should also be moving toward the ball in case it floats away from the intended passer. The students located by the boundary lines should be telling the passer whether the ball is in-bounds or out-of-bounds as well.

Each player should want to pass every serve. This makes for more aggressive passers, and the serve should never hit the ground without someone attempting to make a play on the ball.

When using a five- or four-player serve receive formation (see figure 17.9), the front-row team members open up toward the passer when the serve is too high for them to successfully pass. Many front-row players tend to "duck," which confuses the back-row students and causes the serve to drop onto the court, thereby scoring a point for the opposing team.

TEACHING CUES

- Communication is key!
- Two or three students should move to pass every ball.
- Open passing lanes.

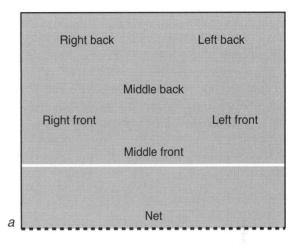

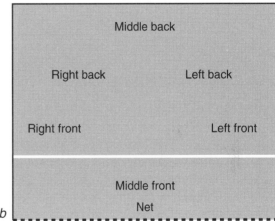

FIGURE 17.9 *(a)* Five-player serve receive formation or "W" formation; *(b)* four-player serve receive formation for advanced students.

Offense

Offense is the most exciting part of the game of volleyball. When the students are in the right position and successfully completing their roles, the entire offense works smoothly. Most offenses are designed to place key players such as the setter and the best hitters in the optimal positions for a successful offensive attack. The formations discussed in this section provide a good basis from which to start placing students in the optimal positions.

Six-Six Offense

A 6-6 offense utilizes every player as a setter and every player as a hitter. This is an easy offense to learn and is best utilized at early high school levels. The player in the middle front position acts as the setter in this type of offense, and the students in the left front and right front positions are the hitters. When the team gains the service and rotates one position, there is a new setter as well as two new hitters (see figure 17.10).

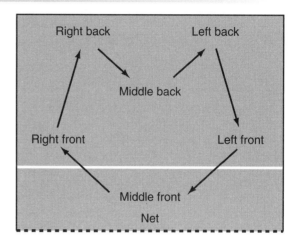

FIGURE 17.10 Rotation for new serve reception formation in 6-on-6 offense.

Four-Two Offense

A 4-2 offense is slightly more complicated and should be taught to high school students once they have mastered the 6-6 offense. A 4-2 offense has four hitters and two setters. The setters are opposite each other in the rotation so that whenever one setter rotates to the back row, the remaining setter rotates into the front row. Thus one setter is always in the front row to set the offense. This specialization allows the best two setters on the team always to set the volleyball. The hitters receive a more consistent set, and the students are not switching back and forth from setting to hitting. The students always know which players are setting and which players are hitters. There is more specialization by position in a 4-2 offense.

The serve receive formations for a 4-2 offense are diagrammed in figure 17.11, *a* through *c.* Only three formations are diagrammed because when the setter from the back row rotates into the front row, the serve receive formation is identical to the formation used with the setter who is rotated into the back row.

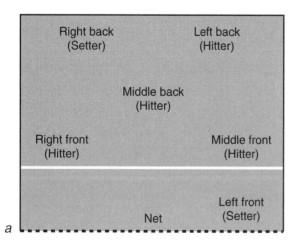

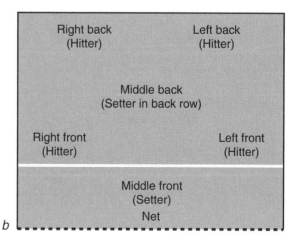

FIGURE 17.11 Four-two offense serve receive with setter in *(a)* left front, *(b)* middle front, and *(c)* right front.

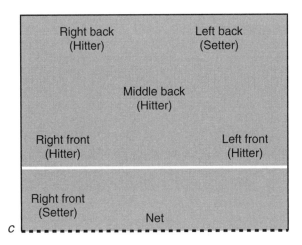

Right back
(Hitter)

Left back
(Setter)

Middle back
(Hitter)

Right front
(Hitter)

Left front
(Hitter)

Right front
(Setter)

Net

c

FIGURE 17.11   *(continued)*

Team Defense

Team defense relies on each player observing what is happening on the opponent's side of the court and responding by moving into the correct position in order to properly defend the ball when it is sent over the net. Each defense is designed to place the students in the optimal position to receive the ball. The location of the ball on the opponent's court determines the optimal placement of the defenders on the court. For a "free ball"—when the ball is passed easily over the net—the formation should be similar to the "W" serve receive formation and is shown in figure 17.9a.

Free Ball Positioning

The defensive formation for a free ball covers the majority of the court and provides the defensive team with ample opportunity to convert the free ball into a means of scoring points.

In team defense, the students need to watch what is happening on the other side of the net and must remember to move accordingly. The students should be in the proper position before the ball crosses the net. The defense must watch where the ball is set because the spiker must move to that location in order to successfully hit the ball. If the set is too far outside of the court, the options available to the spiker change accordingly. However, if the set is too far inside, the options for the spiker change and the defense must adjust their defensive positions. Defenders should automatically react to a ball that is hit in their direction. Calling the ball is also important on defense so that the other students know who will be making the initial contact with the ball.

TEACHING CUES

- Get into a defensive position quickly.
- Adjust to the position of the ball and the hitter's approach.
- React to the ball.

Player-Up Defense

A player-up or a six-up defense is an easy defense to learn. It is also a defense that covers the largest area of the court against teams that do a great deal of tipping the ball over the net and spiking the ball cross-court, as do most beginning teams. In a player-up defense, the player in the six position or the middle back position moves along the 3-meter line and behind the block in order to defend against any tips directed over the block. This player covers all the short tips. In each rotation, a new player becomes the person that defends against tips. Once students have learned the technique of switching positions, a designated back-row player can switch to the player-up position each time he or she is in the back row.

The other students are positioned to either block or defend against the spike. Since the majority of younger students spike the ball cross-court, this defense places two defenders in the cross-court digging position. The area of the court that is left open in this defense is the middle back portion of the court. In theory, the ball must go over the block to reach this particular part of the court, allowing the left and the right back more time to move to play a ball that is directed to that position.

The starting positions for a player-up defense are diagrammed in figure 17.12. These are only the starting positions, and the students must adjust according to the location of the set, the spiker's approach, the spiker's hitting tendencies, and the actual direction of the ball once it is contacted. See these diagrams for proper defensive positioning.

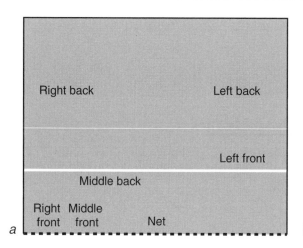
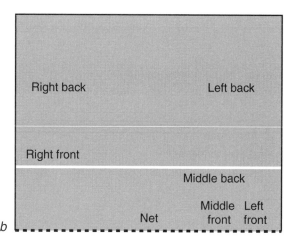

FIGURE 17.12　Player-up defense diagram for *(a)* left-side attack and *(b)* right-side attack.

Player-Back Defense

Player-back defense is used against teams that spike more than tip the volleyball. In this defense, the students start on the perimeter of the court and move into the court as required. The weak area of this defense is located directly behind the block, and players in the left or right back need to be aware of their responsibility to cover tips as well as spikes when playing defense. Also, this defense requires more mobility from the students since the pace of the game is usually quicker.

The starting positions for a player-back defense are diagrammed in figure 17.13. These are the starting positions only, and the students have to adjust depending on the location of the set, the spiker's approach, the spiker's hitting tendencies, and the

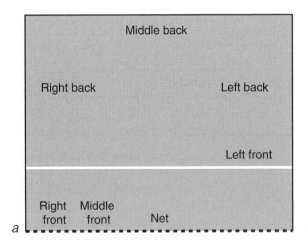 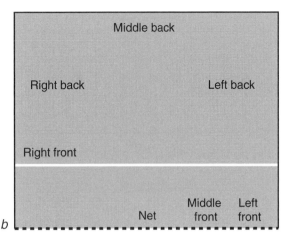

FIGURE 17.13 Player-back defense diagram for *(a)* left-side attack and *(b)* right-side attack.

actual direction of the ball once it is contacted. Remember that the back-row defensive player on the side of the spike is also responsible for covering for tips as well as spikes. If a team is tipping against this type of defense, the back-row player should be adjusted to a location behind the block to cover for the tip. However, this maneuver leaves another area of the court vulnerable to attack. Because the defense needs to "read" what the offense is doing, this defense is more difficult to play.

Wash Drills

Wash drills are used in volleyball to provide more play for the class than the typical scrimmage situation normally provides. The teacher or another student can actually conduct the wash drill, and the students get a maximum amount of playing time during these activities. Wash drills can be used for all skill levels and for all ages.

The problem with a typical scrimmage situation is that many students start the scrimmage with a service error. This does not allow students to contact the ball in that particular rotation. If many students are unable to serve the ball in-bounds, the students end up practicing rotating rather than playing. Of course, the service area can be moved into the court to facilitate more successful serves, but wash drills provide for more volleying of the ball.

In wash drills, the teacher is located off the court and beside the net, where he or she tosses free balls to either team. To initiate a wash drill, one player serves the ball into the opponent's court. This ball is played until one team wins the rally and one "little" point. The winning team then receives a free ball from the teacher, and the rally continues with this second ball until one team wins the rally

and receives one little point. The winning team receives a free ball from the teacher, and the rally again continues until one team wins the rally and receives one little point. The team that has scored at least two out of the three little points receives one "big" point, and that team rotates and starts the drill with a serve. If a team is having trouble in a particular rotation, they have several opportunities to practice in that rotation until they can win a big point and rotate. The wash drill can be continued until one team wins a specified number of big points or for a specified time.

For beginning students, a variation on the wash drill is to have the teacher initiate all balls as free balls, eliminating the serve. For more advanced students, the wash drill begins with the serve, but the teacher initiates the second and third balls with a "down ball" (a spike) to the winning team in order to increase the difficulty of the initial play. In addition, various scoring strategies can be instituted. If the teacher wants to emphasize good passes to the target, each time a team makes a good pass to the setter, that team gets a point in addition to winning the rally. For example, one team might score 6 points after three balls and the other team might score only 4 points, depending on the scoring scheme for the wash drill.

The most important aspect of the wash drill is to keep the students touching the volleyball and not practicing rotating. Wash drills are a great lead-up to actual games while still allowing the teacher to control the activity. Wash drills can even be used to stress particular aspects of the game and to have the students focus on scoring points by accomplishing the specified task.

Skills Assessment

Some of the skill assessments that may be conducted in a volleyball course are the underhand pass, forearm pass, overhand pass, overhead pass or set, and the serve. These assessments can help students determine how their volleyball skills have improved.

Underhand Pass Test

OBJECTIVE

Measures a player's ability to pass the volleyball into the designated target area using the underhand pass

DESCRIPTION

Each player receives 11 trials (trial 1 is practice only) to pass a tossed volleyball into a designated target area. Students pass five official (or "nonpractice") trials from one designated position and five official (nonpractice) trials from the second designated position. Students must pass the volleyball over a string and into the designated target area. The target area has values from 1 to 5 points (see figure 17.14).

SCORING

A player's score is determined by adding together the points awarded for each of the 10 official (nonpractice) trials. Students may catch poorly tossed balls and have those trials repeated. A trial in which the passed ball hits the string or lands outside of the scoring area counts as a trial but receives no points. The designated scorer uses his or her best judgment in awarding a score for each trial.

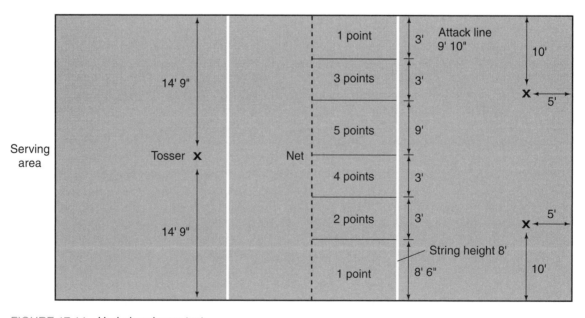

FIGURE 17.14   Underhand pass test.

Overhead Pass (Set) Test

OBJECTIVE

Measures a player's ability to set the volleyball into a designated target area

DESCRIPTION

Each player receives 11 trials (trial 1 is for practice only) to set a tossed volleyball from a designated position into a target area. Students must set the volleyball over a string and into the target area. The target area has values from 1 to 5 points (see figure 17.15).

SCORING

A player's score is determined by adding together the points awarded for each of the 10 official (nonpractice) trials. Students may catch poorly tossed balls and have those trials repeated. If the ball hits the string or the net, or lands outside of the scoring area, it counts as a trial and receives zero points. The designated scorer uses his or her best judgment in awarding a score for each trial.

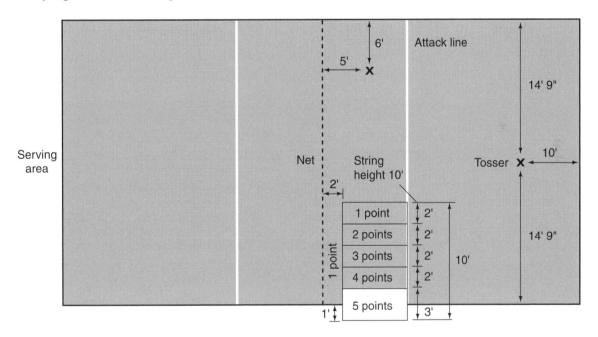

FIGURE 17.15   Overhead pass or set test.

Serve Test

OBJECTIVE

Measures a player's ability to serve the volleyball into a designated target area

DESCRIPTION

Each player receives 11 trials (trial 1 is a practice trial only) to serve a volleyball into a designated target area. Students must serve the volleyball over the net and into the designated target area. The target area has values ranging from 1 to 4 points (see figure 17.16).

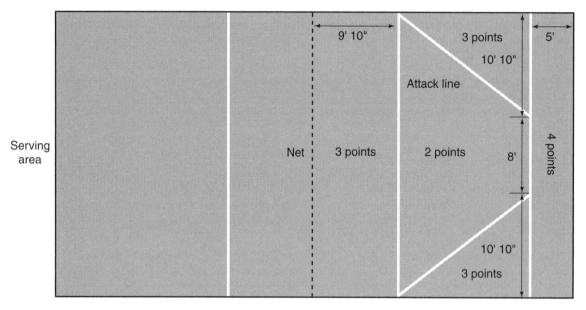

FIGURE 17.16 Serve test.

SCORING

A player's score is determined by adding together the points awarded for each of the 10 official (nonpractice) trials. A trial in which the served ball touches the antenna or an overhead object counts as a trial but receives no points. A trial in which the served ball lands outside of the scoring area counts as a trial but receives no points. The designated scorer uses his or her best judgment in awarding a score for each trial. See table 17.4 for a sample grade scale.

Table 17.4 Grade Scale for Skill Tests

Forearm pass	Overhead pass (set)	Serve	Points
43-50	48-50	34-40	100
38-42	45-47	32-33	96
33-37	42-44	30-31	92
29-32	39-41	28-29	88
25-28	37-38	26-27	84
23-24	35-36	25	80
20-22	32-34	23-24	76

Forearm pass	Overhead pass (set)	Serve	Points
16-19	28-31	21-22	72
11-15	24-27	18-20	68
6-10	20-23	15-17	64
0-5	0-19	0-14	60

Volleyball can be played and enjoyed by all ages and ability levels. The game incorporates teamwork and communication into an enjoyable activity for students. The volleyball course introduces students to the sport, develops individual skills, and fosters team play. Students can enjoy volleyball for many years into the future.

Key Terms

attack—Striking the ball, usually from above net-top level, into the opponent's court.

block—An attempt on the part of one or more players to intercept the ball as it passes over the net toward their court.

cross-court serve—A serve directed across the width of the court.

cross-court spike—A spike directed diagonally across the court.

dig—Passing a hard-struck attack, using one or both hands or arms, while standing, diving, rolling, or jumping.

dink—An attack in which a player strikes the ball using little force and his or her fingertips or fist.

down ball—An aggressive spike by a hitter who is standing on the ground. The down ball is a more aggressive attack than a free ball, but is not as forceful as a spike since the hitter does not jump when hitting the ball.

floater serve—A serve with little or no spin that moves in an erratic path. Floating serves are hit "center of mass" and with very little follow-through.

forearm pass—Playing the ball off of the forearms in an underhand motion. This is the best way to pass a served ball. It is used to pass or dig spikes and balls played close to the court surface.

foul—A failure to play the ball in accordance with the rules.

free ball—A ball called by the defending team when the opposing team cannot effectively attack their third

touch. This signals the defending team's members to assume a serve reception formation to play the ball. Most teams have preselected plays designated for use in free ball situations.

line serve—A serve directed straight ahead of the server.

line spike—A spike directed toward the opponent's sideline, closest to the attacker.

out-of-bounds—Referring to a ball that touches a net antenna, any surface outside the court, or any surface outside the markers on the net antennas, or that passes over the net not entirely between the net antennas.

overhead pass (set)—Playing the ball off of the fingertips from in front of the forehead. The thumb and forefingers of both hands must face in toward one another on a two-handed set.

overlap—A foul committed when players are positioned in incorrect rotational order as the ball is served. No player may infringe on the territory of an immediately adjacent player.

pass—The controlled movement of the ball from one player to another player on the same team.

playover—Putting the ball into play without awarding a point for the preceding play.

roll—A defensive technique used to increase a player's lateral range of motion on the court.

roll shot—A spike hit with less than maximum force to gain a tactical advantage (an off-speed shot).

seam—An area on the court between two serve receivers or defenders. Servers and attackers may try to serve or hit the ball into a seam.

serve—The technique used to put the ball into play. Serves are classified in several ways. They are classified as underhand or overhead serves; when classified by how they move after being struck, they are classified as floater serves or spinning serves.

spike—An attack in which the ball is forcefully struck with an open hand from above net-top level.

Reference

Lenberg, K. ed., (2006). *2006-2007 domestic competition regulations as presented by USA Volleyball.* Boulder, CO: Johnson Printing.

Suggested Readings

American Sport Education Program. (2001). *Coaching youth volleyball.* (3rd ed.). Champaign, IL: Human Kinetics.

Ashton International Media, Inc. (2003). *Volleyball Magazine.* www.volleyballmag.com.

Bertucci, B., & Bertucci, T. (1985). *Championship volleyball drills: Volume 2, Combination and complex training.* Champaign, IL: Leisure Press.

Bertucci, B., & Hippolyte, R. (1984). *Championship volleyball drills: Volume 1, Individual skill training.* Champaign, IL: Leisure Press.

Dearing, J. (2003). *Volleyball fundamentals: A better way to learn the basics.* Champaign, IL: Human Kinetics.

Liskevych, T. (2002). Dominating defensive systems. In D. Shondell & C. Reynaud (Eds.), *The volleyball coaching bible,* 282-299. Champaign, IL: Human Kinetics.

Shondell, S. (2002). Receiving serves. In D. Shondell & C. Reynaud (Eds.), *The volleyball coaching bible,* 178-185. Champaign, IL: Human Kinetics.

Shondell, D., & Reynaud, C. (Eds.). (2002). *The volleyball coaching bible.* Champaign, IL: Human Kinetics.

Suwara, R. (2002). Blocking. In D. Shondell & C. Reynaud (Eds.), *The volleyball coaching bible,* 224-257. Champaign, IL: Human Kinetics.

Volleyball course manual. West Point, NY: U.S. Military Academy, Department of Physical Education.

Wise, M. (Ed.). (1999). *Volleyball drills for champions.* Champaign, IL: Human Kinetics.

Web Resources

www.nfhs.org

www.nagws.org

www.usavolleyball.org

www.usma.edu/dpe/courses/Volleyball/vbhome.htm

Sport-Specific Organizations

The main governing body for volleyball in the United States is USA Volleyball (USAV), which is recognized by the Federation International de Volleyball (FIVB) and by the United States Olympic Committee (USOC). The USAV conducts national championships at all levels of competition for ages 10 to 80. Most championships are conducted from May to July of each year at various locations throughout the United States. In addition, the USAV is responsible for the correct implementation and interpretation of rules for all tournament play. These rules are updated yearly. National and Olympic teams are selected by the USAV, which also provides the coaching staff and training facilities. Membership in the USAV is required to participate in sponsored tournaments and in the national championships.

USA Volleyball
715 S. Circle Drive
Colorado Springs, CO 80910
719-228-6800
Fax: 719-228-6899
Information line: 888-786-5539
www.usavolleyball.org

High school volleyball throughout the United States is governed by the National Federation of State High School Associations (NFHS). The NFHS consists of high school athletic and activity associations throughout the 50 states and in the District of Columbia. Each state association implements the specific rules and certifies the volleyball officials for the respective state.

National Federation of State High Schools
P.O. Box 690
Indianapolis, IN 46206
317-972-6900
Fax: 317-822-5700
www.nfhs.org

Group Fitness

Susan Tendy

Group fitness is a term that encompasses activities in what were formerly termed aerobics classes. The aspect that separates group fitness classes from individual personal workouts is the use of music as the factor that determines and enhances exercise intensity. This is accomplished via control of the speed of the rhythm to which people exercise. Style of music can also be used to set the tone of the class and to motivate the exercisers. For example, a yoga class might employ soothing or soft music to create a relaxed state. A high-cardio aerobics class would need to use faster, high-energy music to mentally and physically energize the participants.

This area includes a wide spectrum of activities. The modalities used in today's group fitness settings include the still-popular aerobics classes, using little or no equipment and employing low-impact, high-cardio, or floor-work activities or some combination of these. There are also step aerobics classes, which have increased in popularity in recent years and have given new meaning to the Harvard Step Test. These classes employ bench stepping and plyometric activities and have been extremely well received. More recently, martial arts–based boxing or kick boxing classes have come to the forefront as very popular conditioning programs that appeal to a large segment of the population.

A national survey that tracked fitness programs over the five-year period from 1992 to 1997 showed which classes were most often requested by members. Kick boxing classes increased by an average of 34 percent across the nation; spinning classes, involving groups exercising as a unit on stationary bikes, increased by 24 percent nationally. Of the programs surveyed, 69 percent offered group circuit training classes. Yoga was the most popular of the new offerings, with 85 percent of the programs surveyed offering yoga-based activities. Pilates evolved from a virtually unknown activity to a 63 percent offering across the country, and water fitness classes maintained their popularity with a 56 percent offering (Ryan, 2003).

The use of music as the key to the activity level of these types of classes is an interesting concept. It allows all participants to work at their own level while "staying with the group." No one is left behind as might happen in a group run or a group cycling trip. This can be a boost to one's self esteem at precisely the time it is needed, when the usual self-doubts about exercise ability kick in. The camaraderie that often develops under the direction of a professionally certified group fitness leader can make a big difference in one's commitment to a lifetime of fitness.

Purpose of the Course

The purpose of our Group Fitness course is to introduce our students to the rapidly expanding world of group fitness classes, introduce them to various activities, and teach them how to lead a group of students safely and effectively. Our students have already taken two Fitness Leadership courses and have a working knowledge of the principles of exercise. We apply this knowledge as we focus on their presentation and leadership skills in a group exercise setting. The students experience music as the key variable concept in the course, and this requires a focus on the rhythmic components that affect exercise intensity. As the course progresses, students get the opportunity to develop and demonstrate their teaching methodology and class-planning abilities.

We also encourage our students to continue to explore and expand their experience in the field of group fitness outside the course by volunteering to teach classes involving training in a group setting with their intramural, club, or varsity athletic team.

To meet specific course goals, students must demonstrate the following:

- The leadership, presentation skills, and technical background necessary to conduct safe, effective, and motivational group exercise classes
- Integration of the components of rhythm, music, and movement
- Awareness of the latest innovative techniques that use music as the controlling factor to improve physical fitness
- Knowledge of planning and goal-setting techniques as evidenced by preparation of a 45-minute written lesson plan
- The ability to use various exercise modes and workout patterns
- Safety awareness while conducting fitness activities

Instructional Area

There are many factors to consider in the selection of an appropriate teaching area. Ventilation and temperature control are important: A closed room with no windows and poor ventilation will foster the growth of mold and bacteria on matted floors, as well as on the equipment handled by students. A standing floor fan can be used in the doorway to aid in air exchange. Floor surface is a second consideration. A suspended hardwood floor allowing for absorption on impact, as opposed to a cement floor covered with carpet, is ideal. A matted floor as found in wrestling or gymnastics teaching areas is ideal for classes that involve high impact or a lot of floor work. Cleanliness of these surfaces is critical. Equally important is the size of your room, which will predetermine the number of students allowed in the teaching area. Students need to be able to take two large steps in any direction, although many sport conditioning classes require more space. If you have a large class, a raised platform enhances teacher visibility. If you have the facility, aqua classes are extremely popular and can greatly add to the variety of conditioning activities.

Equipment

The type and amount of equipment required for group exercise will depend on the specific activity being taught. Group exercise is an activity that can be conducted using little or no equipment or specific equipment for each student.

Sound Equipment

A group exercise class can be well conducted with only one item on your equipment list: a stereo player and sound system of some type. A portable CD or tape player is a good investment, as it allows the class to move from an exercise room location to an aquatics location, or even to an outdoor location. However, many instructors and students desire a more permanent classroom setup, which can be constructed as follows:

1. Obtain a multidisc CD player.
2. Invest in a wireless microphone or headset for the instructor.
3. Utilize a mixer that enables the instructor to vary the sound balance between the music and the instructor's voice.
4. Obtain two to four speakers and permanently mount them in each corner of the room or on the ceiling.

Exercise Equipment

Portable mats will greatly enhance the ability of students to perform floor-work activities involving abdominal, upper body, or kneeling exercises. Simple circuit stations can be set up with a minimal amount of equipment, such as jump ropes, towels, hand weights, and a bench step. Obtaining bench steps for an entire class would be an ideal goal to work toward, as bench step aerobics is very popular. Aqua classes can use flotation equipment such as aqua jogging vests, pool noodles, hand fins, and Styrofoam dumbbells. Kick boxing classes can incorporate boxing gloves, hitting dummies, or simple hand wraps.

Clothing and Personal Equipment

Fashion trends of the day often dictate the types of attire students will wear when participating in exercise classes. Over the years, workout clothing styles have changed from dance-style to more athletic attire as people cross-train from activity to activity. The following are some issues that one should address when recommending the appropriate clothing for a group fitness class.

Clothing Clothing worn during class should allow the body to breathe, as the days of the rubber dehydration suit are long gone. Cotton T-shirts and shorts have replaced the leotard as the standard in exercise wear, as these items are common, comfortable, and affordable.

Footwear Shoes worn during class should be supportive and representative of the activity level of the exerciser. Participants in high-cardio aerobics activities should wear footwear specifically designed for that activity. Running shoes are not good for these classes, as they are made for forward movement only and are not designed for lateral or backward motion support.

Water Bottle A water bottle should be at the very top of a student's equipment list, as hydration is important during exercise. Students should be allowed to bring their water bottle inside the teaching area and should be allowed to hydrate as needed. A water fountain in the area should be identified in case members of the class need to refill their water bottles.

Risk Management

There are many considerations in the realm of risk management, only some of which may apply while your teaching activity is in progress. Conditions such as overuse or prior injury or illness develop outside your purview. For this reason, a prescreening form for each student is necessary.

In the interests of student privacy, your school should have a medical screening form on file that indicates a student's ability to partake in strenuous events. Your part in this process may be a simple "OK" for each student from your administrative office. If you teach in a private setting, for example in home schooling or private classes, consider a medical clearance and release form as part of the general physical education participation requirement, which is signed by both a student's parent or guardian and his or her physician. This form should describe the types of activities to be conducted and should include a statement of potential risks. When screening these forms, every instructor may need to seriously weigh a student's prior medical history versus his or her risk potential before permitting participation in the class. If you are not sure whether your school or setting has liability protection for such activities, see your school's attorney for further guidance.

An instructor certification or review course that keeps instructors informed of the latest issues and trends in teaching methodology is highly recommended for all aerobics teachers so that they may refresh their skills and keep abreast of new trends in exercise activities. Technical skills and pedagogical talent can best be improved under the mentorship of an experienced instructor-trainer. A list of certifying agencies appears at the end of this chapter.

It is every instructor's professional responsibility to establish a proactive approach to injury prevention. Developing a list of potential risk factors and determining the reduction strategies needed to avoid these risks establish not only an educated approach to injury prevention for instructors and students alike, but also a more satisfactory class environment. Table 18.1 lists potential areas of concern and strategies that can be initiated to avoid these dangers.

Skills and Techniques

A number of basic activity themes can be taught as individual units.

Low-Impact Movements and Combinations

Low-impact classes involve movements that are of low intensity and moderate speed, with students keeping at least one foot on the ground at all

Table 18.1 Possible Risks in Group Fitness

Risk identification	Reduction strategies
Muscle strains and ligament sprains	• Teach and enforce warm-up, cool-down, body alignment, and technique as taught in class. • Reinforce proper footwear for class. • Ensure adequate space between students during exercising or active learning drills. • Always check the connecting mat edges for adequate taping (no gaps).
Skin infections	• Ensure proper sanitizing of mats and dry all wet spots prior to class. • Students must report any new or unexplained skin abnormalities (rash, open wounds, infections).
Aggravation of a prior injury	• Any student with a history of injury or a newly acquired injury or ailment will not be able to participate until medically cleared.
Overuse injuries	• Reemphasize the importance of proper technique and body alignment during exercise. • The class is noncompetitive; therefore each student is reminded to work at his or her own level. • Teach and enforce the purpose of each of the class components, as well as the "bell curve" method of exercise intensity and progression.
Dehydration	• Maintain proper room temperature. • Inform students of the location of water fountains and have them use these as needed during class. All students should bring a water bottle to class as well. • Educate as to the need for continuous hydration before, during, and after class.
Clothing	• Clothing should be light and loose, allowing the body to breathe. • Rubber suits designed to make the body sweat must never be worn.

times. To raise the heart rate to a higher training threshold, these classes use larger arm and major muscle movements. A simple rating of perceived exertion (RPE) technique can be used to determine heart rate increase.

Agility and High-Cardiovascular Movements and Combinations

Sessions geared toward agility and more intense cardiovascular work are designed to be more active and employ large arm and major muscle movements for the majority of the class time. The exercises often involve running, skipping, and other movements requiring both feet to leave the ground simultaneously. The purpose is to raise the heart rate to the recommended training zone.

Step Class Activities

Step classes use a bench or a raised box that allows students to step up and down while varying the pattern of their approaches to the bench. Exercises may include low- or high-cardio movements or a combination of both.

Circuit Activities

Circuit classes allow students to move from station to station to perform specific exercises while music is playing. A preset time pattern of music determines the signal for the activity, and the signal to change stations is given when no music is playing. These classes are very popular with athletic teams, as they can be designed using sport-specific exercises.

Aqua Aerobics

In an aqua class, students use the buoyant qualities of the water as both supportive and resistive components of exercise. Both shallow- and deep-water exercises can be incorporated into this type of activity, depending on the ability level of the class.

Fitness Boxing Classes

In fitness boxing classes, martial arts and self-defense techniques are incorporated into an exercise-to-music training regimen. These sport-specific movements, borrowed from various combative activities, provide an exercise opportunity that has become very popular.

Course Overview

Table 18.2 summarizes six major skill themes that can be modified for use as separate lessons or as lesson units within your school setting. In order for students to become proficient in these activities, these six basic lessons should be repeated at least one more time for a 12-lesson unit, or as many as three times each for an 18-lesson unit.

Many activities can be taught by the instructor in a simple "follow the leader" aerobic exercise class. The following group fitness lessons include teaching and leadership opportunities through utilization of a student checklist and small-group and peer teaching activities (see page 401). However, these segments can be eliminated if the instructor plans to lead the entire class.

Sample Lesson Plans

The following lessons are examples of the way in which the Group Fitness course is conducted at West Point. Typically a lesson includes (1) student accountability, (2) introduction to new movements and combinations, (3) demonstration, (4) safety reminders, (5) practice, (6) and cool-down and class closure.

Table 18.2 Overview of Group Fitness Lessons

Lesson	Skill theme	Activities
1	Low-impact movements and combinations	• March: stationary, forward, or backward • Toe tap steps: front, side, or rear • Heel tap steps • Side-to-side step touch • Step and reach: single or double arm • Step and punch: single or double arm • Knee lifts • Half squats • Lunges • Grapevine
2	Agility and high-cardio movements and combinations	• Jumping jacks (limit: two in a row) • Pony or triple step • Step kicks • Jog in place • Hopscotch • Hustle
3	Step class activities*	Directional approaches to the step: • Front • Side • Top • Astride • End • Corner

(continued)

Table 18.2 *(continued)*

Lesson	Skill theme	Activities
4	Circuit activities	With partner or in small groups: • Push-ups • Sit-ups • Bench step movements • Biceps curls • Triceps extensions • Lunges • Modified squats • Rope skipping • Agility footwork drills • Flexibility stations
5	Water fitness	• Basic station exercises • Interval work • Circuit training • Relays and games
6	Fitness boxing	• Jab • Hook • Cross • Uppercut • Bob and weave • Speed bag • Boxer's shuffle

*The following Web page, which contains video clips of many step class skills, can be useful to both students and instructors: www.usma.edu/dpe/courses/Exercise%20Leadership/step/main01.htm.

Low-Impact Movements and Combinations

SEQUENCE (45-MINUTE CLASS)

1. Student accountability.
2. Introduce the principles of low-impact movements and combinations (1 minute).
3. Warm-up exercises employing minor activity and preaerobic stretching (5 minutes).
4. Demonstrate low-impact movements and combinations: Teacher models proper technique (2 minutes).
5. Review key safety and instructional cues while demonstrating (2 minutes).
6. Use a student checklist to reinforce instructional cues during instructor-directed learning activity (11 minutes).
7. Student learning activities:
   - Small-group practice, instruction, and feedback (11 minutes).
   - Partner-to-partner practice, instruction, and feedback (11 minutes).

GROUP FITNESS STUDENT CHECKLIST

Affording students peer-teaching experiences will help make them better learners. These activities can be introduced by utilizing a student checklist during small group practice sessions. This tool will guide proper performance through reinforced instructional cues and feedback among students. The following list presents some of the elements of presentation that can be applied to any of the skills listed in each lesson.

Name	Comments
A. Body language	
1. Mirror image	
2. Sharp movements	
3. Animated expression (smile)	
4. Commanding presence and voice	
B. Technical skills	
1. Proper cadence and rhythm	
2. Verbal cueing and efficiency	
3. Appropriate and safe movements	
4. Transitions/Choreography	
C. Organization	
1. Logical progression and build-up	
2. Group control	
3. Directional balance (symmetrical)	
4. Variety and creativity	

From M. LeBoeuf and L. Butler, eds., 2008, *Fit & active* (Champaign, IL: Human Kinetics).

8. Cool-down and class closure: review of proper techniques, instructional cues, questions (2 minutes).

TEACHING CUES

- Moderate music speed—approximately 120 to 130 beats per minute.
- Use music during active warm-up, low-impact, and cool-down phases of the class.
- Students should maintain one foot in contact with the ground at all times.
- Use the mirror image for the class.
- Students should maintain sharp movements.

SUGGESTED LEARNING ACTIVITIES

The following steps or moves can be combined in many ways for low-impact activities:

- March: stationary, forward, or backward
- Toe tap steps: front, side, or rear
- Heel tap steps
- Side-to-side step touch
- Step and reach: single or double arm
- Step and punch: single or double arm
- Knee lifts
- Half squats
- Lunges
- Grapevine

Agility and High-Cardiovascular Movements and Combinations

SEQUENCE (45-MINUTE CLASS)

1. Introduce the principles of agility and high-cardiovascular movements and combinations (1 minute).
2. Instruct class in warm-up exercises employing introductory lead-up activities and preaerobic stretching (5 minutes).
3. Lead class in agility and high-cardiovascular movements and combinations: Teacher models proper technique (2 minutes).
4. Review key safety and instructional cues during participation (2 minutes).
5. Use a student checklist to reinforce instructional cues during instructor-directed learning activity (11 minutes).
6. Student learning activities:
   - Small-group practice, suggested learning activities, instruction, and feedback (11 minutes).
   - Partner-to-partner practice, instruction, and feedback (11 minutes).
7. Cool-down and class closure: review of proper techniques, instructional cues, questions (2 minutes).

TEACHING CUES

- Faster music speed—approximately 130 to 150 beats per minute.
- Play music during the target heart rate training portion of the class.
- Both feet may leave the ground simultaneously during certain activities.
- Limit jumping activities such as jumping jacks to a preset minimum number.

SUGGESTED LEARNING ACTIVITIES

The following steps or moves can be combined in many ways for high-cardio activities:
- Jumping jacks (limit: no more than two in consecutive order)
- Pony or triple step
- Step kicks
- Jog in place
- Hopscotch
- Hustle

Bench Step Class Activities

The following Web page contains video clips of many step skills that instructors and students may find useful: www.usma.edu/dpe/courses/Exercise%20Leadership/step/main01.htm.

SEQUENCE (45-MINUTE CLASS)

1. Introduce the principles of bench stepping movements and combinations (1 minute).
2. Instruct class in warm-up exercises employing bench step activity–specific lead-up activities and stretching (5 minutes).

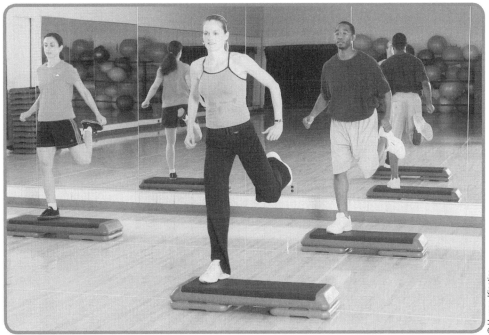

© Human Kinetics

A bench step class in action.

3. Lead class in the six basic directional approaches (front, side, top, astride, end, and corner) involved in bench step movements and combinations: Teacher models proper technique (2 minutes).

4. Review key safety and instructional cues during participation (2 minutes).

5. Use a student checklist to reinforce instructional cues during instructor-directed learning activities (11 minutes).

6. Student learning activities:
   – Small-group practices or suggested learning activities, instruction, and feedback (11 minutes).
   – Partner-to-partner practice, instruction, and feedback (11 minutes).

7. Cool-down and class closure: review of proper techniques, instructional cues, questions (2 minutes).

TEACHING CUES

- Recommended music speed—approximately 125 to 130 beats per minute.
- Class should be positioned so that all steps are visible to the instructor.
- Step height should not exceed 8 inches (20 centimeters)—one platform and two blocks.
- Hands on hips signals students to be ready for a change of pattern.
- Students step up on the center of the step.
- Heel lands, with entire foot, on the top of the step.
- Students should glance at the platform approximately every 4 seconds for safety purposes.
- Toe-ball-heel recovery on the ground.
- Students should maintain a natural body lean—not bend at the waist.
- In case of confusion, students should go back to the basic step.

SUGGESTED LEARNING ACTIVITIES

Practice different directional approaches to the step:
- Front
- Side
- Top
- Astride
- End
- Corner

Circuit Activities

SEQUENCE (45-MINUTE CLASS)

1. Introduce the principles of circuit training movements (2 minutes).

2. Lead class through a brief orientation to the movements for the prearranged circuit stations: Teacher models proper technique (5 minutes).
   – Review key safety and instructional cues while demonstrating.
   – Refer to and use diagrams and pictures to reinforce instructional cues during subsequent learning activity.

3. Instruct class in warm-up exercises employing circuit-specific lead-up and stretching movements (5 minutes).

4. Student learning activities (30 minutes):
   – Organize class into small groups and have students monitor each other.
   – Ensure that class rotates in the same direction after each station.
   – Instructor provides overall monitoring and feedback.

5. Cool-down and class closure: review of proper techniques, instructional cues, questions (3 minutes).

TEACHING CUES

- Music is used as a timer: Silence signals student rotation to the next station.
- Recommended time per station: approximately 1 minute. You may decide to vary this for extra rounds; less time (e.g., 30 seconds) for additional rounds.
- Recommended time between stations: approximately 10 seconds. Younger age groups may need more time to transition to the next station and understand the upcoming task. Remember that less time between stations means less rest for the heart, which equates to more cardiovascular training.
- Each station should be explained individually before activity begins; prepositioned charts will help remind exercisers as they approach each station during the class.
- Introduce warm-up and stretching activities.
- Students divide into groups at each station.
- Organize activities so as to alternate between opposing muscle groups or types of activities.

SUGGESTED LEARNING ACTIVITIES

The following are examples of stations that can be set up so that students rotate with a partner or in small groups:

- Push-ups
- Sit-ups
- Bench step movements
- Biceps curls
- Triceps extensions
- Lunges
- Squats
- Rope skipping
- Agility footwork drills
- Flexibility stations

Water Fitness Activities

SEQUENCE (45-MINUTE CLASS)

1. Introduce the principles of water fitness as an aerobic activity (2 minutes).
2. Relate to prior circuit training activity on land as a frame of reference.

3. Organize class into safety partners who will monitor each other.

4. Demonstrate, with class observing from the deck, the specific water fitness skills to be used that day: Teacher models proper technique (5 minutes).
   - Review key safety and instructional cues while demonstrating.
   - Demonstrate safe pool entry and exit procedures.

5. Class enters pool: Instruct class in warm-up exercises employing activity-specific lead-up and stretching movements (5 minutes).

6. Student learning activities (30 minutes):
   - Provide overall monitoring and feedback at pool-deck level.
   - Refer to and use large diagrams or large movements to reinforce instructional cues and for dealing with auditory impairment due to water environment during subsequent learning activity.

7. Cool-down and class closure: review of proper techniques, instructional cues, questions (3 minutes).

TEACHING CUES

The recommended music speed is approximately 135 beats per minute; however, music speed does not need to be a factor. You can use the music as a timing monitor, as in the circuit class, and as a motivational addition to the atmosphere.

Safety

- Students need to keep track of their swimming partners.
- Students should not exceed their limits.
- Swimmers should stay within arm's length of the pool wall, if necessary.
- Nonswimmers should stay in shallow water.
- Instructors should not permit horseplay in the water.

How to Increase Exercise Intensity

- Start and stop against inertia and momentum.
- Change direction.
- Change speed.
- Apply more force to the movement.
- Increase frontal resistance through body position changes.
- Incorporate travel movements.
- Include moves that use both the arms and the legs and utilize long levers.
- Add equipment as a flotation aid or a workout challenge.
- Change the modality of the exercise session:
  - Basic exercises: The group works together under the direction of the instructor.
  - Interval work: Students do more intense timed elements with rest or cool-down between sets.
  - Circuit training: Students work in pairs or small groups, change stations on a prearranged signal, and perform exercises at each station.
  - Relays: Age- and ability-appropriate races add the element of teamwork and fun.

SUGGESTED LEARNING ACTIVITIES

Each exercise can be performed for 30 seconds, more or less depending on the ability of the class. Use the "aqua jog" movement as a gentle resting activity. The cycle can be repeated, with shorter segments, if time allows. The following suggestions can help the students visualize exactly what the exercises should look like. They are merely suggestions, and any movements that approximate the activity will work well.

- Warm-up activity—moderate movements for 3 to 5 minutes
- Sprint running
- Aqua jog
- Strides
- Flutter kick (side of pool)
- Aqua jog
- Cross-country skier
- Push away–pull back (side of pool)
- Aqua jog
- Gutter push-ups (side of pool or top deck)
- Aqua jog
- Twisting hips (side of pool)
- Aqua jog
- Gutter dips (side of pool or top deck)
- Aqua jog
- Tread water—chest squeeze
- Front flutter kicks (side of pool)
- Sprint run
- Cool-down: moderate aqua jog for 3 to 5 minutes

Fitness Boxing Activities

SEQUENCE (45-MINUTE CLASS)

1. Introduce the principles of fitness boxing as an aerobic activity (2 minutes).
2. Instruct class in warm-up exercises employing activity-specific lead-up and stretching movements (5 minutes).
3. Student learning activities:
   - Lead class through a brief orientation, with class participation, to the basic punch and footwork and punch combinations: Teacher models proper technique (15 minutes).
     - Safety and instructional cues: Knees are slightly bent, and students should not "lock out" (hyperextend) the elbow joint during a punch.
     - Basic body position: Feet are shoulder-width apart; fists, held loosely, cover the nose and cheeks.

- Warm-up: Students marching with arm movements, sidestep with hands held guarding the face, do squats with arm raises.
- Basic boxing footwork movements: sidestep—right to left, forward and back.
- Basic boxing punches: jab, cross, hook, uppercut.
- Basic kicks: front kick, side kick, roundhouse kick.
- Other movements: bob and weave, speed bag, boxer's shuffle.
  - Incorporate combinations of steps and punches, alternating arms (15 minutes):
    - Up and back step with jab.
    - Up and back step with jab and cross.
    - Up and back step with jab, cross, hook.
    - Up and back step with jab, cross, hook, uppercut.
  - Combine bob and weave, speed bag, and boxer's shuffle into the combinations just listed (5 minutes).
  4. Cool-down and closure: review of proper techniques, instructional cues, questions (3 minutes).

TEACHING CUES

- Recommended music speed—approximately 130 to 135 beats per minute.
- Preliminary review of each punch and kick—proper technique and cueing:
  - Moderate music speed at 123 to 128 beats per minute will enhance range of motion.
  - Encourage all students to exercise at their own limits (avoid high kicks, overpunching).
- Body position and alignment (ready position):
  - Feet shoulder-width apart, toes pointing forward.
  - Knees "soft" or slightly bent.
  - Abdominal muscles tight, tailbone pointing to the floor.
  - Shoulders rolled forward slightly.
  - Hands in a fist (not clenched tightly), thumbs out, palms facing each other.
  - Hold elbows in and fists just below eye level. Do not let hands drop below the chin.

SUGGESTED LEARNING ACTIVITIES

Introduce basic movements that use familiar boxing terminology:

- Jab: a punch with the lead arm (closest to an imaginary opponent) and off of the front foot
- Cross: a punch used off of the rear foot; moves across the body with the arm farthest away from the opponent
- Hook: a punch coming from the lead arm and lead leg; comes from the side and is aimed at an imaginary opponent's cheek
- Uppercut: a punch moving upward, with the palm facing in, aimed at an imaginary opponent's chin

- Sidestep: an alternating step-tap movement from side to side or front to back
- Front kick: a kick that can be done from the front leg—lifting the knee first (chambering) and then extending the foot forward, keeping the leg slightly bent at extension
- Side kick: a kick that can be done by chambering (lifting) the hip and kicking out sideward
- Roundhouse: a kick that begins with extending the leg to the side, then moving toward the front, aiming the instep at an imaginary opponent
- Bob and weave: a movement from side to side employing slight squat movements that lower the upper body to the front and side
- Speed bag: small, quick circular movements in the air as if one were hitting a punching bag numerous times
- Boxer's shuffle: slight jumps side to side or up and back

Key Terms

active warm-up—Low-impact activities that allow the heart rate to gradually increase and the body temperature to gradually warm up so as to prevent injury during activity.

cool-down—Activities that allow the heart rate and body temperature to gradually return to normal.

fitness boxing—Activities that incorporate martial arts and aerobic fitness movements.

high-cardio activity—Activities that employ major muscle movements, often allowing both feet to leave the ground (as in running), that are designed to elevate the heart rate to a higher training zone.

low impact—Activities that minimize foot impact, with one foot always on the ground.

postaerobic stretch—Stretching activities after an aerobic workout, designed to relax and elongate muscles that have been forcefully contracted during exercise.

preaerobic stretch—Mild stretching activities before an aerobic workout that are designed primarily to prevent injury.

spinning classes—Group stationary cycling classes that emphasize cadence and are guided by a master instructor.

water fitness activities—Aerobic activities performed in an aquatic environment.

Reference

Ryan, P. (2003). Programs to inspire the world. *IDEA Health and Fitness Source, 21*, 44-49.

Suggested Readings

Books

American Council on Exercise. (1999). *Group fitness instructor manual.* San Diego: ACE.

American Council on Exercise. (2003). *Personal trainer manual.* (3rd ed.). San Diego: ACE.

Bonelli, S. (2000). *Step training.* San Diego: ACE.

Bonelli, S. (2001). *Aquatic exercise.* San Diego: ACE.

Bricker, K. (2000). *Traditional aerobics.* San Diego: ACE.

Hyde, C. (2002). *Fitness instructor training guide.* Dubuque, IA: Kendall/Hunt.

National Dance Exercise Instructor's Training Association. (1992). *Aerobic and fitness instructor's manual.* Minneapolis: NDEITA.

Ordas, T., & Rochford, T. (2000). *Kickboxing fitness.* San Diego: ACE.

Web Sites

Centers for Disease Control and Prevention (2006). Physical activity for everyone: Measuring physical activity intensity: Target heart rate and estimated maximum heart rate. Retrieved 6 June, 2006, from www.cdc.gov/nccdphp/dnpa/physical/measuring/target_heart_rate.htm.

Tendy, S. (2003). Step aerobics video web page. Accessed 6 June, 2006, from www.usma.edu/dpe/courses/Exercise%20Leadership/step/main01.htm.

Videos

Biscontini, L. (2002). *Intro to hi-lo movement.* San Diego: ACE.

Biscontini, L. (2002). *Intro to step instruction.* San Diego: ACE.

Culwell, T. (1991). *Creative Stepps too!* Roswell, GA: Creative STEPPS.

Gasper, G. (1993). *The next step.* Chester, NJ: Xercise Connections.

Whiteside, S. (1991). *Spark, sizzle and step choreography video.* New York: BodyFit Fitness Instructor Training Video.

Sport-Specific Organizations

Aerobic and Fitness Association of America (AFAA)
15250 Ventura Boulevard, Suite 200
Sherman Oaks, CA 91403
877-968-7263 (877-YOURBODY)
www.afaa.com/
E-mail: ContactAFAA@afaa.com

American Council on Exercise (ACE)
4851 Paramount Drive
San Diego, CA 92123
858-279-8227
800-825-3636
Fax: 858-279-8064
www.acefitness.org/
Contact information: www.acefitness.org/aboutace/contact.aspx

International Dance Exercise Association (IDEA)
10455 Pacific Center Court
San Diego, CA 92121-4339
858-535-8979
800-999-4332 (800-999-IDEA)
Fax: 858-535-8234
www.ideafit.com
E-mail: nonmemberquestions@ideafit.com

National Exercise Trainers Association (NETA, formerly NDEITA)
5955 Golden Valley Road, Suite 240
Minneapolis, MN 55422
763-545-2505
800-237-6242 (800-AEROBIC)
Fax: 763-545-2524
www.ndeita.com
E-mail: neta@netafit.org

Cross-Country Skiing

Jeffrey Coelho

Cross-country skiing offers numerous health, fitness, and recreational benefits. Fitness experts consider cross-country skiing one of the best sports for achieving overall physical fitness. It is an activity that develops cardiorespiratory fitness, flexibility, and muscular strength and endurance and requires balance, agility, and coordination. In addition, much of the enthusiasm for this sport comes from the desire to be outdoors enjoying nature. Cross-country skiing is an excellent lifetime fitness and recreational activity and can be enjoyed by people of all ages and abilities. It can also be an excellent competitive experience for the more serious skier.

Purpose of the Course

Cross-Country Skiing is offered in the physical education curriculum at West Point to enhance and broaden the sport interests of future military officers and to encourage students to participate in cross-country skiing as a lifetime recreational and fitness activity. The primary purpose of the course is to teach students the basic skills and techniques of cross-country skiing. Students are also required to exhibit knowledge of cross-country skiing techniques, equipment, and the planning considerations for cross-country ski touring.

To fulfill the objectives of the course, students will be able to do the following:

- Demonstrate the basic concepts of cross-country skiing, including balance, pressure, edging, and turning
- Perform basic skills of cross-country skiing, including diagonal stride, skating, turning, uphill and downhill techniques, and stopping
- Identify and participate in selected cross-country skiing training activities designed to improve physical fitness

- Become aware of the planning considerations for cross-country ski touring
- Name selected features of various types of cross-country ski equipment
- Recognize proper skiing technique and learn to appreciate cross-country skiing as a participant and as a knowledgeable spectator
- Define and practice proper trail skiing etiquette
- Select and adhere to proper safety practices and behaviors necessary for participation in cross-country skiing

Instructional Area

West Point maintains its own golf course and downhill ski slope. When there is sufficient natural snow, most cross-country ski classes are conducted at the golf course. If there is insufficient snow on the golf course, class is held on the lower levels of the ski slope, where snow is produced artificially. A ski lodge, easily accessed from both the golf course and ski slope, provides a comfortable location where students can view videotapes, listen to instruction, and take written assessments. Because changing snow conditions directly affect the instructional area, the daily structure of the course must remain flexible.

Snow-covered athletic fields or any open area can serve as an instructional area for cross-country skiing. Teachers can prepare the instructional area prior to class by breaking trail and setting some tracks for students. Traffic cones can be set up to create boundaries and flow patterns for instruction. Instructional areas that include flat terrain and some hills can also make for an ideal teaching site.

Equipment

The Department of Physical Education at West Point supplies cadets with skis, poles, and boots. Students in the Academy's Cross-Country Skiing course wear issued sweat pants, a sweat top, a parka (if necessary), and a knit cap and gloves. Enough equipment is purchased to fully outfit at least 25 students. This requires the procurement of at least 30 percent more skis, poles, and boots to meet the sizing needs of all 25 students. The equipment suitable for a physical education cross-country ski course consists of light touring, "waxless" skis; fiberglass, bamboo, or aluminum ski poles; and touring boots. Cross-country ski equipment may be borrowed or rented from a local ski shop. Cross-country ski resorts may be willing to donate some of their equipment to a school ski program.

Cross-Country Skis

People can determine the proper length for light touring skis, the most common ski for the average recreational skier, by standing the ski on the floor and raising the arm overhead. The tip of the ski should reach to the wrist of the extended arm. Beginners and young children should consider using a shorter ski. Skis come in a variety of widths. A wider ski provides more support and should be used by heavier skiers.

The term "camber" refers to the bend in the ski. The camber is most noticeable when the skis are placed running surface to running surface. Three factors should be considered in the choice of camber: body weight, ability, and intended use. The ski's camber or stiffness should be in proportion to the individual's body weight. A heavier skier should use a ski with a stiffer camber. A soft-cambered ski is good for a novice. Advanced skiers and racers need a stiffer camber to get a better glide, but must use an aggressive kick to get a grip on the snow.

Many skis must be waxed for maximum performance. A correctly waxed cross-country ski both grips and glides across the snow. The recreational skier is more interested in a reliable grip than in maximum glide. Waxless skis have been developed that grip well and are easier to use and maintain, but they do not glide as well as waxable skis. Despite the poorer gliding capability, waxless skis are the most popular recreational skis available and are a good choice for the beginner through intermediate skier.

Cross-Country Ski Bindings and Boots

Ski bindings and boots, which must be matched, come in a variety of styles based on the type of skiing. The newer "automatic" ski bindings (Rottefella NNN or Solomon Profil) allow the toe of the boots to "click" in, and run the full length of the boot for stability. Older recreational bindings are usually constructed with a three-pin design and with simple heel plates. The heel plates (wedges, stars, "V"s, and metal ridges) are necessary to keep the heels of the boots on the ski. Recreational skiers should choose a high-top, insulated boot with some lateral support.

Cross-Country Ski Poles

Ski poles are critical support items for both novice and advanced skiers because they provide a means of propulsion. Types of ski poles include classical and skating. The length of the classical ski pole is determined by having the skier stand flat; the pole handle should reach snug in the armpit with the shoulders level. The length of the skating ski pole is correct when the skier stands flat and the pole handle reaches between the nose and the chin.

The strap of the ski pole is used to apply pressure during the poling motion. In the follow-through, the hand releases its grip on the pole handle and then the pole becomes an extension of the arm. The basket of the ski pole supports the pole when it is in the snow. There are several types of baskets depending on snow conditions and uses. A round basket is used for touring, while a larger-diameter (8- to 10-inch [20- to 25-centimeter]) basket is for deep snow or backcountry skiing. A basket 4 to 6 inches (10-15 centimeters) in diameter would work well in packed snow. Poles are made from materials ranging from bamboo to carbon graphite. Bamboo will work, but it is heavy and often breaks, so many skiers do not use bamboo poles. Aluminum is strong and lightweight but may bend unless made from the more tempered alloys. Telescopic poles that adjust to different lengths are available and may be a good choice for school programs.

Risk Management

Safety is always a consideration during cross-country skiing. Varying ability levels, constantly changing snow conditions, and the general nature of skiing require strict attention to safety and risk management. Table 19.1 lists some of the primary safety considerations for the West Point Cross-Country Skiing course.

Skills and Techniques

Each cross-country ski class period should begin with a total-body warm-up, which includes basic body positions, balancing skills, basic turning and walking, and stepping and hopping drills. The primary skills taught in the course are (1) basic skills and turns, (2) falling and getting up correctly, (3) flatland track techniques, (4) uphill techniques, (5) downhill techniques, (6) stopping, and (7) skating.

Table 19.1 Possible Risks in Cross-Country Skiing

Risk identification	Reduction strategies
Skiing downhill out of control or too fast for ability	• Execute controlled fall. • Use braking wedge, turn uphill, or hockey stop. • Use pole dragging. • Stay on proper terrain.
Terrain too difficult or dangerous	• Ski on designated trails and areas only.
Collisions with other skiers	• Look uphill before crossing fall line. • Give right of way to downhill skier. • Be aware of others around you.
Exposure, hypothermia, frostbite	• Know danger signs of exposure, hypothermia, and frostbite. • Dress appropriately for conditions. • Dress in layers.
Dehydration	• Carry water. • Consume fluids before, during, and after skiing.

Course Overview

The Cross-Country Skiing course introduces the novice skier to the sport of cross-country skiing (see table 19.2). The students become familiar with, and are able to demonstrate, the diagonal stride, skating, turning, and uphill techniques as well as downhill techniques. The students are also expected to demonstrate baseline knowledge of cross-country skiing techniques, equipment, and planning considerations for cross-country touring.

Sample Lesson Plans

Sample lesson plans are developed based on the outline in table 19.2. However, because of continually changing snow conditions and terrain considerations, lesson plans are regularly modified to fit the conditions and the terrain available. For example, when teaching in hilly locations, it is necessary to teach uphill and downhill techniques before or at the same time as flatland techniques. In icy conditions, it may be necessary to avoid steep terrain and to focus on striding, poling, and skating on the flats. This section is organized by skill theme instead of as a traditional sequence of progressive lesson plans.

Table 19.2   Overview of Cross-Country Skiing Lessons

Lesson	Skills
1	Administration; equipment issue
2	Equipment use; basic body positions, basic skills, basic turns, falling and getting up; trail skiing etiquette
3	Introduction to diagonal stride and poling
4	Continue diagonal stride and poling; introduction to uphill and downhill techniques, turning, and stopping
5	Continue diagonal stride and poling, uphill and downhill techniques, turning, and stopping; introduction to skating
6	Continue skating; review all skills and practice
7	Problem solving; videotaping
8	Ski touring
9	Ski touring and equipment turn-in

Basic Skills and Turns

TEACHING CUES

- Basic body position: The desired body position is one that enables the skier to balance on a point just in front of the heel or just behind the instep. Skiers should assume a slightly flexed, upright stance (see figure 19.1).
- Beginner basic skills: Walking on skis, sidestepping, balancing on one ski, wedge positions, gliding, hopping, and so on.
- Basic turns (stationary):
  - Turning around the tips: Keep tips on the snow, use a high knee lift (may be more difficult in new or loose snow), and open tails of skis. Focus on keeping tips together and try turning in both directions. This turn is the foundation of the wedge position, which will be discussed in more detail in the downhill portion of the class.

- Turning around the tails: Keep tails together and on the snow; keep weight on the heels, flex knees, and then pick up one ski, form a "V," and "match" or bring the skis together.

- Kick turn: Good for narrow trails, in deep snow, or on steep slopes. Also used to change direction at the end of a traverse on steep slopes. Kick the uphill ski out and around. Use the poles for balance. Then repeat with the other ski.

- Bullfighter's turn: Generally used on steep terrain to get skis and body facing straight down the fall line. Plant poles down fall line and step around tails or tips, using poles for support until body and skis face downward.

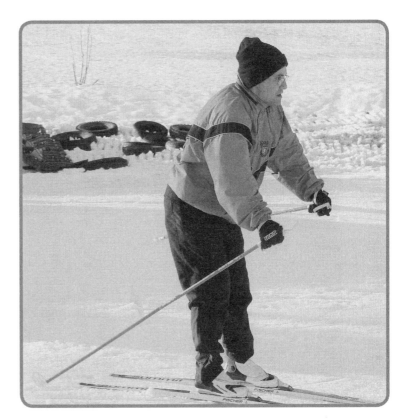

FIGURE 19.1   **Basic body position.**

- Falling and getting up: Falling is a natural occurrence in beginning skiing. Students will learn to execute a controlled fall as a way of stopping.

  - The controlled fall: Sit back on buttocks and lower body to the snow.

  - Getting up: Bring skis together and place them perpendicular to the fall line. Poles can be either on or off. Lean forward to "all-fours" position. Slide downhill ski forward. Use poles and push up to a stand. In deep snow, make an "X" in the snow with the poles on the uphill side of skis just in front of the body. The "X" will act as a platform to push up from. Also, one or both skis may be removed and then remounted.

Flatland Track Techniques

TEACHING CUES

- Diagonal stride introduction: The fundamental Nordic technique for flat or slightly uphill terrain, the diagonal stride is similar to running but has the additional components of gliding on skis and the pole push (see figure 19.2).

  - The kick: The kick is an aggressive downward push on one ski, which propels the other ski forward. A good kick results from a forward-leaning torso.

  - The glide: Upper body remains stationary for a moment, and body weight should be over the gliding ski and centered just behind the ball of the foot.

  - The pole push: A forceful downcompression of the arms, shoulders, and back. With forward elbow slightly bent, plant pole to the side with pole shaft angled forward and slightly into the body. Arms are relaxed and comfortably flexed at the elbow and wrist during planting. Follow through with full arm extension.

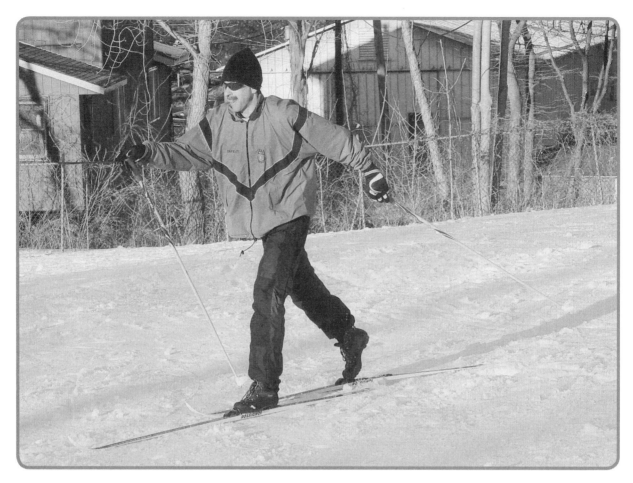

FIGURE 19.2 Diagonal stride.

- Leg-body movement: Alternating push-off from one ski onto a gliding ski. The motion is similar to walking; the heel should come up off the ski at the end of the push-off. Start with a slow shuffling motion that develops into a more powerful compression of body weight on the push-off ski and extension.

- Drills: Walking without poles; exaggerated knee bend; exaggerated arm swing; "quick ski" (running); alternating lifting one ski and then the other out of the track; lifting tips; and practice balancing on one foot.

• Double poling: Used to maintain or increase speed on fast tracks or slight declines. Gives the legs a rest while the upper torso and arms are used for propulsion.

- Practice movement in a stationary position.

- Lean forward, bend trunk, and rise up on toes.

- Plant poles far in front of feet.

- Emphasize pushing the hands past the hips.

- Start off on a flat area, then progress to a gradual downhill.

• One-step double pole: This is a push-off with one leg followed by a double pole, used when terrain is too flat for the diagonal stride and too slow for the double pole. It can be a restful break from a series of double poles or a long section of diagonal striding. The rhythm is similar to that used when skating: push, double pole, push.

Uphill Techniques

TEACHING CUES

- Uphill diagonal stride: This skill can be used on gradual slopes; it is a slight modification of regular stride.
  - Stride length is shortened and tempo is increased to maintain momentum with little or no free glide.
  - The angle of the slope requires a definite weight transfer to the forward ski (that foot is pushed slightly ahead of the knee) to apply maximum pressure on the gripping ski.
  - Push-off is quick and explosive to eliminate time spent on a stopped ski.
  - The hand moves down as the pole is pulled and pushed off in a shorter, more vigorous motion.
  - Use quicker and shorter movements similar to jogging up a hill.
- Herringbone: A technique used to climb straight uphill where the terrain precludes other uphill techniques. This technique is faster than the sidestep and more secure on steep terrain than the uphill diagonal stride.
  - Edging: The skis are placed at an angle ("V" position) with the inside edges turned in. Spread the skis farther apart on steep terrain to prevent sliding back.
  - Poling: The poles move as in diagonal. Plant the pole to the side and behind the feet. Apply pressure on the pole to prevent slipping and move forward for the next step.
  - Body position: Similar to that for diagonal stride with a little more forward lean and knee flex.
  - Students having problems: Those having difficulty should try to avoid steep hills first and emphasize edging and proper use of the poles. They should take larger steps if the tails of the skis are crossing.
- Sidestep: Used to negotiate narrow or steep sections of trail or very deep snow where no other techniques are possible. Can also be used to go down a steep slope.
  - Edging: The skis are kept perpendicular to the fall line, with the edges turned into the hill to prevent the skis from slipping downhill.
  - Body position: Upright, weight over the feet, knees slightly flexed for balance.
  - Arm movement: Arms move simultaneously or alternate, depending on the snow conditions and slope steepness. Arms are used primarily for balance and support.
- Traversing: Cutting diagonally across a slope to reduce slope angle so skis will hold. The preferred method of changing direction at the end of a traverse is to use a herringbone step turn (turn around tails). To change direction on an extremely steep slope, use the kick turn. Upper body faces the direction of travel.

Downhill Techniques

TEACHING CUES

- Straight run: A downhill run with skis directed down the fall line.
  - Body position: Stand up fairly straight, hands at sides, pole baskets on the snow and pointing back. The skis should be shoulder-width apart. Bend the knees and move the hands forward in front of the hips. The center of gravity is over the feet, with the shoulders and back rounded. Faster skiing requires a lower knee bend and center of gravity.
- Problems:
  - Falling backward, which is caused by leaning back too far; skis might be too close together.
  - Skis cross and wobble from side to side during the run, probably because legs are stiff and too tense.
  - Start on fairly level terrain and progress in steepness. Students having difficulty should review the basic body positions and practice moving up and down for balance.
- Gliding wedge: The skis will form a wedge with the tails open or spread apart. This technique is used to control speed and maintain stability on a downhill run.
  - Have skis flat on the snow; ankles and knees control the slight edging of both skis.
  - Push tails out and keep tips together by rotating legs from the hips. Practice on a flat surface and progress to a gentle hill with long, flat run-outs.
  - Use different-sized wedges for varying terrain and steepness.
  - Drills: Jumping jack to wedge, hourglass, assigning numbers to different-sized wedges, sinking and rising, leg rotation from hip.
- Tuck position: A compact aerodynamic position for holding or increasing speed on long downhills. Also used to relax and recover.
  - Go into tuck while standing still. Emphasize staying low in a crouch, back parallel to the ground, elbows in close to the body.
  - Start with a straight run, and then assume the tuck.
  - Use different tuck positions for different terrain.
  - During a resting tuck, the hips are held higher and the elbows are placed on the knees.
  - Best when used on a prepared track.
- Side slipping: On short, steep, or icy slopes, there may be no alternative but to skid the skis sideways down the hill.
  - Stand with skis parallel to fall line.
  - Relax ankles to release edges.
  - To control speed, turn ankles back into the hill for more edge bite.
  - Upper body faces downhill.

Stopping Techniques

TEACHING CUES

- Wedge stop or braking wedge: The skier uses pressure, edging, and width of wedge to control speed, opening tails to a wide wedge and rotating knees and ankles inward (see figure 19.3).
  - Drills: Jumping jack to wedge, hourglass, lifting skis and pivoting leg from hips, setting up stop markers.
- Wedge turn to a stop: A steered turn, with maintenance of a wedge. To execute, shift weight to the downhill ski and continue to turn uphill to a stop.
  - Hip rotation: Rotate legs from hips to steer both skis into the turn.
  - Edging: Keep the inside ski fairly flat, and angle the edge of the turning (downhill) ski more.
  - Apply pressure and stand up straight on downhill ski. Make inside (uphill) ski "lighter."

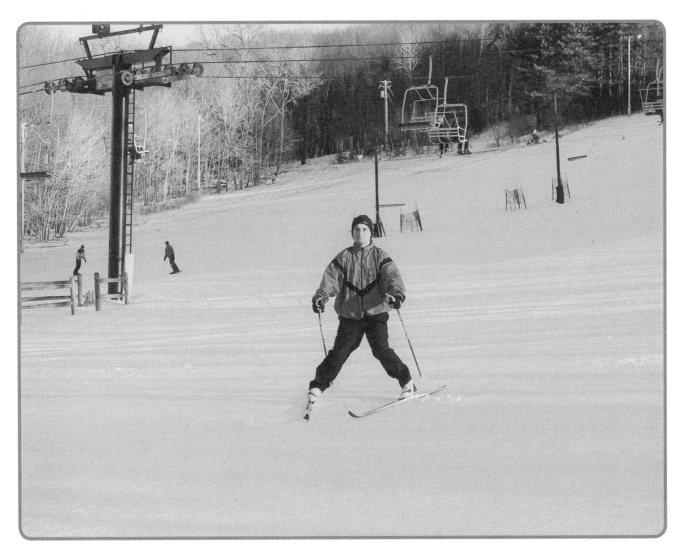

FIGURE 19.3 **Wedge stop.**

- Pole drag: A technique using the ski poles to control speed. Useful for the student who has not yet mastered other downhill techniques. The pole drag, combined with a wedge, may be the safest way down. It is good for steep, narrow, icy trails where controlling speed is a problem.
  - Remove the hands from the straps and hold both poles together. One hand grips the top of the poles, and the other hand grips the poles about three-quarters of the way down the pole shaft.
  - Lower the body by flexing the knees to better utilize the poles as a lever.
  - Weight is equally distributed between the two skis. Use a half-wedge or a full wedge combined with a pole drag for added control.
- Hockey stop: A more advanced stopping technique that the skier performs by turning aggressively while staying in the fall line.
  - Start from a straight run.
  - Stand up quickly to release pressure on the skis.
  - Turn hips, legs, and skis vigorously.
  - Keep upper body and head facing down the fall line.

Skate Techniques

TEACHING CUES

Skating is the most common form of skiing for competition. The motion is similar to ice skating. It is an ideal technique for hard, packed snow. There are several types of skating. The type used most often is V skating, or the V-1 technique.

- Edging: The "pushing" ski is turned on the inside edge, forming a platform from which to push off. The gliding ski is flat on the snow.
- Turn the ankle and knee toward the inside of the turn to edge the ski.
- Repeat with the other ski, forming an alternating push–glide pattern as in diagonal stride.
- Flex the knees to a low crouch, and then extend the leg from an edged ski. The amount of energy exerted in the push-off directly affects the skier's speed in skating.
- Double pole push when skis are brought together.
- Commit the entire body weight to one ski at a time, and ride the gliding ski as long as possible.
- Hips are up and forward over the gliding ski.
- Ankle flexion and knee bend make it easier to glide on one ski.
- Both poles and one ski hit the snow simultaneously (three-point landing).
- Initiate a powerful double pole as soon as pole tips touch the snow.
- Follow through while gliding on the strong-side skating ski.
- Always pole in the direction you are facing, toward the tip of the gliding ski.
- Problems:
  - When the ski slides to the side and does not grip the snow, turn the ankles more to dig the edge in.

- Pay attention to arm movement: Are the arms helping to move the body forward over the gliding ski, or are they simply in the way?

Turning Techniques

TEACHING CUES

- Wedge turns: The skier begins with small, linked deviations from the fall line. These should develop gradually into more refined turns with effective turning, edging, and pressure control skills.
  - Feel one ski become heavier late in each turn.
  - Avoid upper body rotation to turn. Emphasize legs.
  - Practice turning in both directions.
  - Experiment with different-sized wedges and eventually link several turns together.
  - Hip rotation: Rotate skis and legs from hips to steer both skis in the direction of the turn.
  - Edging: Keep the inside ski flat and "light," and angle the edge of the turning (downhill) ski more.
  - Drills: Skiing in pairs, garlands, and applying pressure to big and little toes.
- Step turn: A technique the skier uses to change direction by stepping the skis into a new direction (similar to the stationary step turn around the tails). With skis parallel, flex the knees and commit the body into the turn. Pick up the tip of the inside ski and place it at an angle to the outside ski of the turn, and transfer weight. Bring the outside ski parallel and repeat the sequence to turn.
  - Edging: When performed on the flat, the outside ski is edged to the inside of the turn. The tails are left on the snow, fairly close together. When performed on a hill, both skis are edged to the inside of the turn.
  - Body position: Assume a low position, keeping knees and ankles flexed throughout the turn. Transfer the weight completely from ski to ski throughout the turn, taking short, quick steps.
  - Arms: Hold the arms to the side and forward for balance, poles pointing backward.
  - Keep your feet moving!
  - Add a skate push and double pole.
- Drills:
  - Start the step turn as a series of small steps on flat terrain and progress to a steeper hill.
  - Emphasize weighting the heels, and apply pressure up with the toes to produce a pivoting action on the tail.
- Parallel turn: A more advanced turn. Skis remain parallel as the skier turns and goes across fall line. The turn involves the skidding and matching of skis throughout. The parallel turn originates from a wedge and open parallel turn.
  - Commit to going down and across fall line.
  - Extend body upward to release the pressure of the skis on the snow at the moment the skis change direction.

- Plant inside pole down the hill in front, rise up, lift the outside pole, and turn around the downhill pole.
- Keep upper body facing downhill and anticipate the next turn in the opposite direction.
- Turns should be smooth, round, and linked (S-turns).
- Drills: Garlands, J-turns, skidding and side slipping, skiing on one leg, and so on.

• Telemark turn: The telemark is a functional turn for certain snow conditions and is a stable turn in uneven terrain. It requires a wider ski, with a more stable boot. Skis also have more defined edges that allow the skier to carve turns better.

- Flex the knees; slide one ski forward until the tip of the back ski is halfway between the binding and the shovel of the forward ski.
- Position the front knee over the toes of the front foot. Bend the back knee to form a right angle between the upper and lower leg. Raise the back heel off the ski and support weight on the ball of the back foot.
- When turning, the upper body twists to face downhill throughout. Hands are forward and to the side.
- Edging: At the start of the turn, from a side-hill traverse, transfer weight to the inside ski (downhill), and steer the outside ski out and forward in the direction of the turn. Assume the telemark position. Then transfer weight to the outside ski and turn the ski on edge. Steer the outside ski to control the radius of the turn.

• Drills:

- Start on flat terrain and practice the telemark without moving. Separate feet and bend enough to raise the back heel off the ski.
- Go to a gentle hill and perform a straight run in a telemark position to a gradual stop. Lead with different feet.
- Begin the telemark turn from a half-wedge.
- Beginners should assume a "soft–tall" position and progress to a "hard–short" position.
- Try to link several turns together, or set up a slalom course.

Adapting This Course for Your School

Cross-country skiing involves generating and controlling speed, balance, pressure control, edge control, and turning movements. Skiers must combine these movements in order to ski safely and effectively in varied terrain and snow conditions. Teaching cross-country skiing demands flexibility and creativity from the teacher. Teachers must understand students and their abilities; select appropriate terrain; practice the correct skills for the proper amount of time; and ensure a successful, fun, and rewarding skiing experience for all students.

Teaching This Course at the Elementary Level

Instructional cross-country skiing programs for children should stress the fun of skiing and take a "games approach" to learning. Initial lessons involving equipment familiarization, and basic